Dialysis
and the Treatment of
Renal Insufficiency

Dialysis and the Treatment of Renal Insufficiency

John C. Van Stone, M.D.
Associate Professor of Medicine
University of Missouri Medical School
Columbia, Missouri

With

Anne Campbell, M.S.P.H.

Ted Groshong, M.D.

E. Ann Murray, R.D.

W. Kirt Nichols, M.D.

Michael I. Sorkin, M.D.

Judy C. Webb, B.S.

GRUNE & STRATTON
A Subsidiary of Harcourt Brace Jovanovich, Publishers
New York   London
Paris   San Diego   San Francisco   São Paulo
Sydney   Tokyo   Toronto

Library of Congress Cataloging in Publication Data
Van Stone, John C.
  Dialysis and the treatment of renal insufficiency.

  Bibliography: p.
  Includes index.
  1. Renal insufficiency—Treatment. 2. Hemodialysis.
3. Peritoneal dialysis. I. Title. [DNLM: 1. Kidney
failure, Chronic—Therapy. 2. Hemodialysis. WJ 378
V281d]
RC918.R4V36   1983   616.6'106   83-5595
ISBN   0-8089-1566-5

© *1983 by Grune & Stratton, Inc.*
All rights reserved. No part of this publication
may be reproduced or transmitted in any form or
by any means, electronic or mechanical, including
photocopy, recording, or any information storage
and retrieval system, without permission in
writing from the publisher.

Grune & Stratton, Inc.
111 Fifth Avenue
New York, New York 10003

Distributed in the United Kingdom by
Grune & Stratton, Inc. (London) Ltd.
24/28 Oval Road, London NW 1

Library of Congress Catalog Number 83-5595
International Standard Book Number 0-8089-1566-5

Printed in the United States of America

Contents

Foreword   ix
Preface   xi
Authors   xiii

1. **Systemic Manifestations of Chronic Renal Failure**   1
    John C. Van Stone

    Abnormalities in Calcium, Phosphorus, and Vitamin D Metabolism
    Hematologic Abnormalities
    Cardiovascular Abnormalities
    Gastrointestinal Manifestations
    Neurologic Abnormalities
    Endocrine Abnormalities

2. **Conservative Management of Renal Insufficiency**   43
    John C. Van Stone

    Patient Education
    Diet Therapy
    Blood Pressure Control
    Phosphorus Control
    Treatment of Acidosis
    Initiating Replacement Therapy

3. **Medications in Chronic Renal Failure**   55
    John C. Van Stone

    Antibiotics
    Analgesics

Sedatives and Tranquilizers
Antihypertensive Agents
Diuretics
Digitalis
Antiarrythmic Agents
Anticonvulsants
Antihistamines
Antiinflammatory Agents
Antineoplastic Agents
Miscellaneous Drugs

4. History of Dialysis   71
John C. Van Stone

Hemodialysis
Peritoneal Dialysis

5. Principles and Mechanics of Dialysis   83
John C. Van Stone

Semipermeable Membranes
Ultrafiltration
Solute Transport
Dialysate
Dialyzers
Dialysis Machines
Single-Needle Dialysis

6. Hemodialysis Prescription   119
John C. Van Stone

Determining the Amount of Total Dialysis Needed
Dialyzers
Dialysis Duration and Frequency
Dialysate
Anticoagulation During Dialysis
Determining the Target Weight
Symptoms During Dialysis
Starting Patients on Chronic Dialysis

7. Vascular Access   143
W. Kirt Nichols

Types of Chronic Hemodialysis Access
Immediate Blood Access for Hemodialysis
Vascular Access Complications
Angiographic Fistula Evaluation

8. **Peritoneal Physiology   165**
    Michael I. Sorkin

    Anatomy and Histology
    Factors Controlling Peritoneal Dialysis
    Factors Affecting Peritoneal Dialysis Efficiency
    Measurements of Peritoneal Dialysis Efficiency
    Dynamics of Peritoneal Dialysis
    Alteration of Peritoneal Physiology by Exogenous Agents
    Clinical Applications

9. **Clinical Aspects of Peritoneal Dialysis   179**
    Michael I. Sorkin

    History
    The Peritoneal Catheter
    Techniques for Exchanging Dialysis Fluid
    The Dialysis Fluid
    The Patient
    Nutrition
    Problems
    Integrated Approach to the Patient

10. **Hemofiltration   219**
    John C. Van Stone

    Postdilution versus Predilution
    Hemofiltration Equipment
    Advantages and Disadvantages of Hemofiltration over
        Hemodialysis

11. **Dialysis in Infants and Children   231**
    Ted Groshong

    Causes of Renal Failure in Infants and Children
    Indications for Dialysis
    Peritoneal Dialysis
    Hemodialysis
    Psychological Problems

12. **Acute Renal Failure   259**
    John C. Van Stone

    Pathogenesis of Acute Tubular Necrosis
    Treatment of Acute Renal Failure
    Prognosis

13. Treatment of Drug Intoxication with Dialysis and Hemoperfusion   271
John C. Van Stone

Hemoperfusion
Treatment of Specific Drug Intoxications

14. Education of the Renal Patient: Assistance for Change   287
Anne Campbell

Background of Patient Education
Acute and Chronic Disease Education
Psychosocial Issues of Patients with ESRD
Goals of a Predialysis Renal Education Program
Planning the Education Program
Barriers to Effective Patient Education
Implementation of the Renal Education Program
Evaluation of Renal Education Programs

15. Dietary Management   335
E. Ann Murray, R.D.

The Renal Failure Diet
Nutritional Assessment
Dietary Compliance
Diabetics with Chronic Renal Failure
Predialysis Nutrition
Hemodialysis Nutrition
CAPD Nutrition

16. The Administrative Mandate: Effective Utilization of Human, Professional, and Financial Resources   355
Judy C. Webb

The Team Approach to the ESRD Patient Using a Primary Nurse System
The ESRD Medicare Program
Controlling the Cost of Dialysis

Index   369

Foreword

In the United States more than 60,000 patients are treated annually with some form of chronic dialysis. These patients have many unique problems and needs. Health care professionals caring for these patients must understand the pathophysiology of uremia, the principles and mechanics of dialysis, the adjustments of medications required in dialysis patients, the special dietary needs of dialysis patients, the placement and care of vascular access and peritoneal access, and the selection and preparation of dialysis patients for kidney transplantation.

Those involved in dialysis therapies must be familiar with many medical problems in addition to chronic renal failure. Patients with acute renal failure often require dialysis therapy, and these patients also have unique problems and needs. Dialysis therapy and hemoperfusion can be important in the care of drug intoxication and poisoning. Infants and children present challenging dialysis problems.

There are many methods of providing dialysis therapy. Extracorporeal hemodialysis can be offered in many forms with many different types of equipment. Dialysis therapy may utilize the capillaries of the peritoneum via intracorporeal peritoneal dialysis. Conventional dialysis therapies depend primarily on solute diffusion with some contributions of convection. New approaches to body fluid purification may rely more on convective transport of solutes, such as in hemofiltration. Sorbent systems are increasingly employed, such as in hemoperfusion.

The accumulatng scientific literature in all of these fields is quite vast and is increasing. It is no longer easy to be expert in all aspects of body fluid purification therapies.

In this volume Dr. Van Stone and his associates present an extensive collection of information about renal replacement therapy. Dr. Van

Stone has devoted many years to patient care, teaching, and research in the fields so thoroughly covered in this book, and he is well qualified to coordinate this effort. In these times when multi-authored books are more common, Dr. Van Stone has authored 9 of the 16 chapters presented herein. Dr. Van Stone has always approached dialysis therapies with an appreciation and extensive understanding of the state of the art. He has also pursued research to better understand and to improve this expanding and complicated field of medicine. In this book he and the contributing authors share their experiences, knowledge, and insights in a very readable fashion.

Karl D. Nolph, M.D.
Director, Division of Nephrology
Professor of Medicine
University of Missouri Health Sciences Center
Harry S. Truman Memorial Veterans Administration Hospital
  and Dalton Research Center
Columbia, Missouri

Preface

Over the past 30 years the care of patients with renal insufficiency has become of increasing importance. This is due in large part to the success of hemodialysis in prolonging the life of these patients. In 1982 in the United States alone there were over 70,000 patients being treated for renal failure at the total annual cost of greater than one billion dollars.

The success of this complicated therapy depends on the expertise of members of many disciplines including physicians, nurses, dietitians, social workers, technicians, and others. This book is an attempt to integrate the various aspects of the treatment of renal insufficiency in one volume. (Although renal transplantation is an important aspect in the care of many patients with renal failure, it is not addressed; patients with a successful transplant no longer have renal insufficiency and the treatment of these patients is very different.) The book is intended not only for the practicing physicians, house officers, and medical students involved in the care of patients with renal insufficiency, but also for nurses, dietitians, social workers, technicians, and other paramedical personnel.

In an attempt to avoid excessive duplication and to maintain a relatively consistent style, the majority of this book was written by myself. In order to completely cover the subject, however, I have freely drawn on the expertise of individuals in my own and related disciplines. The theoretical and clinical aspects of peritoneal dialysis are discussed in two excellent chapters by Michael I. Sorkin, M.D. The very important topic of vascular access is covered by W. Kirt Nichols, M.D., who has many years of experience in this field.

The care of the child with renal failure is in many aspects very different from that of the adult and is nicely summarized in the chapter by Ted Groshong, M.D. Diet therapy is of the utmost importance in the treatment of renal insufficiency. The diet therapy of patients before the need for replacement therapy, of patients undergoing different types of replacement therapy, and of special types of patients such as the diabetic, are reviewed by E. Ann Murray, R.D.

For any treatment of renal insufficiency to be successful, it is extremely important that the patient be as actively involved in his or her own care as possible. In order for this to occur, the patient must have as thorough an understanding of the disease and its treatment as possible, and education of these patients therefore has become very important. The various aspects of patient education are covered by Ann Campbell. Finally, in an era when fiscal restraints are becoming greater, the efficient management of a dialysis facility is becoming mandatory, and these problems are addressed by Judy C. Webb.

John C. Van Stone, M.D.

Authors

Anne Campbell, M.S.P.H.
Patient Education Coordinator
Dialysis Clinics, Inc.
Columbia, Missouri

Ted Groshong, M.D.
Associate Professor
Department of Child Health
University of Missouri
Columbia, Missouri

E. Ann Murray, R.D.
Renal Dietitian
Dialysis Clinics, Inc.
Columbia, Missouri

W. Kirt Nichols, M.D., F.A.C.S.
Associate Professor of Surgery
Department of Surgery
University of Missouri Medical School
Columbia, Missouri

Michael I. Sorkin, M.D.
Assistant Professor of Medicine
University of Pittsburgh School of Medicine
Renal Electrolyte Division
Pittsburgh, Pennsylvania

John C. Van Stone, M.D.
Associate Professor of Medicine
University of Missouri Medical School
Columbia, Missouri

Judy C. Webb, B.S.
Administrator
Dialysis Clinics, Inc.
Columbia, Missouri

John C. Van Stone

1
Systemic Manifestations of Chronic Renal Failure

All the organ systems of the body are affected by chronic renal insufficiency. Failure of the kidneys can cause severe problems with the cardiovascular system, gastrointestinal tract, bones, and many other organs. The appropriate management of patients with chronic renal insufficiency requires an understanding of the pathogenesis and treatment of these abnormalities. This chapter will discuss the systemic manifestations of chronic renal failure. It is not meant to be an exhaustive review of all the changes which occur in the body secondary to renal insufficiency, but to be a brief review of the various abnormalities with an emphasis placed on the methods and rationale for treating these abnormalities.

ABNORMALITIES IN CALCIUM, PHOSPHORUS, AND VITAMIN D METABOLISM

Abnormalities in the metabolism of calcium, phosphorus, and vitamin D are important not only because they are one of the earliest changes to occur in progressive renal insufficiency, but also because they are treatable. If appropriate treatment is begun early enough, it is usually successful, but if not, these abnormalities can cause severe morbidity and mortality. If untreated, abnormalities in calcium and phosphorus metabolism will lead to renal osteodystrophy with severe bone pain and pathologic fractures, soft tissue calcification with severe pruritus, and vascular calcification which can lead to ischemia or even gangrene of the extremities. There are three primary abnormalities effecting calcium metabolism which occur in renal insufficiency. These are phosphorus retention from a decrease in phosphorus excretion, decreased calcium absorption secondary to abnormalities of vitamin D activation, and a resistance to the action of parathyroid hormone.

Phosphorus Retention

Phosphorus retention is the earliest problem occurring in chronic renal failure which requires clinical attention.[1] In order to understand phosphorus mtabolism in chronic renal failure it is necessary to briefly review normal phosphorus metabolism. The normal diet contains between 1500 and 2000 mg of phosphorus of which approximately 1000 mg is absorbed from the gastrointestinal tract. To be in neutral phosphorus balance, the normal adult must excrete 1 g of phosphorus each day in the urine. Plasma phosphorus is freely filtered through the glomerulus and variable amounts are absorbed by the renal tubules. Normally, approximately 7 g of phosphorus are filtered through the glomerulus with 85 percent being reabsorbed by the tubules, leaving 1 g to be excreted in the urine.

The two primary methods by which phosphorus balance is normally maintained in the face of differing phosphorus intakes are (1) changes in the total filtered load of phosphorus, mediated through changes in plasma phosphorus concentration and (2) changes in the tubular reabsorption of phosphorus, mediated primarily by changes in parathyroid hormone concentration. As phosphorus intake increases, plasma phosphorus concentration goes up and increases the total amount of phosphorus filtered through the glomerulus. If tubular reabsorption remains constant this in itself will result in an appropriate increase in phosphorus excretion. Phosphorus excretion is also increased, however, by decreasing the amount of phosphorus reabsorbed by the tubules. The major determinant of tubular phosphorus reabsorption is the circulating concentration of parathyroid hormone. As parathyroid hormone levels increase, phosphorus reabsorption by the tubules decreases thus increasing phosphorus excretion.

The effects of renal insufficiency on phosphorus metabolism are schematically illustrated in Figure 1-1. The initial effect of a decline in renal function is a reduction in the filtered load of phosphorus. Filtered phosphorus is equal to the product of the glomerular filtration rate and the plasma phosphorus concentration, therefore, if the glomerular filtration rate decreases by 50 percent, the filtered load of phosphorus

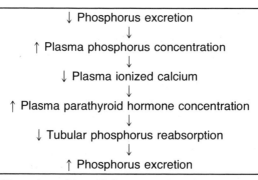

Figure 1-1. Effect of renal insufficiency on phosphorus excretion.

will also decrease by 50 percent. If the tubular reabsorption does not change or even if it decreases in proportion to the decrease in glomerular filtration rate, there will be a reduction in phosphorus excretion with a resultant positive phosphorus balance. The positive phosphorus balance will cause the serum phosphorus to increase. Phosphorus and ionized calcium are in dynamic equilibrium in the plasma and this increase in phosphorus will result in an immediate decrease in ionized calcium concentration. Since the major determinant of parathyroid hormone secretion is the plasma-ionized calcium concentration, there is a rapid increase in parathyroid hormone secretion. The increased plasma parathyroid hormone concentration causes a reduction of tubular phosphorus reabsorption and therefore an increase in phosphorus excretion. This in turn causes plasma phosphorus concentration to decrease and ionized calcium to increase. Early in the course of progressive renal insufficiency this mechanism is sufficient to restore phosphorus balance and maintain both serum phosphorus and serum calcium concentrations in the normal range. These concentrations are only maintained, however, at the expense of a chronic elevation of plasma parathyroid hormone concentration. If untreated, moderate renal insufficiency with a glomerular filtration rate of 20–50 percent of normal, is usually manifested by normal plasma calcium concentration and normal plasma phosphorus concentration, but increased plasma concentrations of parathyroid hormone.[1] These increased parathyroid hormone concentrations have harmful effects on the bones and other organs of patients with renal insufficiency.[2] The chronic stimulation of the parathyroid gland also results in hypertrophy of the gland which makes the later control of secondary hyperparathyroidism more difficult.

Vitamin D Metabolism

Abnormalities of vitamin D metabolism are another major problem in chronic renal insufficiency.[3] Vitamin D is a steroidal compound (Fig. 1-2), normally obtained in the diet: It is also synthesized from cholesterol in the skin after ultraviolet radiation from the sun. The parent vitamin D molecule has very little, if any, direct effects on the body and in order to become activated must have two hydroxyl radicals attached.[4] The first is placed on the 25th carbon position by the liver to form 25 hydroxy vitamin D (Fig. 1-2). The active compound, 1,25 dihydroxy vitamin D ($1,25(OH)_2D_3$), is formed in the kidney by the placement of a second hydroxyl radical on the first carbon position.

$1,25(OH)_2D_3$ can properly be considered a hormone since it is produced by one organ and excreted into the blood stream to have its predominant effects on other organ systems. The rate of production of $1,25(OH)_2D_3$ by the kidney is regulated on the basis of need.[5] The primary function of $1,25(OH)_2D_3$ is to help maintain plasma calcium concentrations in the normal range. The major action of $1,25(OH)_2D_3$ is to increase calcium absorption in the small intestine. $1,25(OH)_2D_3$ stimulates calcium absorption by increasing the synthesis of a calcium carrier protein in the intestinal cells. In the absence of $1,25(OH)_2D_3$ less than 25 percent of dietary calcium may be absorbed, whereas, with high levels of the hormone greater than 75 percent is absorbed.

Vitamin D has other effects in that it plays a permissive role in the action of PTH on bone and may help regulate parathyroid hormone secretion. Vitamin D also affects muscle metabolism, and deficiency can result in severe muscle weakness.[5]

The rate of synthesis of $1,25(OH)_2D_3$ by the kidney is affected in several ways.[6] A low calcium diet, decreased plasma-ionized calcium, increased plasma PTH concentrations, and low serum phosphorus concentration all stimulate $1,25(OH)_2D_3$ synthesis, whereas high plasma calcium and high plasma phosphorus inhibit the synthesis.

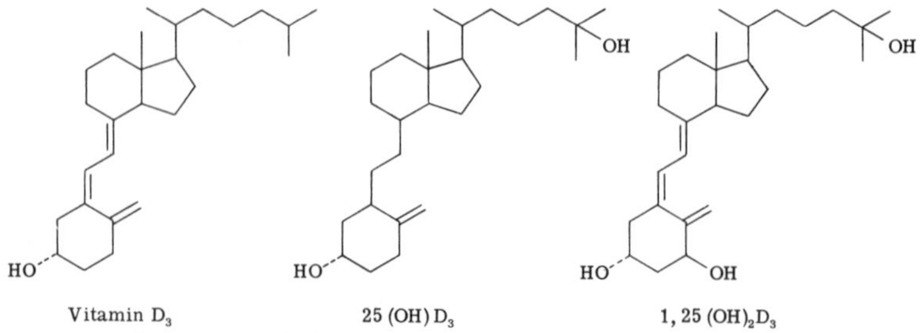

Figure 1-2. Structure of vitamin D and major metabolites.

The synthesis of $1,25(OH)_2D_3$ is reduced in renal insufficiency.[3] Plasma concentrations begin to fall when glomerular filtration rates decrease to 25 ml/min and $1,25(OH)_2D_3$ is absent in the plasma of patients who have had bilateral nephrectomies. Since decreases in gastrointestinal calcium absorption may occur when the glomerular filtration rate is 50–60 ml/min and plasma $1,25(OH)_2D_3$ concentrations are normal, it has been hypothesized that a relative hormone deficiency may occur early in progressive renal failure.[7]

Parathyroid Hormone Resistance

A final abnormality of calcium and phosphorus metabolism which occurs in renal insufficiency is a resistance to the action of parathyroid hormone. Massry and co-workers have demonstrated that patients with chronic renal failure have a reduced response to the skeletal actions of parathyroid hormone.[8] Similar doses of parathyroid hormone result in smaller elevations of plasma calcium in patients with renal insufficiency than in normal controls. This resistance does not seem to be related to phosphorus retention, vitamin D, or renal osteodystrophy and its relative importance to other problems of calcium metabolism in chronic renal failure is not known.

TREATMENT OF ABNORMALITIES IN CALCIUM, PHOSPHORUS, AND VITAMIN D METABOLISM IN CHRONIC RENAL FAILURE

The treatment of abnormalities of calcium, phosphorus, and vitamin metabolism in chronic renal failure is very important because, if properly done and started early enough, it is successful in preventing clinical problems in the vast majority of patients. The first mode of treatment which should be instituted is the reduction of gastrointestinal phosphorus absorption. This should be initiated when the glomerular filtration rate has diminished to 50 percent of normal. When renal function decreases to this level, a phosphorus binding antacid should be prescribed and phosphorus intake should be restricted by limiting the amounts of high phosphorus foods such as dairy products, beans, and chocolate. Generally, 500 mg of aluminum hydroxide or aluminum carbonate with each meal is sufficient. For the reasons described above, it is important that this be done even though the plasma phosphorus concentration is normal. Plasma phosphorus should be monitored closely and if the concentration falls below normal then the phosphorus binders should be decreased and/or phosphorus intake increased. If plasma phosphorus increases above normal in spite of these measures, then the phosphorus binders should be increased and the patient's diet reviewed for possible sources of excess phosphorus.

Oral calcium supplementation should be started at the same time as the initiation of phosphorus restriction. There are two reasons patients with chronic renal failure should receive oral calcium. The first is to counteract the deficiency of $1,25(OH)_2D_3$. The decreased calcium absorption caused by the lack of $1,25(OH)_2D_3$ can be at least partially improved by increasing calcium intake. The second reason for calcium supplementation is to compensate for a calcium deficient diet. Most foods which are high in calcium are also high in phosphorus. When patients are placed on phosphorus restriction, there is a coincidental marked reduction in calcium intake. This dietary calcium deficiency is compensated by the administration of oral calcium. Calcium carbonate is the best calcium supplement because it contains more calcium than the other commonly used calcium salts, such as gluconate or lactate, and is well tolerated by most patients. The usual dose is 1500–2000 mg/day.

Once a patient starts on dialysis treatments, the low gastrointestinal calcium absorption can be partially compensated for with the use of a dialysate with a relatively high calcium concentration. Hemodialysis with a dialysate calcium concentration of 3–4 mEq/liter usually results in a net positive calcium balance of 100 to 500 mg each treatment.[9] It is important that serum calcium be carefully monitored to prevent hypercalcemia.

While there is at least a relative deficiency of $1,25(OH)_2D_3$ in the majority of patients with chronic renal failure, most do not need vitamin D supplementation. Although subclinical changes in bone histology indicative of mild renal osteodystrophy are not prevented by phosphorus restriction and calcium supplementation, it is effective in preventing clinical problems in most patients. If in spite of adequate phosphorus restriction and calcium supplementation, patients develop persistent hypocalcemia and/or clinical evidence of progressive renal osteodystrophy then vitamin D supplementation should be considered. Vitamin D also may be tried in the renal failure patient with muscular weakness.

The most physiologic form of vitamin D is $1,25(OH)_2D_3$ (Rocaltrol). This is the normal active form of vitamin D and does not require metabolism by the kidney. It should be started at 0.125 or 0.25 ng/day and the dose increased every 2 weeks until a clinical response is noted. Serum calcium should be carefully monitored and if hypercalcemia occurs the drug should be stopped until concentrations return to normal. It can then be restarted at lower doses. A major drawback to the use of $1,25(OH)_2D_3$ is the price, with effective doses costing as much as $50–$100 each month.

Dihydrotachysterol is a synthetic vitamin D analog which also does not require activation by the kidney.[10] It is effective in increasing calcium absorption in patients with chronic renal failure. It should be started at a dose of 0.25 mg/day and the dose increased every 2 weeks until the clinical effect is seen. Again if hypercalcemia occurs it usually reverts to normal within 2 weeks and the drug may be restarted at a lower dose. It is somewhat less expensive than $1,25(OH)_2D_3$ and may be as effective. There are at present, however, no controlled comparative studies.

Monitoring Calcium and Phosphorus Metabolism in Renal Failure Patients

It is essential that calcium and phosphorus metabolism be monitored in renal failure patients. There are many parameters which can be used. Serum phosphorus, serum calcium, serum parathyroid hormone concentration, serum alkaline phosphate, and bone roentgenograms are helpful.

The most important measurement is the serum phosphorus concentration which should be determined at least monthly in most dialysis patients. In hemodialysis patients, the predialysis serum phosphorus should be between 3.5 and 5 mg/dl. In peritoneal dialysis patients, the phosphorus concentrations should be maintained between 3 and 5 mg/dl. In compliant patients, these levels can usually be maintained by the appropriate manipulation of the diet and phosphorus binding antacids. In patients who have difficulty in keeping the serum phosphorus concentration in an acceptable range, it is helpful to determine serum phosphorus levels on a weekly basis.

Serum calcium should also be monitored at least monthly. Predialysis concentrations should be kept in the normal range. If available, the measurement of the serum ionized calcium is helpful, as these concentrations are not erroneously affected by changes in serum protein concentration and acid–base conditions. Serum-ionized calcium should be between 1.0 and 1.3 mmol/L. If there is hyperphosphatemia, attempts should not be made to correct hypocalcemia. Serum phosphorus should be reduced first, to avoid causing soft tissue and vascular calcification. In the hypocalcemic patient with normal serum phosphorus concentrations, serum calcium can be increased by increasing dialysate calcium concentration, increasing oral calcium intake, and/or administering vitamin D analogs.

Serum parathyroid hormone concentration, serum alkaline phosphatase, and bone roentgenograms are indicators of the long-term effects of abnormalities in calcium and phosphorus metabolism. There are several different types of plasma parathyroid hormone assays available. Probably the best type of assay to use in the routine management of the dialysis patient is a carboxy terminal assay. Even though this assay measures not only the intact hormone but also its inactive major metabolite, it appears to correlate better with clinical problems in renal failure patients than the N terminal assays which only measure the active hormone. Although serum parathyroid hormone concentrations are sometimes normal in dialysis patients, they are elevated in many patients without clinical problems. Generally with a carboxy terminal assay, if the concentration is not greater than five times the upper limit of normal, patients do not have many problems with secondary hyperparathyroidism.

Excessively high concentrations or progressively increasing PTH levels may be an indication of clinical problems, especially if associated with changes in bone x-rays and/or elevations of serum alkaline phosphatase. Initial attempts at controlling secondary hyperparathyroidism should be made by increasing serum calcium concentrations. If excessively high serum parathyroid concentrations persist inspite of high normal serum calcium concentrations and are causing significant bone problems, then partial parathyroidectomy should be considered. Partial parathyroidectomy is seldom needed in chronic renal failure patients who have had the serum phosphorus and calcium controlled throughout the course of their disease. Although serum alkaline phosphatase can be an indication of the action of parathyroid hormone on bone, other causes of elevation, such as liver disease, must be considered before assuming that elevated levels are an indication of the bone disease.

A complete discussion of bone roentgenography in patients with renal insufficiency is beyond the scope of this text. Ordinary bone x-rays are not a very sensitive indicator of renal osteodystrophy and better methods of monitoring the mineral content of bone in dialysis patients are available such as neutron activation analysis and computerized roetgenography.

With neutron activation analysis, neutrons from a radioactive source, usually ^{241}Am and ^{9}Be, enter the bone and produce the radioistope ^{49}Ca from the ^{48}Ca naturally present.[11] ^{49}Ca emits gamma radiation with the amount of radiation being proportional to the amount of calcium present in the bone. The wrist or the hand is generally studied. This is a reliable technique but the one major drawback of this procedure is that it requires a specially trained personnel and expensive equipment.

Dr. Calvin Cobert has developed a computerized method of determining the mineral content of bone from ordinary roentgenograms.[12] With his method, an x-ray of the hand is taken with a small, standardized aluminum wedge placed next to the forefinger. A computer determines the mineral content of the bone by comparing the optical density of the bone with the optical density of the aluminum wedge. The x-rays can be taken by any standard x-ray equipment and the bone density determined by sending the film to Dr. Colbert's laboratory for analysis. We have found it very helpful to perform this analysis every 6 months on our patients and 80 percent of the expense is covered by Medicare.

Renal Osteodystrophy

The term renal osteodystrophy is a general term used to describe the bone abnormalities which occur with chronic renal failure.[13,14] Renal osteodystrophy is really a combination of at least three and probably five different processes. These are osteomalacia, osteitis fibrosa cystica, osteosclerosis, osteoporosis, and subchrondral resorption. While these different pathologic processes frequently occur simultaneously, much of the time one or two are predominant. Osteomalacia is characterized by a deficiency in the mineral content of the bone with a relatively normal amount of the nonmineral matrix material present. Osteomalacia is the lesion caused in nonrenal failure patients by vitamin D deficiency. Osteoporosis is characterized by a lack of both the mineral content of the bone along with a lack of the matrix. It is impossible to distinguish osteomalacia and osteoporosis by radiography. Osteitis fibrosis cystica is caused by an increase in reabsorption of the bone. It is frequently seen in the cortex of the phalanges and the clavicals. Osteitis fibrosa cystica is usually caused by excessive secretion of parathyroid hormone. Osteosclerosis is manifested by an increase in bone density. It occurs most commonly in the vertebrae, ribs, clavicals, and pelvis. Osteosclerosis appears to be due to an abnormal arrangement of the bone matrix which takes a woven pattern rather than the normal laminar pattern.

The best way to adequately define renal osteodystrophy is by bone biopsy. Bone biopsies need to be processed by special techniques to get an accurate interpretation and are best evaluated by pathologists specially trained in the field of bone histology. These services, unfortunately, are not widely available.

HEMATOLOGIC ABNORMALITIES IN CHRONIC RENAL FAILURE

Anemia

Anemia is the primary hematologic abnormality found in the patients with chronic renal failure. The majority of dialysis patients have significant anemia with hemoglobin concentrations averaging between 6 and 8 g/dl. Although it is impossible to quantitate the clinical significance of this anemia, it undoubtedly has major effects in many if not most dialysis patients. It is likely that the activity tolerance of many of these patients is reduced by the anemia. In patients with underlying heart disease, anemia can also contribute to congestive heart failure and angina and it can aggrevate ischemic symptoms in patients with peripheral vascular disease.

The cause of anemia in chronic renal failure is multifactorial (Table 1-1). A major factor appears to be the decreased production of erythropoietin. Erythropoietin is a hormone normally produced by the kidney which stimulates the bone marrow to produce red blood cells. If anemia develops in normal man, erythropoietin production increases and stimulates the bone marrow to increase erythrocyte synthesis. Even though patients on dialysis may have normal or slightly increased plasma concentrations of erythropoietin,[15] when the degree of anemia is taken into consideration, this level is inappropriately low. Patients with normal renal function with a similar degree of anemia would have erythropoietin concentrations many times higher.

Even in the anuric patient, the diseased kidney is usually still capable of producing some erythropoietin. Bilateral nephrectomy uniformly decreases plasma erythropoietin concentrations and increases the severity of anemia. Although other organs such as the liver and possibly the salivary glands are capable of producing erythropoietin, the amounts produced are apparently less than even the most severely diseased kidney usually produces. For this reason bilateral nephrectomy should be avoided in chronic dialysis patients if at all possible.

Although decreased production of erythropoietin is the major cause of anemia in chronic renal failure, erythropoiesis is also inhibited

Table 1-1
Causes of Anemia in Chronic Renal Failure Patients

Decreased erythropoietin production

Circulating inhibitors of erythropoiesis

Increased red cell destruction
    uremia
    iatrogenic blood loss
    pentose phosphate shunt malfunction
    hypersplenism
    dialysate contaminants
      chloramine
      copper
      zinc

Deficiencies
    iron
    folic acid
? hyperparathyroidism

by toxins present in the plasma of these patients.[16] These inhibitors suppress the synthesis of red cells by the bone marrow. The compound or compounds causing the inhibition have not been well characterized. At least some of them appear to be small, dialyzable molecules, as plasma inhibition titer decreases with dialysis. This probably also explains the fact that there is usually a significant improvement of the anemia in the first several months of dialysis therapy, even though plasma erythropoietin concentrations decrease.

    In addition to the lack of erythropoietin and the presence of erythropoiesis inhibitors, the life span of the red cell is also slightly decreased in chronic renal failure.[17] The normal red cell life span of 115 days is reduced to an average of 73 days. This small decrease in red cell survival would not cause significant anemia in normals, but probably results in a small, significant decreased red cell count in patients with chronic renal failure. The increased red cell destruction appears to be due to a toxin circulating in the plasma, as red cells from patients with chronic renal failure survive normally when transfused into normal controls.[18] It has also been suggested that severe secondary hyperparathyroidism may contribute to the anemia of patients with chronic renal failure.[19] It is hypothesized that increased bone marrow fibrosis inhibits erythropoiesis. Uncontrolled studies show an improvement in anemia after parathyroidectomy in some patients.[19]

Treatment of Anemia

Unfortunately there is as yet no really good therapy for the anemia associated with chronic renal failure. Erythropoietin would appear to be ideal therapy, but as yet the techniques for producing large quantities of the purified hormone have not been perfected.

The first step in the treatment of the anemia caused by chronic renal failure is to eliminate potentially reversible, contributory factors. Iron deficiency is not infrequent in hemodialysis patients.[20] Fifty milligrams or more of iron each week may be lost in the dialyzer and dialyzer tubing. Another source of blood loss and therefore iron loss in chronic renal failure is phlebotomys for blood tests. At the University of Missouri we have developed a plasmaphoresis technique for blood tests, which greatly reduces red cell loss. At the beginning of hemodialysis, blood samples are drawn into heparinized, 20-ml syringes and the syringe is stood up on end. After approximately 30 minutes, most of the red cells have settled into the bottom of the syringe and the plasma can be drawn off the top into a vacuumized test tube. The remaining red cells can then be reinjected into the dialysis tubing. This procedure can prevent the loss of 250–350 ml of red blood cells each year.

Although it was originally thought that patients with chronic renal failure had a decreased ability to absorb iron from the gastrointestinal tract, it is now known that iron absorption in these patients is normal.[20] The amount of iron absorbed from the diet, however, is usually insufficient to replace the iron loss in patients receiving chronic hemodialysis and therefore most patients on chronic hemodialysis should receive replacement iron. The replacement iron can be given orally or can be given systematically in the form of iron dextran. There is some suggestive evidence that iron dextran is preferentially taken up by the liver, spleen, and possibly cardiac muscle, where it is sequestered and not available to the bone marrow for erythrocyte production.[21] For this reason, the best route of replacement iron is orally. Three hundred milligrams of ferrous sulfate 3 times each day is well tolerated and appears adequate in most patients. Phosphate binding antacids decrease iron absorption and should not be administered simultaneously with the iron.

The best method to monitor the iron status of patients with chronic renal failure is to periodically measure plasma ferritin concentration.[20] In contrast to serum iron concentration, serum ferritin has been shown to be a good indicator of bone marrow iron stores in these patients. Serum ferritin concentration should be measured every 6 months and should range between 30 and 300 $\mu g/dl$.

Another potential cause of anemia in chronic dialysis patients is folic acid deficiency.[22] Folic acid, being a small, water soluble compound, is readily removed during dialysis treatments. If not replaced, this removal can lead to folic acid deficiency and macrorytic anemia. Dialysis patients should receive 1 mg/day of supplemental folic acid. This is most easily given by prescribing a prenatal multivitamin preparation which then also supplies the other necessary vitamins.

In the severely anemic dialysis patient or the otherwise stable patient who has a sudden increase in severity of anemia, other contributory factors should be sought. One possible contributing factor in hemodialysis patients is excessive blood loss in the dialyzer and blood tubing at the end of dialysis. This may be due to increased dialyzer clotting from inadequate heparin doses or poor techniques in terminating dialysis.

Some severely anemic renal failure patients have been found to have hypersplenism caused by an enlarged spleen which traps and destroys red blood cells.[23] The enlarged spleen can usually be detected on physical examination, but a more sensitive method is the radionucleotide liver–spleen scan. In these patients removal of the spleen will cause a significant improvement in the anemia. Splenectomy should not be done however, until increased splenic red destruction is demonstrated by ferrokinetic studies.

Many patients with chronic renal failure have an acquired abnormality of the pentose phosphate shunt.[24] This makes them susceptible to hemolysis when exposed to drugs with high oxidizing potential, similar to patients with glucose-6-phosphatase deficiency. Drugs such as primaquin, sulfonamines, and quinidine must be used with caution in uremic patients.

Another factor which can contribute to the anemia in chronic hemodialysis patients is the presence of chloramine in the dialysate.[25] Chloramine is a compound which is added to tap water by some municipalities for bacteria control. Chloramine is an oxidizing agent and can cause red cell hemolysis in the presence of a pentase phosphate shunt abnormality. Chloramines are not removed by water softeners or by reverse osmosis, but are removed by charcoal filters and deionization.

Androgens

One medication which has been shown to improve the anemia in patients with chronic renal failure are the male hormone or androgen compounds.[26] Androgens increase the renal production of erythropoietin and also may improve the response of the bone marrow to erythropoietin. Well-controlled studies have demonstrated that the administration of androgens to chronic hemodialysis patients caused a significant increase in red cell mass. Unfortunately, the improvement is frequently small with an average increase in hemoglobin concentration of about 1 g/dl. In some patients, however, the improvement is much more dramatic. We have seen one patient in whom androgen administration increased hemoglobin concentration from 7 to 13 g/dl on two separate occasions. The effects of androgens on anemia are slow, may not begin for one or two months after starting therapy, and the peak effect may occur as late as 6 months after starting therapy.

Androgens may cause significant side effects. Women may develop acne, increased facial hair, and deepening of the voice. In the male, androgens may cause priapism or aggravate preexisting prostatism. Some of the synthetic androgens also cause liver disease.

The incidence of androgenic side effects (acne, hair growth, voice changes, and priapism) varies greatly with the various androgen preparations and is dependent on the anabolic:androgenic ratio. The testosterone esters have a ratio of 1.0 and because of this have a high incidence of side effects. For this reason they should not be used in females, but may be useful in male patients becase they are effective, they are the least expensive of the androgenic steroids, and they sometimes help with impotence problems.

The 17 methylated steriodal fluoxymesterone (Halotestin, Upjohn Co, Kalamazoo, MI) has an anabolic: androgenic ratio of 2.0 and although it is better than testosterone, it still has a significant incidence of side effects when therapeutic levels are used in women. Another disadvantage is that it can cause liver disease. The main advantage is that it can be given orally.

Nandrolone decanoate (Decadurobulin) has an anabolic:androgenic ratio of 6.0 and does not cause liver disease. It has a low incidence of androgenic side effects. The major disadvantages of nandrolone decanoate are the expense and the fact that it can only be given intramuscularly. In spite of these difficulties, it is probably the best androgenic preparation for dialysis patients, especially female.

Iron Overload

Chronic dialysis patients may also develop an iron overload syndrome. This occurs predominantly in severely anemic patients who require frequent transfusions, such as those who have had bilateral nephrectomy. Each unit of blood or packed red cells contains approximately 200 mg of iron. This iron is deposited in the liver, pancreas, and heart and can cause heart failure, diabetes mellitus, and hepatic dysfunction. These toxic effects are usually seen when the total body iron stores are in excess of 15–20 g as compared to the normal iron stores of 4 g.

Iron overload in chronic hemodialysis can be treated with desferrioxamine.[27] Desferrioxamine is an iron chelating agent which, when given to patients with normal renal function, irreversibly binds iron and it is then eliminated in the urine. When given to hemodialysis patients it binds iron from the plasma and is then eliminated by the dialyzer. Two grams of desferrioxamine given IV with each treatment will remove 45 mg of iron.

Desferrioxamine should be started early in the frequently transfused patient before signs of iron intoxication occur. We routinely give 2 g with each dialysis to such patients. This should be sufficient to maintain a neutral iron balance in patients receiving 3 units of blood each month. Serum ferritin concentrations should be monitored.

We have encountered one patient in whom the administration of desferrioxamine caused a definite increased anemia. The administration of desferrioxamine was associated with an average requirement of 1 unit of blood every 6 days to maintain the hematocrit above 12 percent, compared to a requirement of 1 unit every 12 days both before and after the desferrioxamine therapy.

Immunologic Abnormalities in Chronic Renal Failure

Infection is a major cause of morbidity and mortality in chronic renal failure patients. This is due to a number of immunologic abnormalities which have recently been extensively reviewed by Goldblum and Reed and consist of multiple defects in the various components of the immunologic systems.[28] It is important to realize, however, that in spite of these problems the majority of infections are handled adequately by the chronic renal failure patients.

There is a decrease in both the number and function of lymphocytes in chronic renal failure patients.[29] There is a small but significant decrease in the total peripheral lymphocyte count with an absolute decrease in both the B and T lymphocyte cells. The percentage of T cells is normal, but there is a decrease in the percentage of B cells with a reciprocal increase in the percentage of Null cells.

Cell-mediated immunity is decreased in chronic renal failure as manifested by a high incidence of cutaneous anergy and decreased blastogensis after immunologic stimulation.[29,30] The anergy appears to be related to plasma circulating toxins, as when immunologically capable cells are given to the uremic host the anergy persists, whereas the uremic cells transferred into nonuremic hosts are immunologically competent.[30] There is an improvement, but not normalization of the cellular immunity immediately following hemodialysis treatments,[31] although the anergy appears to be more pronounced in hemodialysis patients treated for greater than 1 year than in patients treated for less than 1 year.[32]

There have been many studies in chronic renal failure patients on the ability to produce antibodies after stimulation with various antigens.[28] Most have found either a normal response or a mild decrease in titer compared to nonuremic controls. Although the response may not be normal, vaccination with tetanus toxoid, pneumococcal capsular polysaccharide, and other vaccines usually result in titers high enough to be protective.

There are also abnormalities of granulocyte function in chronic renal failure. There is good evidence that both granulocyte mobility and chemotaxis are decreased,[33] but the results of studies of phagocytic activity are contradictory.[28] Most find normal granulocyte phagocytic activity in chronic renal failure, however, some studies have shown a small but significant depression.

The hemodialysis treatment itself has a significant effect on the circulating granulocyte count.[34] There is an acute, severe granulocytopenia which occurs early in the hemodialysis treatment. This appears to be due to activation by the dialyzer membrane of circulating complement compounds which results in extensive granulocyte trapping in the pulmonary vascular bed. This is one of the causes of hypoxia during hemodialysis (see Chapter 4). The severity of the granulocytopenia varies with different membranes and is decreased in reused dialyzers.

Platelet Function

Although there is a small, but significant reduction in plasma platelet count in chronic renal failure, it usually remains within the limits of normal. More important, however, are the abnormalities of platelet function which are seen in these patients.[35] Abnormal platelet function is the most consistent and severe hemostatic abnormality in chronic renal failure and is the major cause of the hemorrhagic diathesis seen in uremia.

There is a reduction in both platelet adhesiveness and platelet aggregation in response to various stimuli. The major commonly used clinical coagulation test affected is the bleeding time, which may be markedly prolonged in severe uremia. These platelet dysfunctions appear to be caused by circulating toxins which are dialyzable and marked improvement in platelet function occurs after dialysis. Guanidinosuccinic acid, phenols, urea, and prostaglandins have all been implicated as the culprit in different studies.[36]

There is also an interaction between platelets and the dialyzer membranes during hemodialysis treatments.[37] There is activation and consumption of platelets with a decrease in platelet count across the dialyzer and a release of platelet proteins such as beta-thromboglobulin (BTG), platelet factor 4 and platelet mitogenic factor. Since these platelet proteins are normally cleared by the kidney, nondialyzed chronic renal failure patients have high plasma levels and hemodialysis causes a further increase. Neither the increased platelet protein concentrations nor the mild thrombocytopenia induced by hemodialysis appear to produce, however, any clinical problems and the major coagulation change seen with hemodialysis treatments is that of an improvement due to better platelet function.

CARDIOVASCULAR ABNORMALITIES

There are four major cardiovascular abnormalities which have been associated with chronic renal failure: hypertension, increased atherosclerosis, myocardial dysfunction, and pericarditis. These abnormalities are not completely independent of each other, but are interrelated.

Hypertension

Hypertension is extremely common in renal insufficiency with a majority of patients having increased blood pressure at some time during the course of their disease. Clinically, hypertension is the most important cardiovascular abnormality because appropriate treatment will prevent the grim consequences of uncontrolled hypertension. There are at least two and probably three or four mechanisms causing hypertension in patients with renal insufficiency. These mechanisms include increased extracellular volume, increased renin secretion, increased sympathetically mediated vasoconstriction, and possibly decreased production of vasodilatory prostaglandins.

The most important mechanism causing hypertension in chronic renal failure is probably an increase in extracellular fluid volume.

Excessive extracellular volume increases blood pressure by increasing cardiac output.[38] The increase in cardiac output is the result of an increase of blood flow into the heart (increased preload). The extracellular fluid volume is primarily determined by the total amount of sodium in the body. The inability of the diseased kidney to adequately excrete sodium leads to hypertension through sodium accumulation. It must be recognized, however, that increased extracellular fluid does not always cause hypertension because compensatory mechanisms may prevent an increase in blood pressure.

Renin is a hormone secreted by the kidney which is normally involved in blood pressure regulation.[39] Renin is secreted by the kidney into the vascular system where it converts a circulatory plasma protein, angiotensinogen, into a small peptide called angiotensin I. Angiotensin I is converted into the active compound angiotensin II by the lung. Angiotensin II increases blood pressure by two mechanisms. First, it is a very potent vasoconstrictor which increases peripheral resistance by causing arterial constriction. This results in immediate increase in blood pressure. Second, angiotensin II also indirectly increases blood pressure by stimulating the adrenal secretion of aldosterone. Aldosterone causes sodium retention by the kidney, which increases blood pressure by the mechanism described previously.

Although more poorly understood than the volume and renin mechanisms, it appears that increased sympathetic vasoconstriction is also important in the etiology of hypertension in at least some patients with chronic renal failure.[44] The increase in sympathetic vasoconstriction may be the result of increased central sympathetic outflow, increased circulating catecholamines, or both. Although these mechanisms are very poorly defined at present, there is currently considerable research being conducted in this field which will hopefully increase our understanding. An exaggerated increase in blood pressure in response to placing the hand in cold water (cold pressor test), found in many renal failure patients, is suggestive evidence of this mechanism.

It has been suggested that decreased secretion of prostaglandins by the kidneys also has a role in producing hypertension in some patients with chronic renal failure.[41] Although some of the prostaglandins produced in the kidney have vasodilatory properties, there is no good evidence at present that prostaglandins are involved in normal blood pressure regulation. Any role their deficiency may have in the production of hypertension in renal failure remains speculative at this time.

The treatment of hypertension in chronic renal failure is discussed in Chapter 2 and it needs only be emphasized here that this treatment is one of the most important aspects of the therapy of chronic renal failure.

Increased Cardiovascular Morbidity in Dialysis Patients

Patients on chronic hemodialysis have an increased mortality rate from cardiovascular causes as compared to age-matched controls.[42] This has been interpreted by some to indicate that chronic renal failure and/or hemodialysis is the cause of this mortality, probably through increased atherosclerosis. More recently, however, this interpretation has been questioned.[43,44] Patients with chronic renal failure have a high incidence of risk factors for atherosclerosis. The vast majority have had some hypertension, with many having a history of prolonged periods of severe hypertension. Hyperlipidemia is seen both in renal insufficiency and with the nephrotic syndrome. Many dialysis patients have had periods of the nephrotic syndrome prior to dialysis treatments. Recent studies show that when these risk factors are taken into consideration, the cardiovascular morbidity and mortality rates of chronic hemodialysis patients are not increased.[43,44]

The major risk factor for atherosclerosis in chronic hemodialysis patients appears to be hypertension. Vincenti and co-workers accessed atherosclerosis in 50 nondiabetic hemodialysis patients by examining the iliac artery at the time of renal transplantation.[45] No atherosclerosis was found in patients under the age of 40 without a previous history of hypertension. When the various factors were analyzed there was also a significant correlation between the blood pressure and atherosclerosis, but no correlation between atherosclerosis and plasma lipid level or any of the other metabolic abnormalities of chronic renal failure. The authors concluded that atherosclerosis is not accelerated by hemodialysis and might be prevented by the stringent control of hypertension in uremia.

Myocardial Dysfunction

Between 25 and 40 percent of chronic dialysis patients have evidence of left ventricular dysfunction.[46-49] There are many factors present in chronic renal failure which may contribute to this dysfunction. First of all, chronic dialysis patients have a higher than normal cardiac workload. The primary factors causing this increased workload are anemia, hypertension, and, in hemodialysis patients, the arteriovenous fistula. It has been suggested that a chronic increase in cardiac workload can result in myocardial failure. Experimental work in dogs shows that chronic increases in cardiac work results in permanent changes in ventricular contractility and compliance.[50] Hypertension, in addition to increasing the cardiac workload, also causes myocardial hypertrophy. Excessive myocardial hypertrophy can decrease myocardial function, possibly because the coronary vasculature does not expand sufficiently to supply the increased muscle mass.

It has been suggested that uremia itself can cause myocardial dysfunction (uremic cardiomyopathy) possibly through a direct effect of some uremic toxins.[51] Bailey and co-workers described 5 patients with chronic renal failure treated by conservative methods who developed severe congestive heart failure which did not appear to be the result of hypertension, anemia, or fluid overload.[52] All signs of congestive heart failure disappeared in 1–2 months after intensive dialysis. Others have described similar problems in patients already on dialysis in whom the proposed cardiomyopathy improves after renal transplantation.[53] In none of these studies has it been possible to dissociate the contribution of anemia, fluid overload, and hypertension from the possible contribution of uremic toxins.

Prospective studies of myocardial function in chronic renal failure at first glance appear confusing, but on closer inspection are very informative. When the acute effects of hemodialysis are studied by various techniques, myocardial function may improve, remain unchanged, or deteriorate with the treatments.[48] This apparent confusion is clarified by dividing the patients into groups on the basis of their predialysis myocardial function. In those patients with normal predialysis myocardial function as evidenced by a normal injection fraction, dialysis had either no affect on myocardial function or actually decreased it. This is to be expected since it would be unlikely for dialysis to make myocardial function better than normal and it is frequently necessary to remove large amounts of fluid during the treatment which may reduce blood return to the heart and decrease cardiac output. Patients with myocardial dysfunction prior to dialysis as evidenced by a decreased ejection fraction show, on the other hand, a significant improvement after dialysis treatment. This has been interpreted as suggestive that these patients are operating on an abnormal systolic function curve and that dialysis improves function by decreasing the preload.

The long-term affects of chronic dialysis have also been studied and the results are similar to the acute affects of dialysis.[49] Those patients with evidence of myocardial dysfunction prior to starting dialysis therapy show a significant improvement, while there is no significant change in those patients with normal function at the beginning of treatments. In none of the patients studied was there evidence of progressive decrease in function. It is likely that reduction of chronic fluid overload and improvement in blood pressure are responsible for the improvement in those patients with preexisting dysfunction. While these studies do not completely eliminate the possibility of a unique cardiomyopathy in uremia, the available evidence indicates that it is not a common problem.

Pericarditis

The association between pericarditis and renal failure has been known since it was first described by Richard Bright in 1836.[54] He found signs of pericardial inflammation and fluid in 37 percent of patients dying from uremia. More recent studies are in agreement with careful echocardiographic studies indicating that between 40 and 70 percent of patients have pericardial effusions at the start of dialysis treatment.[55–57] The incidence of symptomatic pericarditis is less, occurring in only about 10 percent of patients treated by conservative management. In patients who develop symptomatic pericarditis prior to starting dialysis, the initiation of dialysis therapy usually results in the prompt resolution of symptoms. For this reason it was originally felt that the availability of dialysis therapy would eliminate or at least markedly reduce the problem of pericarditis in renal failure. This has not been the case and pericarditis not infrequently develops in the otherwise stable dialysis patient. It is now apparent that there are two different types of pericarditis which occur in renal failure patients: *uremic pericarditis,* which usually occurs prior to the onset of dialysis, and *dialysis associated pericarditis,* which occurs in patients on dialysis therapy. The current evidence suggests that these are two distinct, separate entities.

Uremic pericarditis and dialysis-associated pericarditis are compared in Table 1-2. Uremic pericarditis occurs before the initiation of dialysis therapy, is usually associated with other signs and symptoms of uremia, and responds to dialysis. Systemic symptoms such as fever and chest pains are, in addition, less prominant or absent in uremic pericarditis while they can be very severe in dialysis-associated pericarditis. The fluid is usually sanguinous and maybe frankly hemorraghic in dialysis-associated pericarditis while it is serous or serosanguinous in uremic pericarditis. Finally, cardiac tamponade is very rare with uremic pericarditis, but is not uncommon with dialysis-associated pericarditis.

Table 1-2
Comparison of Uremic Pericarditis and Dialysis-Associated Pericarditis

Sign or Symptom	Uremic Pericarditis	Dialysis-Associated Pericarditis
Friction rub	Common	Common
Chest pain	Mild, absent	Severe
Fever	Uncommon	Common
Pericardial fluid	Serous or Serosanguinous	Sanguinous or Hemorraghic
Cardiac tamponade	Rare	Frequent

Uremic pericarditis is thought to be caused by an irritating effect of some uremic toxins on the pericardium and the good response to dialysis is consistent with this hypothesis. The etiology of dialysis-associated pericarditis is less clear. There appears to be no relation to the amount of dialysis, serum urea or creatinine concentrations or other indications of biochemical control. Some studies suggest that chronic fluid overload is contributory, but this is not a consistent finding. Hypercalcemia and hyperparathyroidism have also been implicated, but are clearly not the sole or even major cause. Pabico and Freeman suggest that some, if not most, dialysis-associated pericarditis are infectious in origin.[58] They suggest that renal failure-induced immunologic abnormalities may make these patients more susceptible to the development of infectious pericarditis. Clearly the clinical picture is very suggestive of infection with fever, chills, malaise, and and leukocytosis commonly occurring. Pabico found immunologic evidence suggestive of cytomegalovirus infection in five patients. Other investigators have not been able to find evidence of infection, however.

Pericarditis should be suspected in the chronic renal failure patient who has chest pain, especially if associated with fever. The chest pain is generally substernal in location and is frequently affected by position, most often relieved by sitting up. Pericarditis should also be considered in the previously stable patient who suddenly begins to exhibit unexplained hypotension during dialysis.

A pericardial friction rub is present in the majority of patients with symptomatic pericarditis. The friction rub typically has three ascultatory components during the cardiac cycle. The best confirmatory test for pericarditis is the echocardiogram which will demonstrate significant pericardial fluid in most cases. Pericarditis can occur, however, without demonstrable fluid in the pericardial sac. Also between 10 and 30 percent of asymptomatic patients on chronic dialysis will have pericardial effusion when screened by echocardiography.[55] The significance of this fluid in the asymptomatic patient is unknown. Chest roentgenography and electrocardiography are seldom helpful in the diagnosis of pericarditis.

Pericardial tamponade is a major life threatening complication of pericarditis. It is rare in uremic and asymptomatic pericarditis, but may occur in as many as 20 percent of dialysis-associated pericarditis. Large amounts of fluid in the pericardial sac prevent adequate filling of the heart and decrease cardiac output. Tamponade usually occurs if the fluid accumulation exceeds 1000 ml, but can occur with smaller amounts of fluid if the fluid accumulates rapidly or if the pericardium has been made less distensible by scarring from previous inflammation. A paradoxical pulse, which is a large decrease in pulse pressure occurring with inspiration, is a useful clinical sign indicative of pericardial tamponade. There is also an increase in amplitude of the venous pulsations seen in the neck veins. The diagnosis of pericardial tamponade is best confirmed by cardiac catheterization.

Therapy

The therapy of pericarditis is controversial. To prevent excessive bleeding into the pericardial sac, hemodialysis patients with pericarditis should receive low doses of heparin or regional heparinization during their treatments (see Chapter 4). It has been suggested by some that patients with pericarditis should be preferentially treated with peritoneal dialysis.[59] This eliminates the need for heparin, allows for the gradual removal of any excessive fluid, and avoids acute changes in intravascular volume. The hypothesis that increased removal of middle molecules by peritoneal dialysis may help resolve the pericarditis, although attractive, remains unproven.

Patients with evidence of pericardial tamponade require immediate attention. Pericardiocentesis is recommended by some and can be life saving. Some have experienced, however, a high mortality with this procedure in patients with renal failure.[60] This might be because the very friable pericardium may bleed excessively when touched by the pericardial needle. This can apparently occur even if the needle is monitored with the electrocardiogram. Because of this high mortality rate and because of the usual rapid rate of fluid reaccumulation after pericardiocentesis, a surgical procedure such as a pericardial window or pericardectomy should be strongly considered as the first procedure of choice in patients with pericardial tamponade.

In patients with pericarditis without tamponade, more conservative methods are indicated. Pericarditis in the renal failure patient not on dialysis generally responds favorably to the initiation of dialysis and no other specific therapy is usually needed. Pericarditis developing in the patient on dialysis is frequently more resistant to treatment. It is generally recommended that dialysis time be increased, and although 40 to 50 percent of patients have remissions with this type of therapy, the actual relationship of the response to the increased dialysis is unproven. While it is possible that many of these responses are spontaneous, it may be prudent to initially increase dialysis in patients with dialysis-associated pericarditis. This is especially true if there are other indications of inadequate dialysis. It also appears helpful to remove any extra fluid volume which is frequently present and to prevent overhydration by strict salt and water restriction. Indomethacin has been recommended for those patients who do not respond to increased dialysis. Some observers have noted a good response to 25 mg 4 times each day of Indomethacin.[61] One double-blinded study (reported in abstract form only) could not demonstrate however, any beneficial effect.[62] Although systemic steroids do not appear to have any benefit, the installation of a nonabsorbable steroid (200–900 mg Triamcinolone) directly into the pericardial sac has been reported to be helpful.[63] These are uncontrolled studies and the possibility of complications from the pericardiocentesis needs to be considered.

Surgical therapy is indicated in those patients with resistant or recurrent pericarditis who do not respond to more conservative methods. There are three surgical procedures: pericardial window, subtotal pericardectomy, and total pericardectomy. The pericardial window, where a small opening is made in the anterior or subxiphoid pericardium, should probably be limited to acutely ill patients who are unable to tolerate a more extended procedure. This procedure can be rapidly performed under local anesthesia. Unfortunately, over time the window frequently closes with subsequent fluid reaccumulation. There is also the possibility of incarceration and strangulation of the heart. In the stable patient, subtotal or total pericardectomy with removal of a major portion or the total pericardial sac is the surgical treatment of choice. Patients with marked thickening of the pericardial sac should have a total pericardectomy. These procedures result in an over 97 percent success rate.

GASTROINTESTINAL MANIFESTATIONS OF CHRONIC RENAL FAILURE

Chronic renal failure is associated with changes throughout the entire length of the gastrointestinal tract. Anorexia, especially for high protein foods, is an early sign of the uremic syndrome. As renal failure progresses, nausea and vomiting frequently develop. The nausea and vomiting appear to be caused both by structural changes in the gastric mucosa and from stimulation of the central nervous system. It is typically worse in the morning, frequently causing vomiting after breakfast, and is sometimes associated with a constant metallic taste in the mouth. This bad taste may be secondary to high oral concentrations of ammonia produced locally from urea breakdown. Most of these uremic gastrointestinal symptoms are caused by protein metabolites, since protein restriction will frequently result in marked improvement. All of these symptoms will generally respond to treatment with dialysis or renal transplantation.

Gastroenterocolitis

Uremia causes mucosal alterations seen in all segments of the gastrointestinal tract. These changes include mild edema, submucosal hemorrhage, mucosal ulceration, and necrosis. Hemorrhagic lesions occur most commonly in the esophagus, stomach, ileum, and proximal colon, while ulcerative lesions are more frequent in the ileum and colon. These lesions will result in hematest positive vomitus and are the cause of bloody diarrhea which is not infrequently seen in severe uremia. They appear to be caused by the accumulation of toxic substances and usually respond to treatment by dialysis or transplantation.

Stomach Acid Secretion

Chronic renal failure is associated with variable affects on gastric secretion.[65] Conservatively treated patients with advanced renal failure have markedly impaired acid secretion whereas most patients on chronic hemodialysis have increased gastric acid secretion. This disparity is likely caused by the fact that uremia has differing effects on the multiple factors involved in gastric acidity.

Gastrin is a hormone secreted by the small intestine which stimulates acid secretion in the stomach. Serum gastrin concentrations increase early in the course of progressive renal failure, remain high in chronic dialysis patients, and are the most likely explanation for the increased acid secretion seen in patients in chronic dialysis.[66] There are several possible explanations for the apparent hyposecretion of acid in the face of high serum gastrin levels which is seen in chronic renal failure patients immediately prior to initiation of dialysis. The mucosal structural changes described above may cause a breakdown in the gastric mucosal barrier and allow for increased backleak of acid out of the stomach. There also may be a local conversion of the high levels of urea to ammonia which would then neutralize some of the secreted hydrogen ions. Both of these mechanisms may mask an actual hypersecretion of acid caused by the hypergastrinemia.

It has been suggested that there is an increased frequency of peptic ulcer disease in chronic dialysis patients.[67] This would not be unexpected in view of the increased acid secretion. Prospective studies do not reveal, however, an actual increased incidence[68] and, clinically, peptic ulcer disease does not occur commonly in dialysis patients. There is, however, an increase incidence after renal transplantation,[69] which is probably at least partially caused by the corticosteroid medication.

Constipation

Constipation is an exceedingly common problem in patients with chronic renal failure. The main cause appears to be the administration of phosphorus binding antacids.[70] The addition of a stool softner such as Colace or a stool softner plus a mild laxative such as Pericolace is necessary in most patients. Resistant cases usually respond to the addition of sorbitol, with 1–3 tablespoons a day of 70 percent solution being an average dose. If left untreated, constipation can lead to impacted fecalomas, which cause bowel obstruction and not infrequently lead to perforation.[70]

NEUROLOGIC ABNORMALITIES OF CHRONIC RENAL FAILURE

There are many neurologic syndromes which occur in patients with chronic renal failure.[71,72] They can involve the central, peripheral, and autonomic nervous systems or the muscles themselves. While many of these syndromes are directly caused by the renal insufficiency, some are also the result of its treatment. Most are preventable by an understanding of the pathophysiology of the causation and the institution of appropriate therapy.

Central Nervous System

There are three major central nervous system syndromes which occur in patients with renal insufficiency: uremic encephalopathy, the disequilibrium syndrome, and dialysis dementia. Patients with renal failure also have an increased incidence of cerebral vascular accidents and subdural hematomas. The high incidence of vascular accidents can probably be reduced by the aggressive control of blood pressure.

Subdural hematoma must always be considered when the dialysis patient develops the sudden onset of neurologic symptoms such as persistent headache, confusion, drowsiness, signs of meningeal initiation, hypertension, and/or focal neurologic signs.[73] Predisposing factors in these patients include anticoagulation during dialysis or for maintenance of vascular access, the uremic platelet function defect, and possibly rapid fluid shifts occurring during the hemodialysis treatments. It is not uncommon for there to be bilateral subdural hematomas in these patients. Computerized axiotomography appears to be the best method of diagnosis.

Uremic encephalopathy is usually a sign of severe, advanced renal insufficiency. With sudden, complete loss of renal function, it can occur rapidly within a few days; while with slow, progressive renal insufficiency, the onset is more insidious. The earliest manifestation of uremic encephalopathy is a decreased ability to concentrate. This can be demonstrated clinically by the serial sevens test. In this test, the patient is asked to do serial seven substractions, starting at 100. Many mildly uremic patients who on routine interview do not appear to have any apparent mentation problem, will be completely unable to successfully complete more than one or two steps. That the defect is from uremia is demonstrated by the usually marked improvement in their ability to perform this test after appropriate treatment, such as dialysis. As uremia advances, the uremic encephalopathy progresses from an inability to concentrate, to clouding of consciousness, frequently associated with marked personality changes, and if untreated eventually results in coma. Asterixis, a course tremor provoked by dorsiflexion of the hands, is also frequently seen with uremic encephalopathy.

The cause of uremic encephalopathy is not well understood. It is generally thought that the accumulation of uremic toxins plays a major role. While this is likely true, it is apparent that changes in sodium and water balance are also important. In one perspective study of uremic patients, serum sodium concentration was found to be the most important determinant of uremic encephalopathy.[74] Patients with encephalopathy had significantly lower serum sodium concentrations than patients without encephalopathy, indicating that water intoxication with intracellular brain edema appears to be at least partially responsible. This is important since it is preventable and/or treatable by fluid restriction and/or dialysis treatments.

Uremia is also associated with electroencephalographic changes.[75] Early changes are manifested by a small increase in the percentage of slow wave activity, seen mainly in the fronto-parietal parasaggital area. As severe uremia develops, diffuse spike and wave activity are seen. These EEG changes are best quantified by computer-based spectroanalysis. While dialysis therapy results in marked improvement in the EEG pattern, it remains abnormal in many dialysis patients. The EEG usually becomes normal after renal transplantation. Changes in the EEG correlate with other uremic parameters and therefore the EEG may be useful in determining the adequacy of therapy.

Dialysis Disequilibrium Syndrome

The dialysis disequilibrium syndrome is a complex of symptoms which can occur during or immediately after hemodialysis treatments.[76] It usually only occurs with the initial treatments and rarely, if ever, occurs during chronic hemodialysis. Mild cases of disequilibrium syndrome are manifested by headache, nausea, and vomiting while in more severe cases there may be blurred vision, tremor, muscle twitching, or even generalized convulsions.

Originally the disequilibrium syndrome was thought to be caused by the rapid removal of urea. It was postulated that there was a lag in the removal of uremia from the brain cells which resulted in an osmotic gradiant and caused a shift of water into the cells with the development of intracellular edema. The rapid movement of urea across most cell membranes makes this hypothesis unlikely. Also, Arieff was unable to produce any significant urea gradient in the central nervous system of uremic dogs treated with rapid hemodialysis.[77]

It has also been suggested that the dialysis disequilibrium syndrome was caused by the rapid correction of metabolic acidosis. It is hypothesized that a rapid increase in serum bicarbonate decreases respiration and increases arterial P_{CO_2}. Since bicarbonate crosses the blood brain barrier more slowly than carbon dioxide, this results in an increased acidosis in the central nervous system. The poor correlation between the degree of acidosis and the incidence of disequilibrium syndrome suggests that this is not the primary mechanism.

Arieff hypothesises that the disequilibrium syndrome is the result of the accumulation of idiogenic osmoles in brain cells during uremia.[77] During the development of uremia there is an increase in intracellular brain osmolality which cannot be explained by an increase in the major determinants of osmolality, i.e., sodium, potassium, chloride, magnesium, calcium, or urea. The unknown cause of this increased osmolality has been referred to as idiogenic osmoles and may be related to organic acids and/or changes in protein binding. Arieff suggests that, because of the accumulation of these idiogenic osmoles, rapid hemodialysis does not decrease intracellular osmolality as fast as extracellular osmolality and therefore causes a shift of fluid into the brain cells with the development of cerebral edema.

While the exact pathophysiology of the disequilibrium syndrome is not well understood, it appears to be directly related to the rapid correction of severe uremia. It essentially never occurs with peritoneal dialysis and can usually be prevented in hemodialysis by restricting the intensity of the initial dialysis treatments. In general, the use of a small surface area dialyzer (1 m^2), low blood flows (100–150 ml/min), and short duration (2–3 hours) during the first treatments is advisable. If the patient is severely uremic as evidenced by high serum urea and creatinine concentrations, it is helpful to dialyze the patient daily until the scrum urea concentration is persistently below 100 mg/dl. The intensity of the dialysis treatments can then be gradually increased and the frequency reduced.

Dialysis Dementia

In 1972, Alfrey described a progressive, neurologic syndrome in dialysis patients which had not been recognized before.[78] The syndrome is fairly unique and easy to diagnose when it occurs. It consists of expressive aphasia with slow stuttering speech, myoclonus, asterixis, and apraxia of movement. As the syndrome progresses, which almost inevitably occurs, dementia and psychosis develop. The syndrome is usually fatal with patients dying within one year of diagnosis.

Although there is not universal agreement as to the etiology of dialysis dementia, there is overwhelming evidence which suggests that aluminum intoxication plays a major role in most cases.[79] Aluminum levels in the brain and other tissues are an order of magnitude higher in patients with the syndrome than in normal controls or dialysis patients without the syndrome. Although dialysis patients absorb some aluminum from phosphate binding aluminum salts, the vast majority of cases of dialysis dementia have been associated with increased dialysate aluminum concentrations and the syndrome rarely if ever occurs in patients treated with dialysate aluminum concentrations below 1 mcg/l.

Peripheral Neuropathy

It has long been recognized that chronic renal failure can cause a peripheral neuropathy.[80] Early in the history of dialysis therapy this was a major problem, with patients frequently having severe neuropathy at the start of dialysis and the neuropathy progressing or at least not improving with dialysis therapy. Presently it is very unusual to see clinical problems with peripheral neuropathy in dialysis patients unless there is a secondary cause such as diabetes mellitus. It is likely that this marked reduction in the incidence of peripheral neuropathy is the result of the early initiation of dialysis therapy, before severe uremia develops, more efficient dialysis, and the prevention of malnutrition by not imposing severe dietary restrictions.

Uremia neuropathy is usually confined to the lower extremities and only occurs in the upper extremities after severe involvement of the lower extremities. It commonly starts as a sensory loss in the feet usually involving all sensory modalities. The paresthesia maybe accompanied by pricking, tingling, or painful sensations. On examination, the transition from abnormal to normal sensation occurs more abruptly than with other types of peripheral neuropathy. With progression, weakness of the feet and atrophy of the leg muscles ensue.

Patients with uremic peripheral neuropathy show a marked decrease in motor nerve conduction velocity (MNCV). The large variation in MNCV found in the normal population and the frequent finding of abnormal values in dialysis patients without clinical problems unfortunately make the routine use of this test not very helpful. Periodic routine clinical neurologic testing during physical examination appears adequate for following chronic dialysis patients.

Uremic peripheral neuropathy is manifested pathologically by axonal atrophy and demyelination of the nerve fibers. It is thought that the loss of myelin is secondary to axonal destruction. It is hypothesized, but not proven, that high levels of uremic toxins cause the axonal damage. It is likely, however, that at least in some cases malnutrition from poor dietary intake also contributes to the problem.

Restless Leg Syndrome

Many dialysis patients describe a peculiar creeping, crawling, prickling sensation in their lower legs which is relieved by leg movement.[81] This has been termed the "restless leg syndrome" and may occur in as many as two thirds of dialysis patients. It has also been described in other conditions such as pregnancy, poliomyelitis, vitamin deficiency, and carcinoma. Although the restless leg syndrome has been ascribed to peripheral neuropathy the fact that it occurs with equal frequency in patients without other objective signs of peripheral neuropathy suggests that other etiologies are more important.

ENDOCRINE ABNORMALITIES IN CHRONIC RENAL FAILURE

The affect of chronic renal failure on the various endocrine systems is very complex and in many cases not well understood. There are many mechanisms by which renal insufficiency can affect endocrine function. Since the kidney itself is an endocrine organ, it is not surprising that failure of this organ decreases the synthesis of its hormones: erythropoietin and $1,25(OH)_2D_3$.

The kidney is also a major pathway for the degradation of small peptides. This is accomplished in large part through nonexcretory mechanisms. Many hormones are small peptides and therefore their metabolic clearance decreases during renal insufficiency. This is true for insulin, glucagon, parathyroid hormone, calcitonin, growth hormone, and prolactin. Since the secretion of most hormones are regulated by feedback mechanisms, this decreased degradation should not cause persistently elevated levels. It may result, however, in a delay in the return to normal levels after an acute increase.

Some hormones are degraded in the body into inactive metabolites prior to their elimination. If the excretion of these metabolites are dependent on renal function, they will accumulate in renal insufficiency. These inactive metabolites may retain their antigenicity, and therefore be measured by hormone immunoassay. One reason plasma PTH level concentrations are elevated in uremia by some assays is because of increased plasma levels of inactive metabolites.

Uremia may also directly suppress hormone secretion, as in the case of the testicular secretion of testosterone, or may decrease end organ response to hormones which appears to occur with both insulin and parathyroid hormone.

The lack of understanding of many of the endocrinologic problems which occur during renal failure is not due to lack of research. There have been many studies performed in the last 10 years. Unfortunately, much of the data produced is conflicting and in many cases it is difficult or impossible to draw clinical conclusions. Parathyroid hormone, $1,25(OH)_2D_3$, and erythropoietin have been discussed earlier in this chapter. The remainder of this section will focus on the three endocrine systems in which there are significant clinically relevant data: the thyroid hormones, pancreatic hormones, and reproductive hormones. For a more detailed review of uremic endocrinopathies, the reader is referred to the excellent article by Emmanouel et al. in the June 1981 issue of Seminars in Nephrology.[82]

Thyroid Function

It has been suggested that many patients with renal insufficiency have hypothyroidism. Certainly many signs and symptoms of hypothyroidism are common in the uremic syndrome. Renal failure patients have intolerance to cold, dry coarse skin, anemia, and facial features suggestive of hypothyroidism. These features cause the diagnosis of myxedema to be frequently entertained in these patients.

Different studies of the plasma concentrations of the thyroid hormones in renal failure give conflicting results. The most consistent abnormal finding is that of a decrease in total and free T_3. This has been demonstrated to be caused by a decrease in the peripheral conversion of T_4 to T_3.[83] Both total and free thyroxine (T_4) concentrations are usually in the low normal range, but some studies show them to be abnormally low. The plasma concentrations of thyroxin binding globulin (TBG) are usually normal, but may occasionally be depressed. Thyroid stimulating hormone (TSH) is again usually normal, but may be found on occasion to be elevated.

The clinical relevance of these plasma changes is hard to determine. Spector and co-workers studied the relationship of plasma thyroid tests to the clinical thyroid status in 38 patients on chronic hemodialysis or chronic peritoneal dialysis.[84] Clinical thyroid status was evaluated by the basal metabolic rate (BMR), achilles tendon reflex, pulse wave arrival time, serum cholesterol, and creatinine phosphokinase concentrations. They found that the vast majority of dialysis patients are clinically euthyroid. There was no correlation between either total or free T_3 concentration and the clinical thyroid state. Both serum free T_4 and TSH concentrations, however, appear to be reliable indicators of thyroid state and the authors suggest that if free T_4 is depressed and TSH concentrations are increased that the diagnosis of hypothyroidism should seriously be considered.

Pancreatic Hormones

Chronic renal failure is associated with multiple abnormalities of the pancreatic hormones and glucose metabolism. Patients with renal failure usually have normal fasting blood glucose concentrations, but frequently have an abnormal glucose tolerance curve. This abnormal glucose tolerance curve is not the result of insufficient insulin as patients with chronic renal failure have increased plasma insulin concentrations, both in the fasting and glucose loaded states.[85,86]

The glucose intolerance seen in uremics is caused by a peripheral resistance to insulin. Sophisticated glucose and insulin (clamp) techniques in which both glucose and insulins are simultaneously infused have demonstrated that patients with chronic renal failure need more insulin to transfer a specific amount of glucose across the cell membrane than do normal controls.[86] The exact nature of this insulin resistance is not clear, but it may be related to circulating insulin antagonists, hormone receptor alterations, or abnormalities of the transport mechanisms. The insulin resistance appears to be caused by circulating toxins and significant improvement is seen after intensive dialysis. The metabolism of glucose after it enters the cell appears normal.

Normally, 30 percent of endogenously secreted or exogenously injected insulin is metabolized by the kidney. Renal insulin metabolism is markedly decreased in renal failure which results in an increased insulin half-life. Since insulin secretion is controlled by the serum glucose concentration with a servomechanism, this is not the major cause of the increased insulin levels in nondiabetic patients, but is the reason that insulin requirements in diabetic patients may decrease dramatically as renal insufficiency develops. Insulin requirements not infrequently decrease by 50 percent or greater as the diabetic patient approaches end stage renal disease.

Plasma glucagon concentrations are increased in chronic renal failure.[85] Glucagon is a pancreatic hormone which increases blood glucose concentrations by increasing gluconeogenesis in the liver. The primary cause of increased glucagon levels appears to be impaired glucagon degradation by the kidney. This may contribute to the glucose intolerance seen in chronic renal failure and is probably the cause of the increased hepatic glucose production found in uremia, by some, but not all investigators.

Growth hormone concentrations are also frequently elevated in chronic renal failure.[85] Growth hormone is secreted by the pituitary and increases blood glucose by reducing carbohydrate metabolism in cells and increasing the use of fats for energy. Although the increased growth hormone may contribute to the glucose intolerance, it does not appear to be a major factor as there is no correlation between glucose tolerance and plasma growth hormone concentrations in renal failure patients.

Another problem occasionally seen in uremia is prolonged severe hyoglycemia.[87] Spontaneous hypoglycemia in renal failure was originally described in diabetic patients, but has also now been seen in nondiabetic, renal failure patients. It appears not to be caused by excess insulin, but by decreased gluconeogenesis by the liver. The majority of patients described have been malnourished and the impaired hepatic glucose production is probably the result of insufficient substrate, primarily the amino acid, alanine. Spontaneous hypoglycemia should not occur in the well-nourished renal failure patient, as they usually have normal or increased hepatic gluconeogenesis.

Sexual Dysfunction in Chronic Renal Failure

There are multiple problems in relation to reproductive function which occur in patients with chronic renal failure. Abnormalities of the pituitary and gonadal hormones, psychological problems, drugs which effect sexual function, anemia, and malnutrition all may play a role. While dialysis therapy may result in some improvement, it is seldom completely satisfactory. Transplantation usually, but not always, causes a normalization or at least marked improvement of these problems.

The most easily measured and therefore the most thoroughly studied of the sexual abnormalities are the changes in the plasma levels of the reproductive hormones.[88-90] Plasma luteinizing hormone (LH) concentrations are elevated in the majority of chronic renal failure patients. This hormone is secreted from the anterior pituitary gland. In the normal male LH stimulates the testicular interstitial cells to secrete testosterone. In the female LH causes the ovarian follicular cells to change into lutein cells after ovulation and secrete large amounts of estrogen and progesterones. Normally the secretion of LH is regulated at least partially by the plasma concentration of the gonadal hormones.

There are at least two reasons LH is elevated in chronic renal failure. The first, and probably the most important reason, is because of decreased hormone secretion by the gonads. This is especially true for testosterone secretion which is markedly depressed in renal failure. This appears to be related to a direct suppression of testicular secretion by renal insufficiency. Ovarian hormone secretion is also suppressed in renal failure for, although plasma estrogen and progesterone levels may be in the low normal range, they are inappropriately low in the face of the high plasma LH concentrations. The second reason for elevated LH levels in chronic renal failure is a reduced metabolic clearance rate probably caused by a decrease in the renal metabolism of the hormone.

Plasma follicular-stimulating hormone (FSH) concentration may also be increased in chronic renal failure, but less often and usually to a smaller degree than LH concentrations.[88-90] Follicular-stimulating hormone is another pituitary gonadotrophin. It stimulates the development of the ovarian follicles in the female and spermatogenesis in the male. There apppears to be end organ resistance to FSH in chronic renal failure as, even with high levels of FSH, spermatogenesis is markedly decreased in the male with chronic renal failure and ovulation rarely occurs in the female.

Prolactin is a pituitary hormone which is greatly elevated in most patients with chronic renal failure.[88-90] The primary normal function of prolactin is to produce lactation in the female after delivery. In the nonpuerperal state, hyperprolactemia is associated with galactorrhea in the female and gynecomastia in the male and is probably the cause of these disorders when they occur in renal failure. In nonrenal failure patients, hyperprolactemia is also associated with amenorrhea and infertility in the female and oligospermia and impotence in the male. Since these are very common problems in renal failure patients, it is possible that the increased prolactin contributes to their etiology.

Bromergocryptine is a drug which inhibits the secretion of prolactin. Preliminary studies with this agent indicates that it decreases plasma prolactin levels in uremic patients and is associated with the resumption of menses in some females and improvement in sexual function in some males.[88,90,91] This suggests that prolactin contributes to these problems in chronic renal failure. In view of the high incidence of side effects such as hypotension, the routine use of Bromergocryptine in uremic patients awaits larger, better controlled studies.

It has been suggested that zinc deficiency contributes to sexual dysfunction in chronic renal failure. In patients with normal renal function, zinc deficiency is associated with impotence. Plasma and red cell zinc concentrations are frequently low in hemodialysis patients, possibly from zinc removed during dialysis and/or dietary deprivation.

Mahajan and co-workers performed a double-blinded controlled study which indicated that zinc therapy can increase serum testosterone levels, increase sperm counts, and decrease the incidence of impotence in hemodialysis patients.[92] Because of this and the possible improvement in taste perception, we routinely administer 220 mg of zinc sulfate after each dialysis to our patients.

The administration of testerstone may also improve impotence in the uremic male. Many patients report a marked improvement in function after the administration of 100 mg of testosterone propionate in oil once to twice each week. Impotence in the dialysis population is, however, a complex problem, undoubtedly involving not only physical factors, but also psychological factors.[93] Even with proper counseling and medical management most males on dialysis have decreased libido and sexual performance and a significant number remain completely impotent. Renal transplantation results in marked improvement in this area. The sexual problems of the woman with chronic failure is even less understood than that of the male.

REFERENCES

1. Slatopolsky E, Rutherford WE, Hruska K, et al: How important is phosphate in the pathogenesis of renal osteodystrophy. Arch Int Med 138:848–852, 1978
2. Malluche HH, Ritz E, Lange HP, et al: Bone histology in incipient and advanced renal failure. Kidney Int 9:355–362, 1976
3. Haussler MR, Baylind DJ, Hughes JR, et al: The assay of 1,25 dihydroxy-vitamin D_3: Physiologic and pathologic modulation of circulating hormonic levels. Clin Endocrinol 5:1515–1675, 1976
4. Lawson DEM: Metabolism of vitamin D, in Normal AW (ed): Vitamin D, Molecular Biology and Clinical Nutrition. New York, Dekker, 1980, pp 93–126
5. Henderson RG, Russell RGG, Ledingham JGG, et al: Effects of 1,25-dihydrocholecalciferol on calcium absorption, muscle weakness, and bone disease in chronic renal failure. Lancet 1:379–384, 1974
6. Henry HL: Regulation of vitamin D metabolism, in Norman AW (ed): Vitamin D, Molecular Biology and Clinical nutrition. New York, Dekker, 1980, pp 127–148
7. Goldstein DA, Malluche HH, Massey SG: Management of renal osteodystrophy with $1,25(OH)_2D_3$. Min Electrol Metab 2:35–47, 1979
8. Massey SG, Coburn JW, Lee DB, et al: Skeletal resistance to parathyroid hormone in renal failure. Ann Int Med 78:357–364, 1973
9. Goldsmith RS, Furszyfer J, Johnson WJ et al: Control of secondary hyperparathyroidism during long-term hemodialysis. Am J Med 50:692–699, 1971

10. Szymendra J, Sieniawska M, Bialasik D: Dihydrotachysterol increases absorption and exchangable pool of calcium in uremia. Horm Metab Res 12:418–419, 1980
11. Catto GRD, MacLeod M: The investigation and treatment of renal bone disease. Am J Med 61:64–73, 1976
12. Cobert C, Garrett C: Photodensitometry of bone roentgenograms with an on-line computer. Clin Orthop 65:39–45, 1969
13. Parfitt AM: Clinical and radiographic manifestations of renal osteodystrophy, in Davis DS (ed): Calcium Metabolism in Renal Failure and Nephrolithiasis. New York, Wiley, 1977, p 150
14. Avioli LV, Teitelbaum SL: The renal osteodystrophies, in Brenner BM, Rector FC Jr (eds): The Kidney. Philadelphia, Saunders, 1976, pp 1542–1591
15. Sherwood JB, Goldwasser E: A radioimmunoassay for erythropoietin. Blood 54:885–893, 1979
16. Fisher JW, Ohno Y, Barona J, et al: The role of serum inhibitors of erythroid colony forming cells in the mechanism of the anemia of renal insufficiency, in Murphy MV Jr (ed): In Vitro Aspects of Erythropoiesis. New York, Springer-Verlag, 1978, pp 181–188, 1979
17. Eschbach JW, Korn D, Finch CA: ^{14}C cyanate as a tag for red cell survival in normal and uremic man. J Lab Clin Med 89:823–828, 1977
18. Joske RA, McAlister V, Dige Peterson H, et al: Isotope investigation of red cell production and destruction in chronic renal disease. Clin Sci 15:511–522, 1956
19. Barbour, GL: Effect of parathyroidectomy on anemia in chronic renal failure. Arch Intern Med 139:889–891, 1979
20. Eschbach JW, Cook JD, Scribner BH, Finch CA: Iron balance in hemodialysis patients. Ann Intern Med 87:710–713, 1977
21. Ali M, Fayemi O, Rigolosi R, et al: Hemosiderosis in hemodialysis patients. JAMA 244:343–345, 1980
22. Hampers CL, Streiff R, Nathan DG, Snyder D, Merrill JP: Megaloblastic hematopoiesis in uremia and in patients on long-term hemodialysis. N Engl J Med 276:551–554, 1967
23. Neiman RS, Bischel MD, Lukes RJ: Hypersplenism in the uremic hemodialyzed patient. Am J Clin Path 60:502–511, 1973
24. Yawata Y, Hawe R, Jacob HS: Abnormal red cell metabolism causing hemolysis in uremia. Ann Intern Med 79:362–367, 1973
25. Kjellstrand CM, Eaton JW, Yawata Y, et al: Hemolysis in dialyzed patients caused by chloramines. Nephron 13:427–433, 1974
26. Fried W, Jonasson O, Lang G, et al: Studies of packed cell volume and erythropoietin response. Ann Intern Med 79:823–827, 1973
27. Baker LRI, Barnett MD, Brozovic B, et al: Hemosiderosis in a patient on regular hemodialysis: Treatment by desferrioxamine. Clin Nephrol 6:326–328, 1976
28. Goldblum SE, Reed WP: Host defense and immunologic alterations associated with chronic hemodialysis. Ann Intern Med 93:547–613, 1980

29. Quadracci L, Ringden O, Krzymanski M: The effect of uremia and transplantation on lymphocyte subpopulations. Kidney Int 10:179–184, 1976
30. Bridges JM, Nelson SD, McGeown MG: Evaluation of lymphocyte transfer test in normal and uremic subjects. Lancet 1:581–584, 1964
31. Hanicki Z, Chichocki T, Komorowska Z, Sulawicz W, Smolenski O: Some aspects of cellular immunity in untreated and maintenance hemodialysis patients. Nephron 23:273–275, 1979
32. Sengar DPS, Rashid A, Harris JE: In vitro cellular immunity in vivo delayed hypersensitivity in uremic patients maintained on hemodialysis. Int Arch Allergy 47:829–838, 1974
33. Henderson LW, Miller ME, Hamilton RW, Norman ME: Hemodialysis leukopenia and polymorph random mobility—A possible correlation. J Lab Clin Med 85:191–197, 1975
34. Craddock PR, Fehr J, Brigham KL, et al: Complement and leukocyte mediated pulmonary dysfunction in hemodialysis. N Engl J Med 296:769–773, 1977
35. Harowitz HI, Slein IM, Cohen BD, et al: Further studies on the platelet inhibitory effect of guanidinosuccinic acid and its role in uremic bleeding. Am J Med 49:336–341, 1970
36. Fried, W: Hematologic abnormalities in chronic renal failure. Semin Nephrol 1:176–187, 1981
37. Guzzo J, Niewcarowski S, Musial J, et al: Secreted platelet proteins with antiheparin and mitogenic activities in chronic renal failure. J Lab Clin Med 96:102–113, 1980
38. Guyton, AC: Qualitative Schemas of Principle Arterial Pressure Buffering and Control Mechanisms in Arterial Pressure and Hypertension. Philadelphia, Saunders, 1980, pp 10–30
39. Young DB, Cowley AW, Lohmeier TE: The vasoconstrictor hypertensions, in Guyton AC (ed): Arterial Pressure and Hypertension. Philadelphia, Saunders, 1980, pp 393–402
40. Lilley JJ, Golden J, Stone RA: Adrenergic regulation of blood pressure in chronic renal failure. J Clin Invest 57:1190–1200, 1976
41. Lee JB: Hypertension, natruresis and the renal prostaglandins. Ann Intern Med 70:1033–1038, 1969
42. Lindner A, Chana B, Shenard D, Scribner B: Accelerated atherosclerosis in prolonged maintainance hemodialysis. N Engl J Med 290:697–702, 1974
43. Rostand SG, Greles JC, Kirk KA, Rutsky EA, Andreoli TE: Ischemic heart disease in patients with uremia undergoing maintainance hemodialysis. Kidney Int 16:600–611, 1979
44. Burke JF, Francos GC, Moore LL, et al: Accelerated atherosclerosis in chronic-dialysis patients—Another look. Nephron 21:181–185, 1978
45. Vincenti F, Amend WS, Abele J, Feduska NJ, Salvatierra Jr, O: The role of hypertension in hemodialysis-associated atherosclerosis. Am J Med 68:363–369, 1980

46. Lewis BS, Milne FJ, Goldberg B: Left ventricular function in chronic renal failure. Br Heart J 38:1229–1239, 1976
47. Capelli JP, Kasporian H: Cardiac work demands and left ventricular function in end-stage renal disease. Ann Intern Med 86:261–267, 1977
48. Hung J, Hanis PJ, Uren RF, Tiller DJ, Kelly DT: Uremic cardiopathy-effect of hemodialysis on left ventricular function in end-stage renal failure. N Engl J Med 302:547–551, 1980
49. Ayus JC, Frommer P, Olivero JJ, Young JB: Effect of long-term dialysis on left ventricular ejection fraction in end-stage renal disease. Abst Am Soc Nephrol 13:35A, 1980
50. Pinsky WW, Lewis RM, Hartley CJ, et al: Permanent changes of ventricular contractility and compliance in chronic volume overload. Am J Physiol 237:H575–583, 1979
51. Prosser D, Parsons V: The case for a specific uraemia myocardopathy. Nephron 15:4–7, 1975
52. Bailey GL, Hampers CL, Merrill JP: Reversible cardiomyopathy in uremia. Trans Am Soc Artif Intern Organs 13:267–270, 1967
53. Ianhez LE, Lowen J, Sabbaga E: Uremic myocardiopathy. Nephron 15:17–28, 1975
54. Bright, R: Tabular view of the morbid appearance in 100 cases connected with albuminous urine. Guy's Hosp Rep 1:338, 1836
55. Ayus JC, Frommer JP, Young J: Cardiac and circulatory abnormalities in chronic renal failure. Semin Nephrol 1:112–123, 1981
56. Ayus JC, Frommer P, Olivero JJ, et al: Incidence of pericardial effusion and the effect of dialysis in patients with end-stage renal failure: A prospective echocardiographic study. Clin Res 28:155A, 1980
57. D'Cruz IA, Bhatt GR, Cohen HC, et al: Echocardiographic detection of cardiac involvement in patients with chronic renal failure. Arch Intern Med 138:720–724, 1978
58. Pabico RC, Freeman RB: Pericarditis and myocardiopathy, in Massey SG, Sellers AL (eds): Clinical Aspects of Uremia and Dialysis. Springfield, Charles C. Thomas, 1976, pp 69–99
59. Cohen CF, Burgess JH, Kaye M: Peritoneal dialysis for the treatment of pericarditis in patients on chronic hemodialysis. Can Med Assoc J 102:1365–1370, 1970
60. Singh S, Newmark K, Ishikawa I, Mitra S, Berman LB: Pericardiectomy in uremia. The treatment of choice for cardiac tamponade in chronic renal failure. JAMA 228:1132–1138, 1974
61. Minuth ANW, Nottebohm GA, Eknoyan G, Suki WN: Indomethocin treatment of pericarditis in chronic hemodialysis patients. Arch Intern Med 135:807–813, 1975
62. Spector D, Alfred H, Siedlecki M, et al: Indomethcin treatment of uremic pericarditis. Abstr Am Soc Nephrol 11:30A, 1978
63. Buselmeier TJ, Dovin TD, Simmons RL, et al: Treatment of intractable uremic pericardial effusion. Avoidance of pericardectomy with local steroid instillation. JAMA 240:1358–1359, 1978

64. Zelnick EB, Goyal RK: Gastrointestinal manifestations of chronic renal failure. Semin Nephrol 1:124–136, 1981
65. McConnell JB, Thjodleifsson B, Stewart WK, et al: Gastric function in chronic renal failure, Effects of maintenance hemodialysis. Lancet 1:1121–1123, 1975
66. Sullivan SN, Tustanoff E, Slaughter DN, et al: Hypergastrinemia and gastric acid secretion in uremia. Clin Nephrol 5:25–28, 1978
67. Gordon EM, Johnson AG, Williams G: Gastric assessment of prospective renal transplant patients. Lancet 1:226, 1972
68. Margolis DM, Saylor JL, Geisse, G, et al: Upper gastrointestinal disease in chronic renal failure. A prospective evaluation. Arch Intern Med 138:1214–1217, 1978
69. Owens ML, Passaro Jr E, Wilson SE, et al: Treatment of peptic ulcer disease in the renal transplant patient. Ann Surg 186:17–21, 1977
70. Welch JP, Schweizer RT, Bartus SA: Management of antacid impactions in hemodialysis and renal transplant patients. Am J Surg 139:561–568, 1980
71. Reese GN, Appel SH: Neurologic complications of renal failure. Semin Nephrol 1:137–150, 1981
72. Tyler HR: Neurological disorders seen in renal failure, in Vinkin PJ, Bruyen GW (eds): Handbook of Clinical Neurology, New York, North-Holland Elsevier, 1976, pp 321–348
73. Leonard A, Shapiro FL: Subdural hematoma in regularly hemodialyzed patients. Ann Intern Med 82:650–658, 1975
74. Ahu-Asha H, Ibraham A, Rahman A, et al: Acute uremic encephalopathy in tropical countries. J Trop Med Hyg 81:120–125, 1978
75. Teschan PE, Ginn HE, Bourne JR, et al: Quantitative indices of clinical uremia. Kidney Int 15:676–697, 1979
76. Arieff AS, Massey SG: Dialysis dysequilibrium syndrome, in Massey SG, Sellers AG (eds): Clinical Aspects of Uremia in Dialysis. Springfield, Charles C Thomas, 1976, pp 34–52
77. Arieff AS, Massey SG, Barriento A, et al: Brain water in electrolyte metabolism in uremia: Effects of slow and rapid hemodialysis. Kidney Int 4:177–187, 1973
78. Alfrey AC, Mishell JM, Burks J, et al: Syndrome of dyspraxia and multifocal seizures associated with chronic hemodialysis. Trans Am Soc Artif Int Organs 18:257–261, 1972
79. Alfrey AC, Hegg A, Croswell P: Metabolism and toxicity of aluminum in renal failure. Am J Clin Nutr. 33:1509–1516, 1980
80. Thomas PK: Peripheral neuropathy in dialysis patients. Int J Artif Organs 3:6–8, 1980
81. Nielson VK: The peripheral nerve function in chronic renal failure. Acta Med Scand (Suppl) 573:1–32, 1974
82. Emmanouel PS, Lindheimer MD, Katy AI: Endocrine abnormalities in chronic renal failure: Pathogenetic principles and clinical implications. Semin Nephrol 1:151–175, 1981

83. Linn VS, Henriquez C, Seo H, et al: Thyroid function in a uremic rat model. Evidence suggesting tissue hypothyroidism. J Clin Invest 66:946–954, 1980
84. Spector DA, Davis PJ, Helderman JH, Bell B, Utiger RD: Thyroid function and metabolic state in chronic renal failure. Ann Intern Med 85:724–730, 1976
85. Orskov H, Christensen NJ: Growth hormone in uremia. I. Plasma growth hormone, insulin and glucagon after oral and intravenous glucose in uremic subjects. Scand J Clin Lab Invest 27:51–60, 1971
86. DeFronzo RA, Alvestrand A: Glucose intolerance in uremia: Site and mechanism. Am J Clin Nutr 33:1438–1458, 1980
87. Garber AJ, Bier DM, Cryer PE, et al: Hypoglycemia in compensated renal insufficiency. Substrate limitation of gluconeogenesis. Diabetes 23:982–986, 1974
88. Linn VS, Henriquez C, Sievertsen G, Frohman MD: Ovarian function in chronic renal failure: Evidence suggesting hypothalamic anovulation. Ann Intern Med 93:21–27, 1980
89. Hagen C, Olguard K, McNeilly AS, et al: Prolactin and the pituitary–gonadal axis in male uremic patients on regular hemodialysis. Acta Endocrinol (Kbh) 82:29–35, 1976
90. Gomez F, De La Cueva R, Wauters JP, et al: Endocrine abnormalities in patients undergoing long-term hemodialysis. The role of prolactin. Am J Med 68:522–530, 1980
91. Bommer J, Del Payo E, Ritz E, et al: Improved sexual function in male haemodialysis patients on Bromocriptine. Lancet 2:496–497, 1979
92. Mahajan S, Abbusi A, Prasad A, et al: Effect of zinc therapy on uremic hypogonadism: A double blind study. Abstr Am Soc Nephrol 12:123A, 1979
93. Levy NB: The sexual rehabilitation of the hemodialysis patient. Sex Disab 2:60–65, 1979

John C. Van Stone

2

Conservative Management of Renal Insufficiency

Although this book deals primarily with the care of patients undergoing dialysis treatment, this chapter discusses the care of the patient with renal insufficiency before he or she requires replacement therapy. This predialysis supportive therapy period can be greater than 10 years in duration, and while proper management during this period of time seldom prevents the eventual need for dialysis or transplantation, it can frequently delay the requirement for replacement therapy. The careful management of patients during this period is very important, for it not only has an immediate effect on patient well-being but it also has a very definite effect on the patient's course when he or she undergoes chronic dialysis or receives a kidney transplant.

One of the most important aspects of predialysis management is the elimination of reversible causes of renal insufficiency. While it is not always possible to make a concise diagnosis as to the exact nature of the renal disease, it is very important to exclude all disease processes which are amenable to therapeutic intervention. The major reversible causes of renal insufficiency are obstructive nephropathy, infection, nephrotoxins, and possibly some glomerulonephrities. The estimation of renal size is an important aid in determining whether there are any reversible components to the renal insufficiency. Renal size can be determined by tomonephrography, radioisotopic renal scan, or ultrasound nephrography. Patients with very small kidneys are unlikely to have significant recovery of renal function, whereas patients with a normal or minimally reduced renal mass may well be capable of increasing renal function after appropriate therapy.

Obstructive nephropathy is the most common cause of reversible renal insufficiency and must be eliminated in every patient before the diagnosis of chronic end-stage renal disease is made. Early in the course of progressive renal failure when renal function is 30 percent of normal or greater, urinary tract obstruction can generally be excluded with an intravenous pyelogram. In patients with lesser degrees of renal function, renal scan with radioisotopes and/or ultrasound nephrography is helpful in eliminating the possibility of obstructive nephropathy. It is important to remember that patients with any type of primary renal disease may also develop urinary tract obstruction and the diagnosis should be considered in patients with chronic progressive renal disease who have a sudden, abrupt decrease in renal function.

Pyelonephritis is a rare cause of chronic renal insufficiency in the absence of lower urinary tract disease. It can generally be eliminated by urine culture. If urine cultures are positive, the lower urinary tract should be evaluated by intravenous or retrograde pyelography. Renal tuberculosis, although also a rare cause of renal insufficiency, should be considered if there are clinical indications such as hematuria, fever, weight loss, or urinary tract abnormalities.

A not uncommon cause of renal insufficiency is the nephropathy associated with the excessive use of analgesics. In some parts of the world, analgesic nephropathy is responsible for up to 10 percent of the total cases of renal insufficiency.[1] It is a definitely important cause of renal insufficiency both in the United States and abroad. The diagnosis is usually only made if the clinician maintains a high degree of suspicion. Analgesic nephropathy typically occurs in the middle-aged female who presents with chronic abdominal pains and/or headaches. These patients are frequently very hesitant to admit to the ingestion of large amounts of analgesics and it is important that they be questioned about their analgesic intake in a nonthreatening manner. The diagnosis can usually be confirmed by the typical appearance of papillary necrosis on lower urinary tract evaluation. If the patients can be convinced to stop the excessive intake of analgesics, renal function can frequently be stabilized and may actually improve.

Glomerulonephritis is one of the most common causes of end stage renal disease. Unfortunately with the present available therapies, the majority of chronic, progressive glomerulonephritis do not respond to treatment. However, some cases of glomerulonephritis associated with systemic lupus erythematosis, membranous glomerulopathy, and perhaps other types of glomerulonephritis may improve with the administration of steroids and cytotoxic agents. The diagnosis and therapy of these diseases are beyond the scope of this text.

PATIENT EDUCATION

Education of the patient with renal insufficiency about his disease and its therapy is a very important part of the clinical management. The patient who has some knowledge of his disease and the reasons for the various therapeutic interventions is much more compliant and does better than the patient who has no understanding and is only told what to do and what not to do. It is important that patients with progressive renal insufficiency understand the advantages and disadvantages of the various types of replacement therapy so that a tenative decision as to the type of replacement therapy which is best for him can be made and appropriate actions taken. If the patient is possibly going to be treated with chronic hemodialysis, a subcutaneous AV fistula should be placed sufficiently before the need for dialysis that it has adequate time to develop. Patient education should be started early in the course of progressive renal insufficiency before uremia decreases the patient's ability to comprehend. Patient education is discussed in detail in Chapter 13.

DIET THERAPY

Diet therapy has traditionally been the major treatment of early and moderate renal insufficiency. Chapter 14 is devoted to diet therapy and only a few salient points which are important in the predialysis management of renal failure are emphasized here. It is important to realize that, with the possible exception of phosphorus and/or protein restriction, diet therapy does not affect the course of kidney disease but is used predominately to treat some of the metabolic abnormalities which renal insufficiency produces. Patients must be thoroughly evaluated prior to dietary therapeutic intervention and premature or excessive dietary restriction should be avoided.

Protein Restriction

The primary purpose of protein restriction in renal insufficiency is to decrease the toxic effects of protein metabolites. It is unlikely that these protein metabolites have any harmful effects prior to the development of symptomatology and therefore protein restriction need not be started before patients have symptoms. Protein metabolites can cause mental symptoms which range from the simple inability to concentrate, through lethargy and will eventually result in coma. They also cause gastrointestinal symptoms such as anorexia, nausea, vomiting, and a bad taste in the mouth. In high concentrations, these toxins may lead to the development of peripheral neuropathy and pericarditis.

None of the effects of protein metabolites occur early in the course of progressive renal insufficiency and protein restriction is seldom indicated prior to the time that the blood urea nitrogen exceeds 60 mg/dl or the creatinine exceeds 5 mg/dl. Because severe protein restriction will cause protein malnutrition in uremic patients similar to that seen in nonuremic patients, prolonged treatment with severe protein restriction should be avoided. If limitation of protein intake to 0.5 g/kg body weight each day does not eliminate the toxic symptoms, then it is better to start with some form of replacement therapy rather than restricting protein intake further. If dialysis cannot be started immediately, however, further protein restriction down to 20 g/day will frequently markedly improve the uremic symptomatology. This severe protein restriction probably does not have any major detrimental effects if it is limited to a few weeks.

Sodium Intake

The evaluation of sodium balance in patients with moderately advanced renal insufficiency is a difficult clinical task. Signs of sodium excess such as peripheral edema and pulmonary rales and those of sodium depletion such as postural tachycardia and hypotension usually do not occur until there is a 5 to 7 percent increase or decrease in total body sodium, respectively. Subclinical sodium excess probably does not have significant harmful effects with the exception that it may cause hypertension in some patients. Subclinical degrees of sodium depletion, however, can further decrease renal function. This decrease in renal function is secondary to a reduction in renal blood flow and probably does not have any long-term deleterious effects on the kidney. The decrease in GFR, however, can increase the symptomatology of renal insufficiency. Because of a possible decrease in renal function with mild sodium depletion and the lack of harmful effects of mild sodium excess, it is frequently desirable to maintain a trace of edema in the patient with moderate renal insufficiency as long as the excess sodium does not result in hypertension.

Patients with renal insufficiency have a reduction in the ability to adjust sodium excretion. Normal adults can excrete over 1000 mEq of sodium each day if necessary and in the presence of mild sodium depletion the daily urine sodium excretion can be reduced to 1 or 2 mEq. Most, if not all, patients with chronic renal insufficiency have decreased ability both to excrete excessive amounts of sodium and to conserve sodium. Many patients with renal insufficiency tolerate, however, the usual American diet of 150 to 250 mEq of sodium very well and, similar to protein intake, sodium intake should only be changed if clinically indicated. If a patient is normotensive with no clinical evidence of excess sodium such as peripheral or pulmonary edema or of sodium depletion such as postural hypotension then dietary regulation of sodium is not needed at this time. As mentioned before, sodium restriction in the patient who is unable to decrease sodium excretion to the level of the dietary restriction may cause a temporary decrease in renal function and can result in uremic symptoms. In the absence of hypertension, a small excess of total body sodium as evidenced by trace to 1+ peripheral edema is probably not harmful and may even increase glomerular filtration rate slightly. Renal failure patients, however, with large amounts of peripheral edema or pulmonary rales and hypertensive patients with any peripheral edema should be sodium restricted.

A diet with 2 g or 88 mEq of sodium each day is usually well tolerated by most patients. Sodium restriction below this level necessitates markedly restricting the types of available foods and is best avoided if possible. If a 2-g sodium diet is not sufficient to reduce the sodium excess to a more moderate level then the judicious use of diuretics will generally help. Thiazide diuretics are usually not effective in patients with glomerular filtration rates below 40 ml/min and more potent diuretics such as furosemide or ethacynic acid must be given. The patient with renal insufficiency taking these potent diuretics must be monitored very carefully to avoid sodium depletion and a concomitant decrease in renal function. Frequently it is possible to use the diuretics on a temporary basis to achieve a more ideal sodium balance and then maintain the sodium balance with the use of dietary restriction alone. Patients on sodium restriction or using diuretics should be taught to recognize the clinical signs of sodium depletion so that they can have their diet and/or medications adjusted if this occurs.

A small number of patients with renal insufficiency have major problems with the ability to conserve sodium. This has been referred to as "salt-losing nephritis." It occurs most frequently with the interstitial renal diseases such as chronic pyelonephritis. These patients develop postural hypotension and other signs of sodium depletion while on a normal sodium diet. Their sodium intake must be supplemented with high sodium containing foods and/or sodium chloride tablets. The amount of sodium that these patients need to stay in balance is variable and is best estimated by measuring the 24-hour urinary sodium excretion after any sodium deficit has been replaced and supplying that amount of sodium on a daily basis.

BLOOD PRESSURE CONTROL

The kidney plays a major role in normal blood pressure control and hypertension occurs very commonly in renal insufficiency. Renal disease causes hypertension by at least two different mechanisms: sodium retention and renin secretion.

The control of blood pressure in patients with progressive renal insufficiency is very important. It has been demonstrated that blood pressure control, both before and during replacement therapy of renal insufficiency, is an important determinant of mortality in chronic dialysis patients. Hypertension itself is an important cause of renal insufficiency. Persistently high blood pressure causes a progressive thickening of the arteriolar walls whch restricts blood flow and decreases renal function. This lesion is referred to as arteriolar nephrosclerosis. Nephrosclerosis is the primary cause of renal failure in up to 30 percent of patients with end-stage renal disease and is particularly common in blacks. Uncontrolled hypertension can also increase the rate of progression of renal insufficiency in other types of primary renal disease by similar mechanisms.

Even though the treatment of hypertension in patients with renal insufficiency is sometimes associated with further decreases in renal function, this is not a legitimate reason to leave hypertension untreated in these patients. Renal function may decrease as a result of the fact that the lower pressure is unable to force as much blood through the diseased arterioles and glomerular blood flow decreases. The long-term effects of hypertension, however, are sufficiently bad that, if the renal function decreases to a degree that replacement therapy is necessary, it is best to place the patient on dialysis rather than attempting to prevent the need of dialysis by allowing the blood pressure to be elevated. It is not uncommon for renal function to improve after several months of treatment in these patients and dialysis may no longer be needed. The increase in renal function is probably the result of a decrease in arterial wall thickening, secondary to a reduction of blood pressure.

The treatment of hypertension in renal insufficiency is very similar to that of patients with normal renal function except that excessive sodium depletion must be carefully avoided. The first step is to evaluate the sodium status of the patient. If the patient has evidence of excessive total body sodium, i.e., edema, then the total body sodium should be reduced. This can be done with sodium restriction and/or the administration of diuretics. If diuretics are prescribed it is helpful to have the patients carefully weigh themselves on a daily basis and, if they lose more than a given amount of weight, the diuretics should be discontinued. After this initial reduction in total body sodium, sodium balance can frequently be maintained by dietary restriction.

Although diuretics are useful as the first step of treatment in most hypertensive patients with normal renal function, they should not be used initially in hypertensive patients with renal insufficiency who do not have edema on physical examination. In these patients a beta-adrenergic blocking agent such as propranolol is a good initial antihypertensive agent. It can be started at 40 mg/day in divided doses and increased up to 160 to 320 mg if the blood pressure is not controlled. Propranolol, which affects not only the beta-1 adrenergic receptors in the heart, but also the beta-2 receptors in the lungs, may precipitate bronchospasm in patients with obstructive pulmonary disease.

Metaprolol (Lopressor) is another effective beta-adrenergic agent. It has the advantage over propranolol in that it predominantly blocks the beta-1 adrenoreceptors and therefore affects mainly the cardiac muscle and has little action at normal dosages on the pulmonary receptors. It is therefore advantageous to use metaprolol rather than propranolol if there is underlying pulmonary disease.

If beta blockade does not control the hypertension then the vasodilating drug hydralazine (Apresoline) can be added, starting at 40 mg/day and increasing up to 200 mg daily in divided dosages. Hydralazine may precipitate angina attacks in patients with coronary artery disease and causes headaches in some patients. Previous administration of a beta blocking agent decreases the incidence and severity of these problems.

Beta blockade and vasodilators can cause difficulties in patients with decreased cardiac reserve. Prazosin (Minipress) is a good antihypertensive medication to use in patients with advanced cardiac disease. It decreases blood pressure unaccompanied by clinically significant changes in cardiac output, heart rate, renal blood flow, or glomerular filtration rate and has no measurable negative chronotropic effect on the heart. Prazosin is usually started at 2–3 mg/day in divided dosages and the amount increased up to 20 mg/day as needed to control blood pressure.

Clonidine (Catapress) is also an effective antihypertensive in patients with renal insufficiency. It is usually started at 0.1-mg bid and increased up to 2.4 mg/day as needed. Clonidine unfortunately, tends to cause a dry mouth which for patients with renal insufficiency can be very uncomfortable because of the limited fluid intake. Care must be taken to avoid the abrupt cessation of treatment with clonidine as a rebound severe hypertension can occur.

Minoxidil (Loniten) is a very effective antihypertensive agent whose use at present should be restricted to patients whose blood pressures are not controlled by less potent antihypertensive agents. It is a direct acting peripheral vasodilator which reduces blood pressure by decreasing peripheral vascular resistance. It must be used in combination with a beta blocker such as propranolol or metaprolol to prevent a large reflex increase in cardiac output. It is a long-acting drug and therefore can be given on a twice a day basis. The recommended initial dosage is 5 mg/day which can be increased up to 40 mg/day as necessary. Its major side effect is hypertrichosis which occurs in about 80 percent of patients. The increase in hair growth is noted on the temples, between the eyebrows, the sideburn areas, the upper cheeks, on the back, and legs. This hair growth is especially disturbing to women and they should be thoroughly informed about this effect before minoxidil is begun. Minoxidil is, however, effective in controlling blood pressure in the vast majority of patients with chronic renal failure whose blood pressure cannot otherwise be controlled.

Captopril is a relatively new antihypertensive agent which inhibits the formation of angiotension II from angiotension I. It is especially useful in hypertensive patients with high plasma renin concentration. It must be used with caution, however, since it can cause a large degree of proteinuria in some patients and agranulocytosis in others. These effects are more common in patients with underlying renal disease. The usual starting dose is 25 mg 3 times a day which may be increased to 150 mg TID. It is excreted predominantly by the kidney and the doses should be reduced with renal failure.

PHOSPHORUS CONTROL

One of the most important aspects in the predialysis management of patients with progressive chronic renal insufficiency is that of phosphorus control. A thorough discussion of the abnormalities in calcium, phosphorus, and parathyroid hormone metabolism in chronic renal failure is found in Chapter 1. Prevention of the problems that these abnormalities cause requires that treatment begin early in the course of progressive renal failure before there are any detectable abnormalities in serum phosphorus or calcium levels.

The major abnormality of calcium and phosphorus metabolism which needs early intervention is phosphorus retention. In order to remain in phosphorus balance all of the phosphorus absorbed by the gastrointestinal tract must be excreted in the urine. As explained in Chapter 1, decreased renal function can cause increases in serum parathyroid hormone concentrations without measurable changes in serum calcium and phosphorous concentration. In untreated patients with chronic renal insufficiency, serum parathyroid concentrations begin to rise when the glomerular filtration rate decreases to 50 percent of normal. Although this elevation of serum parathyroid homone initially is able to maintain plasma calcium and phosphorus within normal range, it has the undesirable effect of causing an increased rate of bone reabsorption and should be avoided if possible. The increase can be prevented by decreasing the amount of phosphorus absorbed from the gastrointestinal tract. Slatapolski and co-workers have shown in partially nephrectomized dogs that decreasing the amount of dietary phosphorus proportionately to the decrease in glomerular filtration rate will completely prevent the increase in serum parathyroid hormone concentrations.[2]

Phosphorus absorption can be decreased by two methods: (1) lowering dietary phosphorus intake and (2) the administration of phosphorus binding antacids. Phosphorus unfortunately is an ubiquitous mineral which is present in most foods especially those with high protein content. It is very high in dairy products. It is impractical to attempt to decrease daily phosphorus intake below 800–1000 mg. This can be accomplished by restricting those foods which are very high in phosphorus such as dairy products, chocolate, and beans.

In addition to dietary phosphorus restriction, patients with glomerular filtration rates reduced by 50 percent or greater should also be placed on phosphorus binding antacids. Both magnesium and aluminum, which are found in most antacids, will bind with phosphorus in the gastrointestinal tract and prevent its absorption. Significant amounts of magnesium are absorbed from the magnesium-containing antacids which, in patients with renal insufficiency, cannot be excreted. Therefore, magnesium-containing antacids should be avoided and the aluminum compounds, either aluminum hydroxide or aluminum carbonate, should be used. Generally 1 or 2 tablets or capsules or 1 or 2 tablespoons of the liquid antacid with meals are sufficient early in chronic renal failure. It is important that these should be administered even when the phosphorus is normal since, if they are not, the serum phosphorus will be maintained at a normal level only at the expense of an elevated serum parathyroid concentration. Serum phosphorus, however, should be monitored to prevent the development of hypophosphatemia. It is best to keep the serum phosphorus concentration between 2.5 and 4 mg/dl.

TREATMENT OF ACIDOSIS

Because of the kidney's decreased ability to excrete acid, most patients with renal insufficiency develop metabolic acidosis. Chronic metabolic acidosis has several undesirable effects. It results in chronic hyperventilation and causes a persistent shortness of breath. Acidosis may also contribute to the anorexia and nausea which are frequently present in patients with chronic renal insufficiency. Myocardial contractility is decreased by acidosis which can reduce exercise tolerance. Long-standing acidosis may result in a slow but progressive demineralization of bone.

If the kidney is able to secrete sufficient acid to keep the plasma bicarbonate concentration above 20/mEq liter then no treatment is needed, but if the plasma bicarbonate is persistently below 20 mEq/liter then alkali therapy should be administered. All of the acid which accumulates during renal insufficiency comes from the diet, predominately from the metabolism of protein. The normal American diet produces approximately 60 mEq of acid each day and therefore the administration of 60 mEq of base each day should eliminate the need for any renal acid excretion. Generally considerably less base is usually sufficient. The easiest and cheapest base to administer is sodium bicarbonate. A standard 650-mg sodium bicarbonate tablet contains approximately 8 mEq of bicarbonate. The administration of 4 to 8 of these tablets each day will usually maintain good acid–base balance in patients with renal insufficiency. Occasionally at the beginning of alkali treatment there will be a fairly large acid accumulation and higher doses may be needed initially to neutralize this acid.

Some patients are unable to tolerate sodium bicarbonate because of gastric discomfort. In these patients Scholl's solution, which is a mixture of citric acid and sodium citrate, may be given. One milliliter of Scholl's solution is metabolized to produce 1 mEq of bicarbonate and therefore the administration of 30–60 ml/day is sufficient to maintain acid–base balance. We have found that if the citric acid is reduced to 15 g/liter and the salts are dissolved in 50 percent Fanta cherry syrup a much more pleasant tasting solution is obtained and patient compliance is increased. Although there may be some hesitancy to administer sodium bicarbonate or sodium citrate because of fear of increasing sodium retention, studies indicate that sodium bicarbonate does not lead to increased edema or hypertension in sodium-restricted patients with renal insufficiency.[3] Since sodium citrate is metabolized to sodium bicarbonate it can be reasonably inferred that this also should not lead to fluid retention.

INITIATING REPLACEMENT THERAPY

Deciding when renal insufficiency has advanced to the degree that replacement therapy is needed is a difficult clinical task. It is important that dialysis is initiated or transplantation performed before uremia has produced irreversible damage to other organ systems. Patients were treated in the past with conservative management by severe dietary restriction until it was felt that they could no longer survive without replacement therapy. Patients who were starting dialysis frequently had severe malnutrition, muscle wasting, and uremic complications such as peripheral neuropathy and pericarditis. At the present time, dialysis usually is initiated before the development of these problems.

The decision to place a patient on dialysis or perform a kidney transplant should not be made solely on the basis of the patient's serum chemistry values or degree of renal function impairment, but should be primarily made on the basis of the clinical status of the patient. There is some advantage, however, for some symptoms of uremia to be present prior to starting dialysis, so that the improvement in these symptoms which occurs with dialysis therapy will make the undesirable aspects of chronic dialysis therapy somewhat more tolerable.

Although initially protein restriction will relieve most uremic symptoms, as mentioned before prolonged severe protein restriction should be avoided. Usually replacement therapy should be started if uremic symptoms such as anorexia, nausea, vomiting, or mental confusion occur on a 0.5 g/kg/day protein diet. The development of uremic pericarditis or peripheral neuropathy are also indications to initiate replacement therapy.

Although glomerular filtration rate and serum chemistries are not used as indications for starting dialysis, the creatinine clearance is generally below 10 ml/min and the serum urea nitrogen concentration above 75 mg/dl before dialysis is needed. If symptoms suggesting uremia are occurring when renal function is greater than this, other causes of these symptoms besides renal insufficiency should be eliminated before dialysis is started.

REFERENCES

1. Burry AF: The evolution of analgesic nephropathy. Nephron 5:185–189, 1967
2. Slatopolsky E, Coglar S, Gradowska L, et al: On the prevention of secondary hyperparathyroidism in experimental chronic renal disease using "proportional reduction" of dietary phosphorus intake. Kidney Int 2:147–151, 1972
3. Husted FC, Nolph KD, Maher JF: $NaHCO_3$ and NaCl tolerance in chronic renal failure. J Clin Invest 56:414–419, 1975

John C. Van Stone

3
Medications in Chronic Renal Failure

One of the most important aspects of the clinical management of patients with renal insufficiency is the avoidance of certain medications and the adjustment of the dosage of medications which are wholly or partially metabolized by the kidney. While most medications can be administered to patients with renal insufficiency, if they are normally metabolized by the kidney then the dosage may need to be adjusted. Generally the initial amount administered is the same but subsequent doses need to either be reduced in amount or the interval between their administration increased so that toxic accumulations are avoided. Dr. William Bennett has developed from the literature and personal studies, guidelines for prescribing most commonly used medications in patients with chronic renal failure. These guidelines are continuously updated and published periodically, the most recent at the time of publication of this book being in the 1980 July and August issues of the Annals of Internal Medicine.[1] Whenever any medicine is given to a patient with renal insufficiency, unless the physician is sure of the proper dosage for the patient's degree of renal function, the appropriate dosage should be looked up. Table 3-1 lists some common medications that can be administered normally to patients with renal failure. Medications which require special consideration in renal failure patients are discussed in the following section.

Table 3-1
Drugs that Can Be Used Normally in Patients with Renal Failure

Generic Name	Brand Name	Manufacturer
Anti-Infective Agents		
Amphotericin B	Fungizone	Squibb, Princeton, NJ
Chloramphenicol	Chloromycetin	Parke-Davis, Morris Plains, NJ
Clindamycin	Cleocin	UpJohn Co, Kalamazoo, MI
Cloxacillin	Tegopen	Bristol Laboratories, Syracuse, NY
Dicloxacillin	Dynapen	Bristol Laboratories, Syracuse, NY
Erythromycin		
Metronidazole	Flagyl	Searle, Chicago, IL
Miconazole	Monistat	Janssen, New Brunswick, NJ
Nafcillin	Unipen	Wyeth, Philadelphia, PA
Oxacillin	Prostaphlin	Bristol, Syracuse, NY
Pyrimethamine	Daraprim	Burroughs Wellcome Co, Research Triangle Park, NC
Rifampin	Rifadin	Merrell Dow, Cincinnati, OH
Sedatives and Tranquilizers*		
Amitriptyline	Elavil	Merck Sharp & Dohme, West Point, PA
Chlordiazepoxide	Librium	Roche, Nutley, NJ
Chlorpromazine	Thorazine	Smith, Kline & French, Philadelphia, PA
Desmethylimipramine	Norpramin	Merrell Dow, Cincinnati, OH
Diazepam	Valium	Roche, Nutley, NJ
Ethchlorvynol	Placidyl	Abbott, North Chicago, IL
Flurazepam	Dalmane	Roche, Nutley, NJ
Haloperidal	Haldol	McNeil Pharmaceutical, Spring House, PA
Imipramine	Tofranil	Geigy, Ardsley, NY
Methaqualone	Quaalude	Lemmon, Sellersville, PA
Nortriptyline	Aventyl	Eli Lilly, Indianapolis, IN
Pentobarbital	Nembutal	Abbott, North Chicago, IL
Secobarbital	Seconal	Eli Lilly, Indianapolis, IN
Cardiovascular Agents		
Alprenolol		
Clonidine	Catapress	Boehringer Ingelheim, Ridgefield, CT
Diazoxide	Hyperstat	Schering, Kenilworth, NJ
Guanethidine		
Hydralazine	Apresoline	CIBA, Summit, NJ
Lidocaine		
Methyldopa	Aldomet	Merck, Sharp & Dohme, West Point, PA
Metoprolol	Lopressor	Geigy, Ardsley, NY

Table 3-1 (continued)

Minoxidil	Loniten	UpJohn, Kalamazoo, MI
Prazosin	Minipress	Pfizer, New York, NY
Propranolol	Inderal	Ayerst, New York, NY
Quinidine		
Reserpine		

Antineoplastic Agents

Cytosine arabinoside	Cytosar	UpJohn, Kalamazoo, MI
Doxorubicin	Adriamycin	
5 - Fluorouracil	Adrucil	Adria, Dublin, OH
Melphalan	Alkeran	Burroughs Wellcome, Research Triangle Park, NC
Vinblastine	Velban	Eli Lilly, Indianapolis, IN
Vincristine	Oncovin	Eli Lilly, Indianapolis, IN

Corticosteriods

Cortisone		
Dexamethasone	Decadron	Merck Sharp & Dohme, West Point, PA
Hydrocortisone		
Methylprednisolone	Medrol	UpJohn, Kalamazoo, MI
Prednisolone		
Prednisone		

Miscellaneous Drugs

Bromocriptine	Parlodel	Sandoz, East Hanover, NJ
Carbidopa-levodopa	Sinemet	Merck Sharp & Dohme, West Point, PA
Cholestryamine	Questran	Mead Johnson, Evansville, IN
Heparin		
Levodopa	Larodopa	Roche, Nutley, NJ
Phenytoin	Dilantin	Parke-Davis, Morris Plains, NJ
Pyridostigmine	Mestinon	Roche, Nutley, NJ
Succinylcholine	Anectine	Burroughs Wellcome, Research Triangle Park, NC
Sulfinpyrazone	Anturane	CIBA, Summit, NJ
Theophylline		
Tolazamide	Tolinase	UpJohn, Kalamazoo, MI
Tolbulamide	Orinase	UpJohn, Kalamazoo, MI
Trihexphenidyl	Artane	Lederle, Wayne, NJ
Tubocurarine		
Valproate	Depakene	Abbott, North Chicago, IL
Warfarin	Coumadin	Endo, Manati, Puerto Rico

*Patients with renal failure taking sedatives need to be clinically monitored carefully because they may develop excessive sedation in spite of apparently normal drug metabolism.

There are two methods of reducing the amount of drug given because of renal failure. With the first method the quantity of drug given each time is reduced and the frequency of administration is kept the same. The amount of reduction varies for each individual drug and is generally adjusted on the basis of the glomerular filtration rate. In the adult patient with stable, reduced renal function the glomerular filtration rate can be estimated with the serum creatinine concentration by dividing 100 by the serum creatinine, i.e., if serum creatinine is 2 mg/dl the approxmate glomerular filtration rate (GFR) is 50 ml/min, for 4 mg/dl—25 ml/min, and for 10 mg/dl—10 ml/min. In children and adult patients with rapidly changing renal function, the GFR should be determined by timed urine collection. In patients with markedly reduced renal function, an average of creatinine clearance and urea clearance is a better estimate of GFR than creatinine clearance alone.[2]

With the second method of dosage adjustment, the quantities administered are maintained the same and the intervals between doses are increased. In the patient with stable decreased renal function, the serum creatinine concentration can be used to calculate the interval by multiplying its value by a constant. For example, for gentamicin the constant is eight. Therefore if the steady-state serum creatinine is 2.5 mg/dl, the maintenance dose of gentamicin should be administered every 20 hours. If renal function is not stable then glomerular filtration rate must be determined (see above). The steady-state serum creatinine concentration can be approximated by dividing 100 by the creatinine clearance and this value used to determine the interval.

ANTIBIOTICS

As listed in Table 3-1 many antibiotics do not require adjustment in chronic renal failure. Because of an inability to concentrate the drug in the urine, however, none of the antibiotics are as effective for urinary tract infections in patients with renal insufficiency. Drugs which do not achieve systemic bacteriostatic or bactericidal levels such as nalidixic acid (NegGram, Winthrop, New York, NY) and nitrofurantoin (Furadantin, Norwich-Eaton, Norwich, NY) are not useful when the GFR falls below 40 ml/min.

Aminoglycosides

The aminoglycoside antibiotics pose special problems for patients with renal failure. They are solely excreted by the kidney and therefore need extensive dose modificaion. They have a fairly low toxic-to-therapeutic ratio with auditory and nephrotoxicity being major threats. Toxic levels can further decrease already compromised renal function. The aminogloycosides are removed by both hemodialysis and peritoneal dialysis. Therapeutic concentrations can be maintained in peritoneal dialysis patients by loading systemically and then placing therapeutic concentrations in the dialysate. Therapy with these agents is greatly enhanced by the frequent estimation of serum antibiotic concentration.

Amikacin (Amikin, Bristol, Syracuse, NY). Therapeutic blood levels of amikacin are 15–25 ng/ml and toxic blood levels are greater than 35 ng/ml. Hemodialysis patients should be given a 7.5 mg/kg loading dose and 4 mg/kg after each dialysis. For peritoneal dialysis, give a 7.5 mg/kg loading dose and place 20 mg/liter in the dialysate. For predialysis renal failure, load with 7.5 mg/kg and then give 5 mg/kg every (9 × steady-state serum creatinine) hours.

Gentamicin (Garamycin Schering, Kenilworth, NJ). Therapeutic blood levels of gentamicin are 3–5 ng/ml and toxic blood levels are greater than 10 ng/ml. Hemodialysis patients should be given a 1.5 mg/kg loading dose and 0.75 mg/kg after each dialysis. For peritoneal dialysis, administer a loading dose of 1.5 mg/kg and place 6 mg/liter in the dialysate. For predialysis renal failure, give a loading dose of 1.5 mg/kg and then give 1 mg/kg every (8 × steady-state serum creatinine) hours.

Tobramycin (Nebcin, Eli Lilly, Indianapolis, IN). Use the same adjustments for tobramycin as for gentamycin (see above).

Cephalosporins

The cephalosporins have a very high toxic-to-therapeutic ratio and problems with toxicity are rare. They may, however, be nephrotoxic when given with aminoglycosides or to the volume-depleted patient. Although their primary route of excretion is the kidneys, most can also be metabolized by the liver and they need minimal adjustment in renal failure. For simplicity they are divided into two groups; Group I, those needing a moderate reduction of dosage and Group II, those needing a minimal reduction of dosage.

Group I: Cefador (Ceclor Eli Lilly, Indianapolis, IN), cefamandole (Mandol, Eli Lilly, Indianapolis, IN), cephalothin (Keflin, Eli Lilly, Indianapolis, IN), cephalexin (Keflex Dista, Indianapolis, IN), cephapirin (Cefadyl, Bristol, Syracuse, NY), cephradine (Velosef, Squibb, Princeton, NJ). If the patient's GFR is greater than 50 ml/min, give the usual doses of the these drugs. If the GFR is less than 50 ml/min, but the patient is not on dialysis, give 50 percent of the usual dose. In hemodialysis and peritoneal dialysis patients, give 25 percent of the usual dose.

Group II: Cefadroxil (Duricef, Mead Johnson, Evansville, IN), cefazolin (Kefzol, Eli Lilly, Indianapolis, IN), cefoxitin (Mefoxin, Merck Sharp & Dohme, West Point, PA). If GFR is greater than 50 ml/min, give the usual dose of these drugs every 8 hours. If the GFR is less than 50 ml/min, but the patient is not on dialysis, give the usual dose every 12 hours. In hemodialysis and peritoneal dialysis patients, give the usual dose every 12 hours.

Penicillins

Penicillin and most of its derivatives can be given in normal doses to patients with renal failure. Although the kidney is the major route of excretion of most of the penicillins, in absence of renal function they are readily metabolized by the liver. Massive doses are not well tolerated and may cause central nervous system toxicity. No more than 10 million units or 6 g of any penicillin each day should be given in advanced renal failure.

Penicillin G, cloxacillin, dicloxacillin, nafcillin, and oxacillin. Can be given in the usual doses. Amoxicillin, ampicillin, carbenicillin (Geopen, Roerig, New York, NY), methicillin (Staphcillin, Bristol, Syracuse NY), and ticorcillin (Ticar, Beecham, Pittsburgh, PA) can be given in normal amounts to patients with a GFR above 20 ml/min but those with a GFR below 20 ml/min and dialysis patients should be given a dose reduced to 25 percent of normal.

Sulfonamides

With the exception of sulfamethoxazole and sulfoxazole, the sulfonamides should be avoided in patients with renal failure. The combination sulfamethoxazole–trimethoprim and also sulfoxazole are well tolerated by patients with renal failure. Normal doses are needed to obtain high urine concentrations but will result in high blood concentrations. The high blood concentrations are well tolerated but if normal blood concentrations are desirable the dose should be reduced to 50 percent for a GFR below 20 ml/min and to 25 percent for a GFR below 10 ml/min. In dialysis patients the dose should be reduced to between 25 and 50 percent. Determination of blood concentration is not helpful.

Tetracylines

The tetracylines inhibit the anabolic pathways and therefore result in a relative increase in catabolism with the accumulation of catabolic end products such as urea. The administration of tetracycline to patients with stable chronic renal failure may precipitate marked uremic symptoms. There are very few infections in which the tetracyclines are the only effective antibiotics, and it is best to avoid these antibiotics in patients with renal insufficiency. If they are administered the dose should be reduced 50 percent in patients with a GFR below 20 ml/min.

Miscellaneous Anti-Infective Agents

Vancomycin (Vancocin, Eli Lilly, Indianapolis, IN). This agent is metabolized predominantly by the kidney and is not removed by dialysis. Therapeutic blood levels are 5–20 ng/ml and toxic blood levels (ototoxicity and nephrotoxicity) are above 80 ng/ml. Patients with renal failure before dialysis should receive a 20 mg/kg loading dose and then 10 mg/kg every (20 × steady-state serum creatinine) hours. Hemodialysis patients should receive a loading dose of 20 mg/kg and then should receive 10 mg/kg every week.

Lincomycin (Lincocin, Lincoln, Miami, Florida). If the serum creatinine is above 2 mg/dl reduce the dose by 50 percent; if the serum creatinine is above 4 mg/dl reduce to 25 percent of normal dose.

Isoniazid (INH, CIBA, Summit, NJ). If the serum creatinine is above 10 mg/dl, or if the patient is on dialysis, reduce the dose to 200 mg/day.

Ethambutal (Myambutol, Lederle, Wayne, NJ). Give normal doses of 15 mg/kg/day if the serum creatinine is below 4 mg/dl. If the serum creatinine is between 4 and 10 mg/dl, give 10 mg/kg/day. If serum creatinine is above 10 mg/dl or if the patient is on dialysis, give 15 mg/kg every other day.

Flucytosine (Ancobon, Roche, Nutley, NJ). If the serum creatinine is above 2 mg/dl, give 25 mg/kg twice a day. If serum creatinine is above 10 mg/dl, give 25 mg/kg/day. It is removed by dialysis and the daily dose should be given after the hemodialysis treatment.

ANALEGESICS

Aspirin. Both the kidney and the liver metabolize aspirin, and usual doses are well tolerated by patients with renal insufficiency. If high doses are to be used (as for arthritis) then blood concentrations must be monitored. Therapeutic levels are 10–20 mg/dl and toxic levels are greater than 30 mg/dl. There is an increased incidence of gastrointestinal symptoms and bleeding in renal failure patients and aspirin is best avoided in these patients if possible.

Acetaminophen (Tylenol, McNeil, Fort Washington, PA). Acetaminophen is metabolized by the liver and normally the metabolites are excreted in the urine. The metabolites are also removed, however, by dialysis. Dialysis patients and patients with advanced renal failure should not take more than 4 g/day.

Narcotics

All of the narcotics are rapidly tissue bound and therefore the pharmokinetics are difficult to study and of questionable significance. Although scientific documentation in the literature is lacking, it is the clinical impression of many nephrologists that the effect of narcotics lasts much longer in patients with severe renal failure. While the current recommendations are that codeine, morphine, and talwin can be used normally in these patients, it would appear prudent to observe these patients closely and to repeat the administration of these agents as little as possible.

Propoxyphene (Darvon, Eli Lilly, Indianapolis, IN). In patients with severe renal failure decrease the dose to 50 percent because of increased serum levels from increased bioavailability.

Meperidine (Demerol, Winthrop, New York, NY). Active metabolites accumulate in renal failure and may cause seizures. Prolonged administration should be avoided.

SEDATIVES AND TRANQUILIZERS

Similar to the narcotics, many sedatives and tranquilizers seem to cause excessive sedation in patients with renal failure in spite of seemingly normal metabolization. Although no dosage adjustment is recommended for many sedatives and tranquilizers, (Table 3-1), they all must be used with caution in renal patients. The following drugs need dosage adjustment in patients with renal faiure.

Phenobarbital. Administer normal doses of phenobarbital until the GFR is below 20 ml/min or until the serum creatinine is above 5 mg/dl; for these patients and dialysis patients, reduce the dose by 50 percent.

Meprobamate (Miltown, Wallace, Cranbury, NJ). When the GFR is below 20 ml/min or when the serum creatinine is above 5 mg/dl, reduce the dose of meprobamate by 50 percent or increase the interval between doses from 6 hours to 12 hours.

Glutethimide (Doriden, USV, Tuckahoe, NY). Use normal doses of glutethimide until the GFR is below 10 ml/min or until the serum creatinine is above 10 mg/dl; avoid using the drug at those levels because of the accumulation of metabolites.

ANTIHYPERTENSIVE AGENTS

Although many of the antihypertensive agents are metabolized by the kidney, the dose in chronic renal failure patients, as in patients with normal renal function, should be adjusted on the basis of blood pressure.

Nitroprusside. This agent needs special consideration in patients with renal failure. The dose is the same but the metabolite, thiocyanate, may accumulate and cause severe toxicity. If the drug is administered for more than 24 hours serum thiocyanate levels should be monitored and the concentration should not be allowed to rise above 10 mg/dl. Thiocyanate is readily removed by hemodialysis.

DIURETICS

All diuretics are less effective in patients with renal insufficiency. The thiazides, spironalactone, triamterone, acetazolamide, and chlorthalidone are ineffective when the GFR is below 30 ml/min or when the serum creatinine is above 3.5 mg/dl. Ethacrynic acid may cause permanent ototoxicity and should be avoided in patients with severe renal impairment. Furosemide (Lasix) and metolazone (Zaroxolyn) may be effective in high doses in patients with less than 8 percent of normal renal function.

DIGITALIS

The digitalis preparations may enhance uremic gastrointestinal symptoms and doses have to be carefully adjusted for renal function. Serum levels are helpful but immunoassay may overestimate levels in severe renal failure. Cardiac toxicity may be precipitated during hemodialysis by rapid potassium removal. The rate of potassium removal is more important than the actual serum potassium concentration. Magnesium removal may have a similar effect.

Digoxin (Lanoxin, Burroughs Wellcome, Research Triangle Park, NC). Normally 85 percent of digoxin is excreted by the kidney and 15 percent by the liver. Excretion is markedly reduced in severe renal failure and there is also a decreased volume of distribution. In patients with a GFR greater than 50 ml/min, give a loading dose of 0.75–1.25 mg in divided doses and then give 0.25 mg/day. Patients with a GFR between 10 and 50 ml/min should receive a loading dose of 0.5–1.0 mg, with maintenance of 0.125 mg/day. Those with a GFR below 10 ml/min and dialysis patients should receive a loading dose of 0.5–1.0 mg. with maintenance of 0.125 mg/day or every other day. Monitor serum levels for dosage adjustment.

Digitoxin. Digitoxin is metabolized predominantly by the liver. In patients with a GFR greater than 10 ml/min, normal doses can be used. In patients with GFR below 10 ml/min, including those on dialysis, the dose should be reduced 50 to 75 percent.

ANTIARRHYTHMIC AGENTS

Alprenolol, lidocaine, propranolol, quinidine. These drugs require no dosage adjustment for renal failure.

Procainamide (Pronestyl, Squibb, Princeton, NJ). In patients with a GFR above 50 ml/min, give normal doses; those with a GFR of 10–50 ml/min should receive 12.5 mg/kg every 6–12 hours; and patients with a GFR below 10 ml/min and dialysis patients should receive 12.5 mg/kg every 12–24 hours.

Disopyramide (Norpace, Searle, Chicago, IL). When the patient's GFR is greater than 40 ml/min, give 100 mg every 6 hours; when the GFR is 30–40 ml/min, give 100 mg every 8 hours; when the GFR is 15–30 ml/min, give 100 mg every 12 hours; and when the GFR is less than 15 ml/min and for dialysis patients, give 100 mg every day.

ANTICONVULSANTS

Phenytoin (Dilantin, Parke-Davis, Santurne, PR) and *valproic acid* (Depakene, Abbott, North Chicago, IL). These drugs require no dosage adjustment for renal failure.

Carbamazepine (Tegretol, Geigy, Ardsley, NY). Carbamazepine can be given in normal amounts if the patient's GFR is above 10 ml/min. In patients with a GFR below 10 ml/min and in dialysis patients, reduce the dose to 75 percent.

Primidone (Mysoline, Ayerst, New York, NY). When the patient's GFR is greater than 50 ml/min, give 250 mg every 6 hours; when the GFR is 10–50 ml/min, give 250 mg every 8–12 hours; and when the GFR is less than 10 ml/min and for dialysis patients, give 250 mg every 12–24 hours.

ANTIHISTAMINES

Chlorpheniramine (ChlorTrimetron, Schering, Kenilworth, NJ) and *diphenhydramine* (Benodryl, Parke-Davis, Santurce, PR). Although neither chlorpheniramine nor diphenhydramine are metabolized by the kidney, clinical experience suggests that prolonged administration may cause excessive sedation in renal failure patients. Daily doses should be limited to 12 mg of chlopheniramine or 100 mg of diphenhydramine.

ANTI-INFLAMMATORY AGENTS

Corticosteroids

All of the corticosteroids can be given in usual doses in renal failure (Table 1). In high doses they cause an increase in BUN from increased protein catabolism.

Nonsteriodal Anti-inflammatory Agents

Most of these agents may decrease renal function and cause sodium retention in patients with renal insufficiency, possibly by inhibition of prostaglandin synthesis. They should be used with caution in patients with mild to moderate renal failure but these agents do not cause a problem in patients on dialysis. Renal failure patients may be more susceptable to GI bleeding from these agents.

Ibuprofen (Motrin, UpJohn, Kalamazoo, MI). When the patient's GFR is greater than 50 ml/min, give 400 mg every 6 hours; when the GFR is between 10 and 50 ml/min, give 400 mg every 8 hours; and when the GFR is below 10 ml/min, give 400 mg BID. Ibuprofen may decrease renal function (see above).

Naproxin (Naprosyn, Syntax, Palo Alto, CA). When the GFR is greater than 10 ml/min, give 375 mg BID; when the GFR is less than 10 ml/min, give 250 mg BID. This agent may decrease renal function (see above).

Other agents. For patients with renal failure, no adjustment of dosage of the following nonsteroidal anti-inflammatory agents is needed; these agents, however, may decrease renal function:

- fenoprofen (Nalfon, Dista, Indianapolis, IN)
- indomethacin (Indocin, Merck Sharp & Dohme, West Point, PA)
- phenylbutazone (Butazolidin, Geigy, Ardsley, NY)
- sulindac (Clinoril, Merck Sharp & Dohme, West Point, PA)
- tolmetin (Tolectin, McNeil, Fort Washington, PA)

ANTINEOPLASTIC AGENTS

Azathioprine (Imuran, Burroughs Wellcome, Research Triangle Park, NC). If the GFR is below 10 ml/min, the dose should be reduced to 75 percent of usual.

Bleomycin. When the GFR is greater than 50 ml/min, give 0.25–0.50 units/kg twice weekly; when the GFR is between 10 and 50 ml/min, give 0.2–0.3 units/kg twice weekly, and when the GFR is below 10 ml/min, give 0.1–0.2 units/kg twice weekly.

Cisplatin (Platinol, Bristol, Syracuse, NY). This agent causes severe nephrotoxicity and should be avoided in patients with renal insufficiency if possible.

Cyclophosphamide (Cytoxin, Mead Johnson, Evansville, IN). When the GFR is greater than 10 ml/min, this agent may be given in the usual doses. If the GFR is below 10 ml/min, reduce the dose to 50 percent.

Methotrexate (Mexate, Bristol, Syracuse, NY). When the GFR is greater than 50 ml/min, use the usual doses, when the GFR is between 10 and 50 ml/min, reduce the dose to 75 percent; and when the GFR is below 10 ml/min, reduce the dose to 50 percent.

MISCELLANEOUS DRUGS

Acetohexamide (Dymelor, Eli Lilly, Indianapolis, IN). When this drug is given to patients with renal failure, active metabolites accumulate and may cause prolonged hypoglycemia. Acetohexamide is best avoided if the GFR is below 50 ml/min.

Amantadine (Symmetrel, Endo, Manati, Puerto Rico). Amantadine may cause central nervous system toxicity if the dose is not decreased in renal failure. When the GFR is greater than 50 ml/min, give 100 mg every 12 hours; when the GFR is 10–50 ml/min, give 100 mg every 24 hours; and when the GFR is less than 10 ml/min and for dialysis patients, give 100 mg every 5 days.

Chlorpropamide (Diabinase, Pfizer, New York, NY). This drug is excreted by the kidneys and may accumulate in renal failure and cause prolonged hypoglycemia. It is best avoided if the GFR is below 50 ml/min.

Cimetidine (Tagamet, Smith, Cline & French, Philadelphia, PA). Cimetidine may increase serum creatinine from decreased tubular creatinine secretion. In renal failure usual doses of the drug produces high plasma cimetidine concentrations that cause CNS toxicity with mental confusion. When the GFR is greater than 50 ml/min, give 300 mg every 6–8 hours; when the GFR is 10–50 ml/min, give 300 mg every 8–12 hours; and when the GFR is below 10 ml/min and for dialysis patients, give 300 every 12 hours.

Clofibrate (Atromid-S, Ayerst, New York, NY). If the clofibrate dose is not reduced in patients with renal failure, it can cause severe myalgia with increased concentrations of serum muscle enzymes. When the GFR is greater than 50 ml/min, give 500 mg every 6–12 hours; when the GFR is 10–50 ml/min, give 500 mg every 12–24 hours; and when the GFR is less than 10 ml/min and for dialysis patients, give 500 mg every 24–72 hours.

Insulin. Insulin is partially metabolized by the kidney and the dose needs to be reduced as renal function decreases. As in patients with normal renal function, the blood glucose concentration should be used to adjust dose.

Methimazole (Tapazole, Eli Lilly, Indianapolis, IN). When the GFR is greater than 50 ml/min, give 5–20 mg every eight hours; when the GFR is 10–50 ml/min, give 5–20 mg every 12 hours; and when the GFR is less than 10 ml/min, give 2.5–15 mg every 12 hours.

Neostigmine (Prostigmin, Roche, Nutley, NJ). When the GFR is greater than 10 ml/min, give 15–60 mg every 4–6 hours. When the GFR is less than 10 ml/min, give 15 to 60 mg every 6 to 24 hours.

Propylthiouracil (Eli Lilly, Indianapolis, IN). When the GFR is greater than 50 ml/min, give 50–150 mg every 12 hours; when the GFR is 10–50 ml/min, give 50 to 100 mg every 12 hours; and when the GFR is less than 10 ml/min, give 25–75 mg every 12 hours.

Terbutaline (Brethine, Geigy, Ardsley, NY). Oral terbutaline is metabolized predominately by the liver and the dose does not need adjustment. Systemic (intravenous or subcutaneous) terbutaline is excreted by the kidneys. When the GFR is greater than 50 ml/min, give the usual doses; when the GFR is 10–50 ml/min, reduce the dose by 50 percent. Avoid repeated doses in patients with a GFR below 10 ml/min.

REFERENCES

1. Bennett WM, Muther RS, Parker RH, et al: Drug therapy in renal failure: Dosing guidelines for adults. Ann Intern Med 93:62–89, 286–325, 1980
2. Bauer J, Brooks CS, Burch RN: Renal function studies in man with advanced renal insufficiency. Am J Kidney Dis 2:30–35, 1982

John C. Van Stone

4
History of Dialysis

Dialysis utilizing membranes to allow the passage of small molecules through them but not large molecules was first described by the Scottish chemist, Thomas Graham in 1854.[1] He prepared membranes from an ox bladder and performed many studies of the movement of various solutes through this membrane. During the second half of the nineteenth century various investigators studied the properties of dialysis using membranes made of parchment paper or collodion. Collodion was found to be particularly useful because it prevents the passage of substances with a molecular weight greater than 5000 with the relatively free passage of molecules smaller than this. The first description of the dialysis of human blood is by the English researcher, B. W. Richardson in 1889.[2] Using collodion membranes, he separated the substances of blood and other body fluids into two groups: "crystalloid substances" which readily pass through the membranes and "colloidal substances" which do not pass through colloidal membranes.

HEMODIALYSIS

Abel, Rowntree, and Turner, working at the Johns Hopkins University in Baltimore, are accredited with performing the first true hemodialysis.[3] They designed an apparatus which looks remarkably similar to today's hollow fiber capillary dialyzers (Fig. 4.1). It consisted of a series of tubes made of collodial membrane which were encased in a large glass tube. They designed this apparatus primarily in

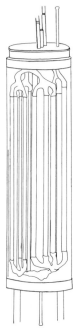

Figure 4-1. The first hemodialyzer which was developed by Abel, Rowntree, and Turner in 1914.

an attempt to remove salicylates from blood but demonstrated the effective removal of urea and other nitrogenesis substances. Their dialyzer was only used for animal experiments. The animals were first anticoagulated with nirudin obtained from leeches. Blood was removed from the animal, introduced into the dialyzer with the fluid, and after a suitable period of time, returned back to the animal.

The first hemodialysis in the United States was performed by Hess and McGuigan at Northwestern University Medical School in Chicago, Illinois.[4] They developed a device very similar to that of the English investigators and used it to study the condition of sugar in the blood. Their device, however, used a continuous flow of blood obtained from the carotid arteries of dogs and returned into a suitable vein. The coating of the tubing with petrolatum and a rapid, pulsatile blood flow prevented the need for anticoagulation in their system. All of their studies were performed in the canine and their device was never used clinically.

The first hemodialysis done in humans was done in Germany in 1915 by George Haas at the University Clinic of Giessen.[5] He used a device very similar to that of Abel, utilizing colloidal membranes. In order to obtain sufficient surface area, he connected as many as six such devices in parallel. In contrast to the intermittant filling and draining of the device used by Abel, Haas used a continuous flow system with the use of a blood pump to propel the blood through his many devices. Haas at first also used hirudin as an anticoagulant in his early experiments, however, later he used heparin and found it a much more preferable anticoagulant.

Another German researcher, Heinrich Necheles, working at Peking University in China designed a dialyzer using sheep peritoneum for the membranes.[6] His device consisted of a series of membrane packages which were compressed between screens in the dialyzing compartment. Necheles' device had the advantage of having a relatively large surface area while maintaining a relatively small blood volume. Necheles may well be the only person to have ever performed extracorporeal peritoneal dialysis.

Love from Chicago designed a device which used chicken intestines as the dialyzer.[7] This, because of the small surface area, was not very successful.

In 1937 in Germany, Thalhimer discovered that material made for packaging sausages could be used as a dialyzing membrane.[8] This material, cellophane, made from cellulose rapidly became used in most dialysis for the ensuing 40 years. He demonstrated effective urea removal through these membranes from anephric dogs with a device similar to that of Abel.

The clinical adaptation of the use of dialysis for the treatment of renal insufficiency has to be credited to Willem Kolff.[9,10] Kolff attacked the problem of developing a functional artificial kidney in a scientific manner, initially performing in vitro experiments studying the relationship of urea removal to tubing size and time. Using data from these experiments he designed the first truly functional artificial kidney. Although his rotating drum artificial kidney was designed in 1940, problems caused by the war in Europe prevented its clinical use until 1943. This device (Fig. 4-2) consisted of 25 to 30 m of 1-inch-wide cellophane sausage tubing wound around a 2-foot aluminum cylinder. The tubing was filled with blood and the whole device rotated in a large 100-liter tank containing dialysis fluid. Initially dialysis was discontinuous in that the blood was removed from the patient, dialyzed, and then returned to the patient. Kolff soon modified the device so that blood ran continuously from an artery through the dialyzer and back into the patient. Kolff initially used his device in patients with chronic irreversible renal failure. The patients showed more clinical improvement with the treatments, however, all eventually died because the treatments required cut down arteriotomy for blood access and

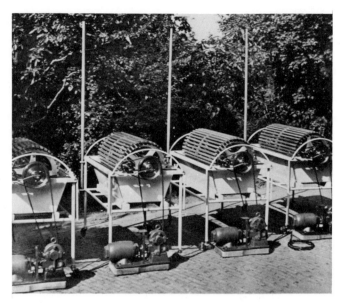

Figure 4-2. Four rotating drum kidneys made during the war and during the German occupation of the Netherlands. During the war these devices were hidden in various places in town to reduce the risk of destruction. After the war in 1946 one was sent to London, England, one to New York and one to Montreal.

eventually blood access was impossible. After his initial experiences, Kolff limited his dialysis efforts to patients with reversible acute renal failure.

There were multiple problems with these initial attempts including membrane leaks, hemolysis, blood line disconnections, and hemorrhages. Fourteen of the first fifteen patients with renal failure whom Kolff treated did not survive. The one patient who survived had a urinary obstruction relieved after one dialysis treatment and probably would have survived without dialysis. The first patient whose life actually was prolonged by hemodialysis was a 67-year-old woman with acute renal failure secondary to glomerulonephritis and/or sulfonamide drugs. This woman awoke during the dialysis treatment from an unconscious uremic state and eventually recovered from her acute renal failure. She died 6 years later from an unrelated disease.

After the war, models of the Kolff rotating drum artificial kidney were sent all over the world, to Montreal, New York, London, and Boston among other places, and the era of treatment of renal insufficiency with hemodialysis had truly begun.

Shortly after the development of the Kolff kidney, Nils Alwall in Lund, Sweden independently designed a dialyzer in which the cellophane tubing was wrapped around a 8-inch coil.[11] The cellophane tubing was compressed with metal grids similar to the Necheles dialyzer previously described, suspended into a large glass tank, and the dialysate fluid circulated around it. The Alwall dialyzer had many advantages over the Kolff rotating drum. The encasement of the dialysate tubing within the grid allowed the use of positive hydrostatic pressure for the removal of fluid, whereas the Kolff dialyzer necessitated increasing the osmolality of the fluid with glucose to remove access fluid. The grid also decreased the incidence of blood leaks. The keeping of the dialysis tubing stationary and circulating the dialystate fluid made for a quieter, less complicated operation and an increased efficiency from the continuous contact of the tubing with dialysate. In later models, Alwall completely encased the dialyzer in the dialysate compartment and created a negative pressure on the dialysate to remove fluid (Fig. 4-2). In spite of these advantages and the fact that the dialyzer was commercially marketed, it never gained much popularity.

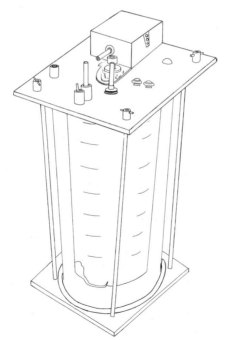

Figure 4-3. Hemodialyzer developed by Alwall in 1947.

The first clinical hemodialysis in North America was performed using a dialyzer, also independently developed, by Dr. Murray in Toronto, Canada.[12] The Murray kidney was very similar in design to that of the Alwall kidney and was used in 1947 to successfully treat a patient with acute renal failure who eventually recovered normal renal function. It was the first system to incorporate a blood pump with blood being obtained from the great veins so that arterial puncture was not required.

In 1947 Malinow and Korzon at Michael Reese Hospital in Chicago developed the forerunner of hemofiltration with a device utilizing the properties of semipermeable membranes for fluid removal.[13] Cellophane tubing was placed in closed tubes and a negative pressure was applied to draw water and small molecules out of the blood. The device was used in anephric dogs using lactated ringers solution to replace fluid loss. Although significant urea removal was obtained, the method was abandoned because of the superior efficiency of dialysis.

In 1948 MacNeill and co-workers in Buffalo, New York designed a dialyzer which consisted of multiple short lengths of flat, cellulose tubes.[14] These tubes were stacked together and separated by specially prepared screens made from nylon mesh. The blood flowed through the tubes in a parallel type configuration with the dialysate running between the tubes. The device was not used clinically until 1954, but then was used both as a dialyzer to treat renal failure and intoxication and as an ultrafilter to treat intractable edema.

Also in 1948, Skeggs and Leonard at Western Reserve University in Cleveland, Ohio described the first parallel plate dialyzer.[15] Their dialyzer consisted of variable numbers of pairs of flat cellulose sheets. Each pair of cellulose sheets was separated by a flat rubber pad which had its surfaces finely grooved. The device was designed so the blood flowed between the two cellophane sheets and the dialysate flowed between the rubber pads and the cellophane sheets.

The size of the dialyzer could be adjusted by the number of units which was placed together and the dialyzer had the advantages of a low volume to surface area ratio and a very low resistance which allowed it to be used without the use of a blood pump.

The Skeggs design was further perfected by Fredrik Kiil in Norway in 1960, who introduced a parallel plate dialyzer which was very popular in the late 1960s and early 1970s.[16]

The first hollow fiber dialyzer was described in 1966 by Richard Stewart.[17] After unsuccessfully attempting to produce a hollow fiber blood oxygenator for use in cardiopulmonary bypass procedures,

Stewart changed directions and used these capillary fibers to produce a parallel dialyzer. His original device contained 800 fibers with a internal diameter of 30 μ and a surface area of $0.17m^2$. The first clinical unit contained 11,000 fibers which provided 1 m^2 of surface area. These were encased in a 3-inch plastic tube. It has proved to be a very efficient dialyzer design and rapidly gained acceptance to become a very popular clinical dialyzer.

Blood Access

Initially the total number of dialysis which could be performed in any patient was limited by the number of sites available for blood access. Prior to 1960, most hemodialysis was performed with the placement of cannula directly into an artery. After each procedure the cannula was removed from the artery and the vessels could be performed. Various efforts were attempted to provide a permanent access, but clotting usually resulted. In 1960 Drs. Wayne Quinton and Belding Scribner described the first useful device for maintaining permanent access to the circulation.[18] Their device was made of polytetrafluoroethylene (Teflon) tubing. A piece of this tubing was placed in an artery and an adjacent vein so as to supply blood access and blood return during dialysis. At the end of each dialysis treatment, the two Teflon tubings were connected with a small section of Teflon tube using reducing unions thus allowing blood to continuously flow through the tubings between dialysis to prevent clotting. This device revolutionized the field of dialysis by allowing repeated dialysis of patients with irreversible renal failure. Shortly thereafter much of the rigid Teflon was replaced with softer, more flexible silicone rubber which allowed the shunt to be moved without stressing the vessels.

Although the Quinton, Scribner arterial venous shunt allowed for the initiation of chronic hemodialysis, it was not without problems. The continuous protrusion of the foreign body through the skin made it very susceptible to infection and clotting of these devices was also not infrequent. In 1962 Drs. Cimino and Brescia in New York described a method which provided adequate blood flow without the implantation of foreign material.[19] They created an arteriovenous fistula between the radial artery and adjacent vein. In addition to increasing blood flow through the vein, the arteriovenous fistula has two additional effects. One, the increased flow and pressure through the veins causes them to enlarge in size making venopuncture with the large bore needles needed for dialysis easier; and two, the increased pressure in the veins causes a thickening or arterialization of the veins providing a stronger vessel wall. The arteriovenous fistula is still considered the most preferable route of access for chronic hemodialysis.

In some patients, however, the venous system of the arm does not expand enough to be adequate for chronic hemodialysis. In 1969, May described implantation in the arm of saphenous veins removed from the leg which were connected from an artery to a vein to provide access for hemodialysis.[20] In 1972 Chinitz described the similar use of bovine carotid arteries, previously treated with formalin so as to make it relatively inert, and in the mid 1970s synthetic grafts made of Dacron or polytetrafluoroethylene came into common use for subcutaneous arteriovenous conduits.[21]

PERITONEAL DIALYSIS

The first reported account of use of the peritoneal cavity for lavage is by the German investigator, Wegner, who noted that when hypertonic solutions containing sugar, salt, or glycerin were injected into the peritoneal cavity of a dog, there was an increase in the volume of fluid which could be removed.[22] In 1894, Starling and Tubby demonstrated that the rate of fluid transfer from the body into the peritoneal cavity is directly related to the osmolality of the peritoneal fluid.[23] They also demonstrated that some substances such as methylene blue and indigo carmen were absorbed from the peritoneal cavity into the blood. The first study demonstrating the transfer of substances from the body into peritoneal fluid were reported by Putnam in 1922 when he demonstrated that urea, glucose, protein, and various dyes which had been injected into the body could be recovered in peritoneal fluid.[24] The first use of this principle for the treatment of uremia was in Germany by Ganter in 1923.[25] He originally performed peritoneal dialysis in guinea pigs and rabbits in whom uremia was caused by bilateral ureteral ligation. He reported moderate clinical improvement in these animals. He also performed the first recorded use of this technique in patients in 1927 when he instilled 1.5 liters of normal saline into the peritoneal cavity of a woman with acute uremia and noticed transient improvement. In 1934 Balazs found an improvement after peritoneal lavage in three patients with acute renal failure secondary to mercury poisoning.[26]

The first reported attempts to keep patients with chronic renal failure alive by the use of peritoneal dialysis was by Rhoads and co-workers in 1938.[27] Multiple complications plagued their attempts.

Sporadic attempts of peritoneal dialysis were made in the 1940s and 1950s, however, the preparation of special fluids, difficulties in catheter placement, and high infection rates prevents its widespread use. In the late 1950s, catheters which could be inserted percutaneously and solutions which became commercially available increased the popularity of the method for acute renal failure. In spite of these advances most investigators found that patients with irreversible renal insufficiency maintained chronically by peritoneal dialysis experienced recurrent infections, malnutrition, and a poor rate of rehabilitiation. In the late 1960s silicone rubber catheters with Dacron cuffs to prevent infections were developed which could be placed permanently into the peritoneal cavity. Machines for the automatic preparation of dialyzing fluid also were designed so that patients could receive prolonged periods of peritoneal dialysis while at home and asleep. Henry Tenckhoff in Seattle demonstrated that, with the use of these catheters and machines, patients could be trained to successfully undergo maintenance peritoneal dialysis at home and that this was a successful alternative to hemodialysis for some patients with end-stage renal failure.[28]

In 1976 Popovich and co-workers described the method of continuous ambulatory peritoneal (CAPD) dialysis.[29] In this technique peritoneal fluid is placed in the abdomen and allowed to dwell for 4–8 hours. During this period of time patients are free to carry on normal daily activities. At the end of each exchange, the fluid is removed and fresh solution is instilled into the abdomen. These workers demonstrated that three to five 2-liter exchanges each day maintained patients in excellent metabolic conditions. In the past 6 years this technique has gained wide acceptance and in 1982 there were 5000 patients on CAPD treatment.

REFERENCES

1. Graham T: The Bakerian lecture on osmotic force. Phil Trans R. Soc Lond 144:177–228, 1854
2. Richardson BW: Practical studies in animal dialysis. Asclepiad (London) 6:331–332, 1889
3. Abel JJ, Rowntree LG, Turner BB: The removal of diffusible substances from the circulating blood of living animals by dialysis. J Pharmacol Exp Ther 5:275–316, 1914
4. Hess CL, McGuigan H: The condition of the sugar in the blood. J. Pharmacol Exp Ther 6:45–55, 1914

5. Haas G: Uber blutwaschung. Klin Wochenschrift 7:1356–1365, 1928
6. Lim RKS, Necheles H: Demonstration of a gastric secretory excitation in circulating blood by VIVI-dialysis. Proc Soc Exp Biol 24:197–198, 1926
7. Love GH: Med Rec (NY) 98:649, 1920
8. Thalhimer W: Experimental exchange transfusions for reducing azotemia. Use of artificial kidney for this purpose. Proc Soc Exp Biol Med 37:641–643, 1938
9. Kolff WJ, Berk H, Welle M, et al: The artificial kidney: A dialyzer with great surface area. Acta Med Scand 117:121–134, 1944
10. Kolff WJ: First clinical experience with the artificial kidney. Ann Intern Med 62:608–619, 1965
11. Alwall N: On the artificial kidney. I. Apparatus for dialysis in the blood in vivo. Acta Med Scand 128:317–325, 1947
12. Murray G, Delorme E: Development of an artificial kidney. Arch Surg 55:505–522, 1947
13. Malinow MR, Korzon W: An experimental method for obtaining an ultrafiltrate of the blood. J Lab Clin Med 32:461–471, 1947
14. MacNeill AE, Bowler JP: Irrigation and tidal drainage. N Eng J Med 223:128–132, 1940
15. Skeggs LT, Leonard JR: Studies on an artificial kidney. I. Preliminary results with a new type of continuous dialyzer. Science 108:212–213, 1948
16. Kiil, F: Development of a parallel-flow artificial kidney in plastics. Acta Chir Scand[Suppl] 253:142–150, 1960
17. Stewart RD, Baretta E, Cerny JC, Mahon HI: An artificial kidney made from capillary fibers. Invest Urol 3:614–624, 1966
18. Quinton W, Dillard D, Scribner BH: Cannulation of blood vessels for prolonged hemodialysis. Trans Am Soc Artif Intern Organs 6:104–113, 1960
19. Brescia MJ, Cimino JE, Appel K, Harwich BJ: Chronic hemodialysis using venipuncture and surgically created arteriovenous fistula. N Eng J Med 275:1089–1094, 1966
20. May J Tiller D, Johnson J, Stewart J, Sheil AGR: Saphenous-vein arteriovenous fistula in regular dialysis treatment. N Eng J Med 280:770–774, 1969
21. Chinitz JL, Yokoyama T, Bower R, Swartz C: Self-sealing prosthesis for arteriovenous fistula in man. Trans Am Soc Artif Intern Organs 18:452–455, 1972
22. Wegner G: Chirurgische bemerkungen uber die peritonealhohle mit besonderer berucksichtigung de ovariotome. Arch Fur Klin Chir 20:51, 1877
23. Starling EH, Tubby AH: The influence of mechanical factors on lymph production. J Physiol 46:140, 1894
24. Putnam TJ: The living peritoneum as a dialyzing membrane. Am J Physiol 63:547, 1922

25. Ganter G: :Uber die beseitigung giftiger stoffe aus dem blute durch dialyse. Munch Med Wochenschr 70:1478, 1923
26. Balazs J, Rosenak S: Zar behandlung der sublimatanurie durch peritonealdialyse. Wein Klin Wschr 47:851–854, 1934
27. Rhoads JE: Peritoneal lavage in the treatment of renal insufficiency. Am J Med Sci 196:642–647, 1938
28. Tenckhoff H, Curtis FK: Experience with maintenance peritoneal dialysis in the home. Trans Am Soc Artif Intern Organs 16:90–95, 1970
29. Popovich RP, Moncrief JW, Nolph KD, et al: Continuous ambulatory peritoneal dialysis. Ann Intern Med 88:449–456, 1978

John C. Van Stone

5
Principles and Mechanics of Dialysis

SEMIPERMEABLE MEMBRANES

All dialysis involves the use of one type or another of a semipermeable membrane that allows the passage of small molecules while preventing the transfer of large molecules. Although semipermeable membranes actually do not have pores and the passage of substances through them involves complex intermolecular action, conceptually it is helpful to view the membranes as having submicroscopic pores. The size of these theoretical pores varies with different membranes and determines the size of the molecules which can pass through. The permeability of membranes does not have a single discrete molecular cutoff size. For most membranes there is a molecular size below which molecules freely pass, a size above which molecules are completely unable to pass, and usually a fairly large intermediate zone in which the membrane partially inhibits the passage of molecules. In hemodialysis the membrane is generally man-made, commonly from cellulose. The peritoneal membrane, the interstitial tissue, and capillary endothelium act together as the membrane in peritoneal dialysis. During dialysis both the solvent (fluid phase of the solution) and the solutes (dissolved particles) can cross the membranes.

ULTRAFILTRATION

Solvent, which in the case of clinical dialysis is water, can be transported from one side of a semipermeable membrane to the other side. Clinically, it is usually necessary to remove fluid from the blood into the dialysate. This is called ultrafiltration and is accomplished by creating a pressure gradient across the membrane. This pressure gradient can be either hydrostatic or osmotic in nature.

In hemodialysis ultrafiltration is done hydrostatically, either by creating a negative pressure on the dialysate, as is done in most single-pass parallel flow dialysis, or by increasing the positive pressure in the blood compartment as is used in coil dialysis. The rate of ultrafiltration is dependent on the pressure gradient across the membrane, the surface area of the membrane, and the ultrafiltration properties of the membrane. Each membrane has a unique ultrafiltration coefficient which is dependent on the structure of the membrane and the membrane thickness. The thicker the membrane, the lower the rate of ultrafiltration. Some modern hemodialyzers are capable of removing greater than 3 liters of water each hour. Patients, however, rarely tolerate such high rates of fluid removal.

Fluid removal during peritoneal dialysis is done by osmotic pressure. The osmolality of the fluid is dependent on the total number of dissolved molecules in each unit of solvent. Fluid moves across semipermeable membranes from solutions of low osmolality to solutions of higher osmolalities. In peritoneal dialysis the osmolality of the fluid is usually increased by dissolving large amounts of glucose in the dialysate. The glucose concentration of peritoneal dialysate is typically between 1 and 5 g/dl (1000–5000 mg/dl). The rate of fluid removal during peritoneal dialysis is slower than hemodialysis and usually does not exceed 300 ml/hour.

SOLUTE TRANSPORT

Diffusive Transport

Solutes cross semipermeable membranes by two basic mechanisms referred to as diffusive transport and convective transport. In diffusive transport, the molecular motion of the solute results in its movement across the membrane. The energy source for transportation of the molecules is obtained from the molecular motion of the substance itself. There are four major determinants of the rate of diffusive transfer across semipermeable membranes.

1. *Membrane permeability*. This is a unique property for each individual membrane and is dependent not only on the size of the "pores" but also on the relative total area of the pores in the

membrane and the membrane thickness. A membrane which has a large number of small pores will allow the faster passage of small molecules than a membrane that has a small number of small pores. Membranes which are highly permeable and allow the rapid passage of solutes (and solvent) are referred to as "high-flux" membranes.
2. *Surface area.* The rate of diffusion of solutes across membranes is directly proportional to the surface area of contact of the solution. For this reason large surface area dialyzers are more efficient.
3. *Concentration gradient.* Diffusive transport of a solute is directly proportional to the concentration gradient of the solute across the membrane. It is important in the design of dialyzers to quickly remove diffusing substances from the downstream side of the membrane so as to maintain the concentration gradient as large as possible.
4. *Molecular weight.* The movement of molecules by diffusive transport is inversely proportional to their molecular weight. This means that even if the membrane will allow free passage of molecules with molecular weights of 100 and 200, the molecule with a molecular weight of 100 will cross the membrane by diffusion at a rate of twice that of a molecule with a molecular weight of 200.

Conductive Transport

Conductive transport is the movement of solute across a membrane caused by the passage of the solvent containing the solute. It is also called "solvent drag." The rate of convective transport of a solute is affected by three basic properties:
1. *The rate of solvent transport.* Conductive transport is directly proportional to the ultrafiltration rate.
2. *The concentration of the solute in the solvent.* Conductive transport of any individual solute is directly proportional to its concentration in the solvent.
3. *The sieving properties of the membrane.* A membrane's sieving coefficient is a measurement of the size of the theoretic pores. Membranes have individual sieving coefficients for each individual solute. A sieving coefficient of one means that the membrane does not inhibit the passage of the solute and therefore the solute will pass through the membrane at a concentration equal to its concentration in the solvent. A sieving coefficient of zero indicates that

the pores are sufficiently small that the solute is unable to cross the membrane in any significant quantities, while a sieving coefficient of 0.5 means that the pores inhibit the passage of the solute sufficiently to prevent half of the molecules from crossing the membrane. With a 0.5 sieving coefficient the solute therefore, crosses the membrane in a concentration of one-half its concentration on the initiating side of the membrane.

The sieving coefficient of a membrane for a solute can be expressed mathmatically as $S = C_F/C_W$, where S is the sieving coefficient, C_F is the concentration of the solute in the ultrafiltrate passing through the membrane, and C_W is the concentration of the solute in the original solution. The sieving coefficient of a solute for a membrane is directly related to the theoretical pores in the membrane and the molecular size and shape of the solute. If the membrane has an electrical charge then the electrical charge of a solute will also affect the sieving coefficient.

The basic differences in diffusive and conductive transport cause a relative difference in the importance of these two mechanisms for transport of solutes of different molecular weights. The pore size or sieving of a membrane affect both processes similarly, decreasing both diffusive and convective transport proportionally to the sieving coefficient. Since increasing molecular weight, however, decreases diffusive transport independent of membrane sieving properties but not conductive transport, conductive transport becomes more important as molecular weight increases. Finally, since the transport of substances by conductive forces is independent of the concentration gradient, the removal of the solute from the downstream side of the membrane does not affect conductive transport. Conductive transport is therefore independent of dialysate flow and not as much effected by dialyzer design as is diffusive transport.

DIALYSATE

The fluid on the side of the membrane opposite from the blood is referred to as dialysate. The composition of the dialysate determines which and how much of the diffusible blood solutes are removed during the dialysis procedure. If the concentration of the solute is lower in the dialysate than in the blood, then there will be net diffusive transport of the substance from the blood into the dialysate but, if the concentration in the dialysate is greater than in the blood, the diffusion will be from the dialysate into the blood. If the blood and dialysate concentrations are equal there will be no net diffusive transport. It must be remembered, however, that the total net transfer of solutes depends not only on diffusive transport but also convective transport.

Since it appears desirable to remove as much of the nitrogenous waste products such as urea, uric acid, and creatinine as possible, the dialysate contains none of these substances. While patients generally need a net removal of most of the major cations and anions of the blood such as sodium, potassium, magnesium, and chloride, if the dialysate did not contain substantial quantities of these ions, too much would be removed. Most dialysates for either hemodialysis or peritoneal dialysis contain sodium, potassium, calcium, magnesium, chloride, glucose, and some form of base such as acetate, lactate, or bicarbonate. The concentrations of these solutes vary and can be individualized on a patient to patient basis or even be changed during the dialysis procedure (see Chapter 6).

Hemodialysis Dialysate

Hemodialysis dialysate is usually prepared by diluting with water a commercially manufactured concentrate which contains all the solutes in a concentration of 35 times that of the final dialysate. An important consideration in the development of dialysates has been the compatibility of the basic constituents in this concentrated form.

Water Preparation

The quality of the water used in the preparation of dialysate is important. During the typical dialysis treatment the patient's blood is exposed to over 30 gal of water, being separated from it by only a thin membrane. Any solute present in the water with a molecular weight below 10,000 daltons will be transferred in significant quantities from the dialysate into the blood. Dialysate was originally prepared with ordinary tap water. It soon became evident that, because of the varying amounts of the divalent cations calcium and magnesium, it was advantageous to use water which had been treated with a water softener. Water softeners contain cation exchange resins which remove these divalent cations and replace them with sodium ions. Although some dialysate is still being made with softened water, most nephrologists feel that further purification is necessary.

There is no universal agreement as to the degree of purity of water needed for the preparation of dialysate. The recommendations of the Association for the Advancement of Medical Instrumentation (AAMI) are shown in Table 5-1.[1] There are two methods in use to obtain water with this degree of purity, ion exchange resin and reverse osmosis. Ion exchange resins work similarly to water softeners except that they contain both cation exchange resins and anion exchange resins. The cation exchange resins remove the positively charged cations and replace them with hydrogen ions and the anion exchange resins remove the negatively charged anions and replace them with hydroxyl ions. The final result is the substitution of water for the salts. A drawback of this method is that it does not remove uncharged compounds such as many organic compounds. These can usually be removed by passing the water through an activated charcoal bed.

The reverse osmosis process of water purification uses semipermeable membranes, similar to dialyzer membranes. These membranes have small "pores" which allow the passage of water

Table 5-1
Maximum Allowable Chemical Contaminant Concentrations in the Water Used for Preparation of Dialysate as Recommended by the AAMI

Contaminant	Maximum Concentration
Calcium	0.1 mEq/liter
Magnesium	0.3 mEq/liter
Sodium*	3.0 mEq/liter
Potassium	0.2 mEq/liter
Fluoride	0.2 mg/liter
Chlorine	0.5 mg/liter
Chloramines	0.1 mg/liter
Nitrate nitrogen	2.0 mg/liter
Sulfate	100.0 mg/liter
Copper	0.1 mg/liter
Barium	0.1 mg/liter
Zinc	0.1 mg/liter
Aluminum	10.0 μg/liter
Arsenic	5.0 μg/liter
Lead	5.0 μg/liter
Silver	5.0 μg/liter
Cadmium	1.0 μg/liter
Chromium	14.0 μg/liter
Selenium	90.0 μg/liter
Mercury	0.2 μg/liter

*10 mEq/liter of sodium is allowed if the sodium concentration of the concentrate has been reduced to compensate for excess sodium and if conductivity of the water is monitored continuously.

molecules but inhibit the dissolved impurities. The passage of pure water through the membrane creates an osmotic gradient which favors water flow in the opposite direction. To overcome this osmotic pressure, hydrostatic pressure is used to force water through the membrane. Greater than 90 percent of impurities can be removed by the reverse osmosis process. When purifying large amounts of water, reverse osmosis is usually more economic than ion exchange treatment. The water produced by reverse osmosis can be further purified by deionization and activated charcoal if desired. Removing the majority of the contaminants with reverse osmosis reduces the cost of deionization.

Although clinically patients dialyzed with dialysate made from raw or softened water frequently appear to do as well as those in which more purified water was used, there is ample evidence that impurities present in the water can cause untoward effects. Kjellstrand and co-workers have demonstrated that chloramines present in the water used for dialysate preparation can cause hemolysis and significantly increase the anemia seen in patients on hemodialysis.[2] Chloramines are produced from chlorine and ammonia which are added to the water by many municipalities for bacterial control. Chloramine causes oxidative injury and results in an acute hemolytic anemia which is characterized by Heinz bodies present in the red blood cells. Chloramine is removed by either deionization or activated charcoal but not reverse osmosis.

Excessive amounts of copper in the dialysate can also cause hemolytic anemia. Although copper is occasionally added to municipal water supplies to control algae, more often excessive amounts of copper in the water has been leached from copper plumbing. When water with a pH below 6 is passed through copper plumbing, significant amounts of copper are dissolved into the water.[3] Acidic water can occur naturally or may be produced by exhausted deionization equipment. Since the pH of ultrapure water is frequently below 6 from the absorption of carbon dioxide, the water used for the preparation of dialysate should not be exposed to copper plumbing after purification.

There is increasingly accumulating evidence that more than trace amounts of aluminum in the dialysate can cause dialysis dementia. Dialysis dementia is a syndrome characterized by a progressive dementia, ataxia, and fecal incontinence. It is discussed further in Chapter 1 but it should be noted here that it is imperative to keep dialysate aluminum concentrations to a minimum.

The water used for dialysis need not be sterile or pyrogen free. The dialyzer membrane provides an effective barrier to the passage of bacteria and pyrogens. Excessively high dialysate bacterial counts, however, can cause febrile reactions. The AAMI recommends that the total bacteria count of the water used for the preparation of dialysate not exceed 100/ml and that the bacteria count of dialysate not exceed 2000/ml.[1]

Dialysate Temperature

Dialysate must be heated to body temperature in order to prevent excessive heat loss during the treatment. Heating the dialysate to 38°C generally allows for some cooling between the machine and dialyzer. In the febrile patient, lower dialysate temperatures can be used to reduce the fever. The effect is similar to placing the patient on a cooling water blanket.

It is very important to prevent overheating of the dialysate.[4] If the dialysate temperature rises above 51°C, there is an immediate and massive hemolysis which can result in fatality. Dialysate temperatures below 44°C are not associated with deleterious effects. Dialysate temperatures between 47°C and 51°C cause damage to red cells which results in delayed hemolysis. If it is discovered that a patient has been dialyzed with a dialysate in this temperature range, it is important that the patient be hospitalized for several days and carefully monitored for signs of hemolysis and hyperkalemia.

Overheated dialysate is usually caused by a defective thermostat in the dialysis equipment. There generally is a gradual rise in dialysate temperature and the conscious patients will report an increased sensation of warmth. An alert dialysis staff will recognize these symptoms and detect the error in dialysate temperature before any harmful effects. Most modern dialysis equipment, in addition, is protected by an extra temperature-sensing mechanism which alarms when the temperature rises above 40°C.

Dialysate Sodium

The major cation of dialysate is sodium. There is no common agreement as to the proper sodium concentration of the dialysate. Sodium concentrations at different dialysis units vary from 130–155 mEq/liter. At the University of Missouri Medical Center in an effort to determine the consequences of changing dialysate sodium concentration, we studied the effects of different sodium concentrations on changes in distribution of body fluid during dialysis.[5] The dialysate sodium concentration was found to have major effects on the distribution of total body water. There are major intercompartmental fluid shifts which follow classical physiologic theory. Low sodium dialysate decreases extracellular osmolality and results in a shift of water into the cells. The converse happens with a high dialysate sodium, which increases extracellular osmolality and shifts water out of the cells. Fluid removed by ultrafiltration comes predominantly from the extracellular space, which is what would be expected since it is removed isonatremically. The effects of dialysate sodium concentration and fluid removal are independent of each other.

While these studies demonstrate the effects of changing the dialysate sodium concentration, they are not necessarily helpful in determining what the ideal dialysate sodium concentration should be. Gotch points out that ideally the dialysate sodium concentration should be adjusted so as to remove water and sodium during dialysis in amounts equal to that gained since the last dialysis treatment. He studied a small group of patients in whom fluid and sodium gain between dialysis was estimated from changes in serum sodium and total body weight.[6] The dialysate sodium and ultrafiltration rate was then adjusted so as to remove a similar amount of sodium and water. Because of the varying proportions of sodium and water intake in different patients, the dialysate sodium concentration varied between 140 and 147 mEq/liter. He found that these adjustments in dialysate sodium concentrations significantly decreased the number of side effects during dialysis. At the present time it unfortunately does not appear practical to adjust the dialysate sodium concentration for each dialysis, but this may be helpful in selected patients who have excessive symptoms during dialysis.

There is no doubt that changes in the dialysate sodium concentration produce significant objective and subjective differences in patients undergoing chronic hemodialysis. Several studies have demonstrated that increasing the dialysate sodium concentration significantly reduces the incidence of untoward symptomatology such as muscle cramps, nausea, and headaches during dialysis. This is especially true if one goes from a dialysate concentration which is hyponatremic compared to the patient's plasma sodium concentration to one which is isonatremic. There is a trade-off with the high dialysate sodium, however, and most studies show that predialysis blood pressure and interdialysis weight gain are significantly increased. The average increases are small (blood pressure 5 mm/Hg, weight gain 0.5 kg) and are probably not clinically significant in most patients. Robson, Oren, and Ravid described, however, a group of 6 patients in which an inadvertent increase in the dialysate sodium from 130–143 mEq/liter resulted in excess hypertension and recurrent episodes of pulmonary edema.[8] While it is probable that at least some of these problems may have been prevented by increasing the ultrafiltration during dialysis, it is possible that some patients are not able to tolerate the higher dialysate sodium concentrations. At the University of Missouri we routinely use a dialysate sodium of 142 mEq/l and have not found any patients in which the dialysate sodium needed to be reduced because of hypertension or fluid overload.

It has been suggested that it may be helpful to begin with a high dialysate sodium concentration of 150 mEq/liter for the first 3 hours of the dialysis treatment and then reduce the concentration to 130 mEq/liter during the later part.[9] With some of the newer dialysis machines such as the Cordis Dow 7000J® (Cordis Dow Corporation, Miami, Fl) or the Cobe Century II® (Cobe Laboratories, Inc., Lakewood, Co), this is easily accomplished. With this regimen the majority of the ultrafiltration is performed during the initial part of the treatment and after completion of the ultrafilration the dialysate sodium concentration is lowered in an attempt to prevent the increased thirst, weight gain, and blood pressure caused by the higher sodium concentrations. We have tried this suggestion on several problem patients and have not been impressed with the results.

Dialysate Potassium

There is a dearth of data that can be used to objectively determine the optimal concentration of potassium in the dialysate. The concentrations used generally vary between 0 and 4 mEq/liter. Several studies have shown that when patients are dialyzed with low potassium dialysate they may become potassium depleted.[10] This, of course, also depends on the potassium intake. Low potassium dialysates also can cause an increased incidence of cardiac arrythmias, especially in patients receiving digitalis preparations. The rate at which potassium is removed during dialysis is more important than the total amount removed and causes an increased incidence of arrythmias with shorter, more efficient treatments.[10] Although measurement of erythrocyte potassium content may be a better indication of total body potassium than serum potassium,[11] routine monitoring of erythrocyte potassium in chronic dialysis patients does not appear to be practical at this time.

At the University of Missouri we individualize the dialysate potassium concentration in an attempt to keep the predialysis serum potassium concentrations between 4.5 and 6.0 mEq/liter. Even though serum potassiums between 5.4 and 6.0 mEq/liter are above that usually found in the normal population, there does not appear to be any serious harmful consequences of such values in the chronic dialysis patients. We are able to accomplish these values in the majority of our patients with a dialysate potassium concentration of 0, 1, or 2 mEq/liter.

Patients taking digitalis preparations are particularly sensitive to the shifts in potassium which occur during hemodialysis. Use of low dialysate potassium concentrations can result in serious ventricular arrythmias in digitalized patients and in these patients we usually use a dialysate concentration of 2 or 3 mEq/liter and attempt to control the serum potassium concentration by stricter dietary restriction.

Dialysate Calcium

Calcium is present in the plasma in three forms: (a) protein bound calcium, (b) calcium complexes, and (c) ionized calcium. The physiologic important form of plasma calcium is the ionized calcium. This is true for both the beneficial actions such as nerve function, muscle function, and bone structure and also the harmful effects of soft tissue calcification and central nervous system toxicity. Although it requires specialized equipment, it is now not difficult to measure plasma-ionized calcium. At the University of Missouri we routinely measure ionized calcium and find it helpful in the clinical care of the patient. A more complete discussion of the complex abnormalities of calcium metabolism in hemodialysis patients is found in Chapter 1. Decreased absorption of calcium by the gastrointestinal tract results in negative calcium balance in many patients with chronic renal failure. It is therefore desirable to have a positive flux of calcium from the dialysate to the patient during the dialysis treatments. Diffusive transport of calcium during dialysis depends on the relationship between the calcium concentration of the dialysate and the ultrafilterable calcium concentration of the plasma. Ultrafilterable calcium is made up of ionized calcium and calcium complexes. It usually equals 50–60 percent of total plasma calcium and averages 2.5–3.0 mEq/liter. Therefore dialysate concentrations of 3.0–3.5 mEq/liter (6.0–7.0 mg/dl) usually result in a net flux of calcium from the dialysate into the patient.[12] The process is self-regulatory in that increases in plasma calcium concentration decreases the diffusion gradient. With dialysate calcium concentrations of 3.25 and high normal plasma calcium concentrations (10–11 mg/dl) result in minimal net calcium transfer but in the hypocalcemic patient the net transport of calcium with this dialysate during a 4-hour hemodialysis treatment may exceed 500 mg.

Some patients, especially surgically anephric patients, have persistent hypocalcemia. In these patients dialysate calcium concentration can be further increased to levels between 4.0 and 4.5 mEq/liter. Because of the risk of soft tissue and vascular calcification, these higher dialysate calcium concentrations should not be used unless the predialysis serum phosphorous is 5.0 mg/dl or lower.

Serum calcium needs to be carefully monitored in the dialysis patients, especially those in which the higher dialysate calcium concentrations are used. Although the serum calcium in the majority of dialysis patients is either normal or low, hypercalcemia is not rare. Hypercalcemia can present in the dialysis patients as an acute central nervous system syndrome with disorientation, dysarthria, seizures, myoclonic jerks, hallucinations, irritability, confusion, memory and judgment defects, plus bizarre behavior.[13] In patients in which the higher dialysate calcium concentrations are used it is important to monitor not only the predialysis serum calcium but also the postdialysis serum calcium.

Total serum calcium increases significantly during most hemodialysis treatments. This increase in serum calcium is not due entirely to a net transfer of calcium from the dialysate, but is also the result of a combination of other contributing factors:

1. During most hemodialysis treatments plasma protein concentration increases. This is a result of fluid removal. Although usually less than 10 percent of total body water is removed during a treatment, a disporportionately large amount is lost from the plasma volume and plasma protein concentrations may increase greater than 25 percent. Since total serum calcium is approximately 50 percent bound to protein this 25 percent increase in protein concentration will increase total serum calcium concentration 10–15 percent (1–1.5 mg/dl) without any net increase in total plasma calcium.
2. The correction of metabolic acidosis during the hemodialysis treatment causes an increase in protein binding of calcium and further increases total serum calcium concentration independent of calcium balance.

Therefore one cannot assume that increases in serum calcium concentration are an indication of positive calcium balance during dialysis.

Dialysate Magnesium

In normal man total body magnesium stores appear to be completely controlled by the kidneys. With high magnesium intakes, normal kidneys are capable of excreting large amounts of magnesium and in magnesium depletion they are capable of conserving magnesium to the extent that excretion is less than 1 mEq/day. In chronic renal failure, plasma magnesium concentrations and erythrocyte magnesium increase.[14] Unless intake is excessive, however, plasma magnesium concentrations do not increase above 3–3.5 mEq/liter (normal 1–2 mEq/liter). There is no evidence that these mild increases in plasma magnesium have any deleterious effects. It is important to remember, however, that the administration of magnesium-containing drugs, such as magnesium antacids or magnesium sulfate, to patients with renal insufficiency can cause marked increases in plasma magnesium with considerable morbidity and even mortality.

There is some evidence that higher plasma magnesium concentrations can suppress parathyroid hormone secretion and that hypomagnesemia stimulates secretion of PTH. Pletka and co-workers demonstrated that increasing dialysate magnesium concentrations from 1.5–2.5 mEq/liter can decrease plasma PTH concentration and decreasing the concentration to 0.5 mEq/liter increases plasma PTH.[15] Lowering the dialysate magnesium concentration has been reported to improve peripheral nerve conduction.[16] Since peripheral nerve conduction, however, is no longer a major problem in most chronic hemodialysis patients (see Chapter 1), it does not appear necessary to decrease dialysate magnesium concentration for this reason.

The dialysate magnesium concentration is currently a matter of personal preference with little sound scientific data to support one choice over another. At the University of Missouri Medical Center we are currently using 1–1.5 mEq/liter.

Dialysate Base

Originally the base used in the hemodialysis dialysate was the major plasma buffer, bicarbonate. In 1964 Mion and co-workers at the University of Washington substituted acetate for bicarbonate to facilitate the preparation of a dialysate concentrate without the precipitation of the divalent cations, calcium and magnesium.[17] Acetate is transferred from the dialysate to the patient and is metabolized to produce bicarbonate. They demonstrated that a dialysate acetate concentration of 35–40 mEq/liter results in the production of sufficient bicarbonate to replace the bicarbonate that is lost through the dialyzer and correct the bicarbonate deficit which develops between dialysis treatments. Although there was no critical appraisal of the effect of the acetate infusion, it was felt that acetate dialysate was as well tolerated as bicarbonate and it rapidly became used in essentially all hemodialysis treatments throughout the world.

In 1978 workers at the University of Washington suggested that the use of acetate dialysate with the newer, more efficient, large-surface-area dialyzers can cause problems.[18] In a series of studies they demonstrated that with these dialyzers, acetate dialysate was associated with more untoward symptoms and the tolerable rate of ultrafiltration was less than with bicarbonate dialysate. They also found that the correction of acidosis was smoother with bicarbonate dialysate.

During a routine 4-hour hemodialysis treatment over 1000 mEq of acetate are infused, which is an amount nearly twice the total body bicarbonate stores. Acetate occupies a pivotal point in human metabolic pathways. It can be used to produce protein by incorporation into amino acids, diverted into carbohydrates from the formation of pyruvate, incorporated into either cholesterol or fatty acids, or can be metabolized to CO_2 and H_2O through the Krebs cycle. The majority of acetate infused during dialysis is metabolized to CO_2 and water but significant quantities do enter some of these other pathways.

The rate of acetate metabolism is best defined by a Michaelis-Menten model.[19] This implies that at low rates of acetate infusion there is a first-order reaction, with the rate of metabolism increasing as plasma acetate concentration increases. At moderate and high acetate infusion rates, however, more is a limit to the rate at which acetate can be metabolized. The mean maximum rate of acetate metabolism (V_{max}) in man has been estimated to vary from 2–18 mol/min. It has also been suggested that tissue hypoxia decreases acetate V_{max}. If the rate of acetate infusion exceeds the maximal rate of acetate metabolism, no steady-state condition can occur and plasma acetate concentrations will increase as long as the infusion continues.

This limit in the rate of acetate metabolism places potentially serious limitations on the use of acetate as a dialysate base. If the rate of bicarbonate removal during dialysis exceeds the rate at which acetate is metabolized into bicarbonate, there will be a progressive fall in plasma bicarbonate with the worsening of metabolic acidosis during the dialysis treatment. Normally the rate of acetate metabolism during the majority of dialysis treatments is well below V_{max}. However, the development of arterial hypoxemia or hypotension during dialysis, both of which cause tissue hypoxia, may decrease acetate metabolism and increase plasma acetate concentration at critical times.

Acetate has two major effects on the cardiovascular system: first, it produces peripheral vasodilation; second, it has marked depressant effects on the myocardial contractility.[20] Both of these actions cause arterial blood pressure to fall. Whether the amount of acetate infused and the resultant plasma levels during hemodialysis treatments are sufficient to have significant effects is not certain at this time. There is evidence strongly suggesting, however, that acetate infusions from dialysate can at times cause cardiovascular instability.

In 1976 Novello and co-workers described three patients in whom plasma concentrations rose to greater than 15 mEq/liter during dialysis with acetate dialysate.[21] Two of the patients experienced repeated hypotensive episodes during these treatments, but not when bicarbonate dialysate was used.

In 1978 Graefe and co-workers reported a group of patients with symptomatic hypotension when treated with large surface area dialyzers and acetate dialysate who had a marked decrease in untoward symptoms with the substitution of bicarbonate for acetate in the dialysate.[18]

In 1978 we performed a double-blinded study of 9 randomly selected, stable hemodialysis patients at the University of Missouri Medical Center to determine if bicarbonate dialysate was of any benefit in patients without a history of excessive symptoms during dialysis treatments.[22]

All untoward symptoms occurring during treatments were evaluated by the dialysis staff without knowledge of the type of dialysate, and rated as mild, moderate, or severe. Although the incidence of symptoms was low with both types of dialysate, twice as many total symptoms and two and a half times as many moderate or severe symptoms occurred with acetate dialysate as compared to bicarbonate. When evaluated blindly by questionnaire, patients stated they felt significantly better after dialysis with bicarbonate dialysate than with acetate (Table 5-2). Although there were no significant differences in the blood pressures during or after the dialysis treatments, we concluded that even stable, chronic hemodialysis patients have less symptoms during, and feel better after dialysis with bicarbonate dialysate than with acetate dialysate.

During dialysis with acetate dialysate, arterial blood Po_2 and Pco_2 usually fall, and plasma bicarbonate concentration and pH are relatively stable. It has been suggested that the cause of this hypoxia is hypoventilation secondary to carbon dioxide loss from the blood into the dialysate. The rate of direct carbon dioxide lost by this mechanism compared to the rate of carbon dioxide production is relatively minor, however, and should not significantly depress respiration.[23] There is

Table 5-2
Comparison of Acetate and Bicarbonate in Stable Chronic Hemodialysis Patients*

	All Symptoms*	Moderate or Severe Symptoms*	State of Well-Being Index
Acetate	44	22	−13
Bicarbonate	22†	9†	+14†

*Adapted from Van Stone JC, Cook J: The effect of bicarbonate dialysate in stable chronic hemodialysis patients. Dial Transplant 8:703–709, 1979.
*Percent of treatments with symptoms.

another mechanism of carbon dioxide loss during acetate dialysis. As previously mentioned, large amounts of bicarbonate are removed by the acetate dialysate. This bicarbonate is replaced by the reaction of carbon dioxide and water ($CO_2 + H_2O \rightarrow H_2CO_3 \rightarrow HCO_3^- + H^+$). The hydrogen ion produced enters acetate metabolism and the CO_2 is no longer available for respiratory excretion. Sargent and co-workers calculate that as much as 30 or 40 percent of metabolic CO_2 production during the dialysis treatment may be lost by this mechanism.[23] This should significantly depress respiration and decrease arterial Po_2. If this is the mechanism of hypoxia, it should not occur with bicarbonate dialysate, since there is no net loss of bicarbonate.

We evaluated the effect of dialysate base on arterial blood gas concentrations.[22] Arterial Po_2, Pco_2, pH, and bicarbonate concentrations were measured after 1 and 3 hours of dialysis with both acetate and bicarbonate dialysate. Treatment with acetate dialysate caused a significant decrease in arterial Po_2 (Table 5-3). The use of bicarbonate dialysate completely prevented this hypoxemia and corrected the metabolic acidosis faster.

Acetate can be metabolized to produce cholesteral and fatty acids. It has been suggested that the infusion of large amounts of acetate 2 or 3 times each week may increase lipid synthesis and contribute to the hyperlipidemia and accelerated atherosclerosis seen in hemodialysis patients. Although there were no truly long-term studies (6 months or greater), short-term controlled studies do not demonstrate any difference in plasma lipids between bicarbonate and acetate dialysate.[24,25]

In conclusion, the best evidence available today indicates that, in at least some patients, bicarbonate dialysate is associated with better cardiovascular stability, decreased symptoms during dialysis, and better dialysis tolerance than acetate dialysate. This is true for critically ill patients, patients with acute renal failure, and patients with stable chronic renal failure. It is likely that there is a reduction in the rate of acetate metabolism during hypotensive episodes, which may lead to increased plasma acetate concentrations and further aggravate the already present vascular instability. We currently use bicarbonate dialysate for acutely ill patients and patients prone to hypotension during routine dialysis.

Glucose

There currently is a debate on whether or not the dialysate should contain glucose. Glucose is one of the more expensive constituents of the dialysate. Glucose-free dialysate results in the loss of 20–30 g of glucose during a 4-hour hemodialysis procedure and diabetics with

Table 5-3
Comparison of Acetate and Bicarbonate Dialysate on Arterial Blood Gas Determination

	P_{O_2}		P_{CO_2}		HCO_3^-		pH	
	1 hr	3 hr	1 hr	3 hr	1 hr	3 hr	1 hr	3 hr
Acetate dialysate	88 ± 6	86 ± 4	38 ± 1	37 ± 1	17 ± 1	18 ± 1	7.37 ± .02	7.40 ± .02
Bicarbonate dialysate	93* ± 4	96† ± 4	39 ± 1	38 ± 1	21† ± 1	23† ± 1	7.40* ± .02	7.433† ± .02

*$p < 0.05$ compared to acetate dialysate.
†$p < 0.01$ compared to acetate dialysate.

moderate hyperglycemia may lose two to three times this amount. Glucose loss during dialysis stimulates gluconeogenesis and results in increased protein catabolism and urea production. Glucose in the dialysate prevents the glucose loss and the resultant increased gluconeogenesis.[26,27] It has been suggested that glucose in the dialysate may cause or at least aggravate the hyperlipidemia which is seen in many hemodialysis patients. Swamy and co-workers showed in an uncontrolled study that 50 percent of patients had a significant decrease in mean serum cholesterol and 25 percent of the patients had a decrease in the serum triglyceride when the dialysate glucose concentration was decreased from 500 mg/dl to zero.[28] Other studies, however, suggest that lower dialysate concentrations of 100–200 mg/dl do not have any significant effect on plasma lipid concentration.[29] Intuitively, it does not apepar wise to induce a catabolic state during the dialysis procedure. At the University of Missouri we use 200 mg/dl of glucose in all of our dialysate. It is especially important that insulin requiring diabetics be treated with a dialysate containing glucose since they are unable to decrease serum insulin concentrations in response to decreases in blood glucose concentration and may develop severe hypoglycemia with the use of glucose-free dialysate.

DIALYZERS

Dialyzer Membrane

Since the dialyzer membrane is the main determinant of what and how much is removed during dialysis, it is the most important component of the dialyzer. The original dialysis experiments used membranes of collodion made from a solution of cellulose nitrate in an organic solvent. The dialyzer membranes were made by coating glass tubes with this solution and allowing the organic solvent to evaporate. These membranes were not of a consistent quality and were very difficult to handle because of poor strength. In the early part of the century other materials were tried as membranes, such as visceral animal peritoneum and chicken intestines, without much success.

In the 1930s cellophane was developed for the specific purpose to use as sausage casings. Similar to collodion, cellophane is also made from cellulose. Native cellulose is used, however, rather than the nitrate derivative. Cellophane is a "regenerated cellulose" which is produced by initially dissolving the cellulose in sodium hydroxide. The dissolved cellulose material is then aged, treated with carbon disulfide, and excess sodium hydroxide added. The cellulose is then "regenerated" and the membrane formed by extruding this solution into an acid bath. Membrane properties such as ultrafiltration rate and sieving qualities can be changed markedly by changing the various conditions during the production. Rigid control of these conditions are required to produce a membrane of predictable qualities.

Cuprophan is a regenerated cellulose membrane which is produced by the Bemberg Corporation of Germany. It is currently the most commonly used membrane in hemodialyzers. It is produced by a slightly different method than that described above for cellophane in that the cellulose is dissolved in an ammonia solution of cupric oxide, rather than sodium hydroxide. A cuproammonium–cellulose complex is formed, which when extruded into an acid bath yields a cellulosic membrane which has the cuproammonium radical incorporated into its structure. Cuprophan has slightly better diffusion and ultrafiltration properties than ordinary regenerated cellulose membranes and the Bemberg Corporation maintains rigid control of the manufacturing process in order to keep variation at an acceptable level.

Another membrane currently commercially available for hemodialyzers is the cellulose acetate membrane in which the cellulose is acetylated prior to membrane formation. These membranes have permeabilities that are somewhat greater than ordinary regenerated cellulose or cuprophan and have higher ultrafiltration rates.

The only other membrane currently in use in the United States for hemodialysis is the polyacrylonitrile membrane. This membrane is produced by the copolymerization of methylvinyl pyridine and sodium methallyl sulfonate. They have increased diffusive permeabilities, especially for higher molecular weight substances (middle molecules) and have very high ultrafiltration coefficients. Fluid removal with dialyzers made from these membranes can be extremely rapid and is not entirely predictable. For this reason the Hospal Company has developed the Cotral® (Hospal SA, Meyzieu, France) which is a special apparatus which can be attached to most dialysis machines and allows fluid to be removed during dialysis at a controlled steady rate.

Membrane–Blood Interaction

During the initial part of dialysis treatments with most commonly used dialyzers there is a marked fall in circulating neutrophil count. The cause of this neutropenia is not the removal of neutrophils by the dialyzer but their sequestration in the pulmonary vascular bed. This pulmonary sequestration is the result of blood–membrane interaction.

Upon contact with blood, regenerated cellulose membranes activate the compliment system which in turn causes the margination of neutrophils in pulmonary small vessels. It is not unusual in the initial 15 minutes of dialysis for the circulating neutrophil count to fall below 1000 cells/mm^3. The neutropenia is short lived and neutrophil counts return to normal within 1−2 hours following the initiation of dialysis. It is not certain whether there are any deleterious effects of the neutropenia. Evidence suggests, however, that the pulmonary neutrophil sequestration contributes to the hypoxia which occurs early during dialysis and it has also been implicated in causing chest pain during dialysis in some patients.

While the development of neutropenia is universal with the use of regenerated cellulose membranes, it does not occur with all membranes. Hemodialysis with cellulose acetate membranes also results in a significant decrease in neutrophil count early in dialysis, but the decrease is much less than that seen with regenerated cellulose, and polyacrylonitrate membranes cause very little if any significant decrease in white cell count. Another interesting phenomenon which has been observed with regenerated cellulose is that when the dialyzers are reused, the decrease in neutrophil count is significantly less than that seen with the initial use.

Dialyzer Evaluation

With the current wealth of dialyzers available and each manufacturer claiming superiority for his product, it is very difficult for the clinician to decide which dialyzer(s) to choose. Because of different needs of the individual patients, it is unlikely that the prudent physican will be able to choose a single dialyzer for use in all instances. Table 5-4

Table 5-4
Important Attributes in Dialyzer Evaluation
- Ultrafiltration rate
- Small solute clearance rate
- Large solute clearance rate
- Blood compartment volume
- Blood compartment compliance
- Residual blood volume
- Thrombogenicity
- Reusability
- Cost

lists important attributes which must be taken into consideration in dialyzer evaluation.

The ultrafiltration coefficient of the dialyzer is an important factor. For the patient who tends to gain large amounts of weight between treatments, it is necessary to use a dialyzer with an ultrafiltration capability high enough to allow the removal of fluid gained. The use of a dialyzer with a high UF coefficient in a patient with minimal interdialysis weight gains may necessitate, however, the administration of large amounts of normal saline to prevent excess weight loss.

Since the removal of small- and medium-sized toxins is a major objective of dialysis, the clearance rates of these molecules is of obvious importance. When comparing dialyzers in relationship to either small or middle molecular weight solute clearances, it is important that the blood flow rate be in the range that you expect to use clinically. As discussed in Chapter 6, there unfortunately is very little sound information available to help the physican decide how much solute clearance is necessary for an individual patient.

The extracorporeal blood volume is the volume of blood contained in the dialyzer and lines during dialysis. It is an important consideration in choosing a dialyzer. Since patients have an increased susceptability to hypotension during dialysis, it is desirable to keep this volume as low as possible. In addition to the priming volume of the dialyzer it is equally important to take into consideration the dialyzer compliance, i.e., the change in blood compartment volume which occurs with change in transmembrane presssure. In a dialyzer with a high compliance the increase in transmembrane pressure causes a large increase in blood compartment volume. Since transmembrane pressures are highest during high fluid removal rates and this is the time when patients are most likely to develop hypotension it is desirable to keep the dialyzer compliance as low as possible.

Residual blood volume refers to the amount of blood left in the kidney at the end of the dialysis procedure. Anemia is a major problem in patients on chronic hemodialysis. Although the primary cause of the anemia is not blood loss (Chapter 1), a large dialyzer residual loss of blood can increase the anemia. Reliable data on the residual blood volume of most available dialyzers unfortunately are not readily available. Dialyzer blood loss is dependent not only on the dialyzer but also the rinse back technique used at the termination of dialysis. It is important that as much blood as possible be returned to the patient.

Thrombogenicity refers to the tendency of the dialyzer membrane to initiate clotting on its surface. Most, if not all, dialyzer membranes cause some degree of clotting which necessitates the use of anticoagulation during the procedure. Although there is no doubt that this is more of a problem with some dialyzers than with others, there is very little comparative information available on this at this time. Although there are scattered reports of being able to dialyze some patients with certain dialyzers without the use of anticoagulates, there are at present no dialyzers with which patients can consistently be dialyzed without anticoagulation.

Although there are currently no dialyzers marketed with a FDA approval for reuse, many dialysis centers both in the United States and abroad, currently reuse dialyzers. The number of times a dialyzer can be used before its performance deteriorates to a point that it has to be discarded varies from dialyzer to dialyzer. Some dialyzers such as the Cordis Dow 2.5® can only be used two or three times before many of its fibers are blocked and unuseable while other dialyzers can be used up to ten times without significant loss of function. There also is very little data available on this subject in the literature. Table 5-5 illustrates the average number of reuses found for different dialyzers in our dialysis unit.

A final consideration in choosing a dialyzer is cost. With current economic conditions, both in the United States and abroad, this is becoming an important factor. Dialyzer reuse decreases the importance of initial dialyzer cost.

Table 5-5
Average Number of Treatments for each Dialyzer with Reuse Program

Brand of Dialyzer	Average
Travenol 1211*	6.3 ± 0.8
Travenol 1511*	7.1 ± 1.8
Travenol 2308*	4.3 ± 0.3
CDAK 1.3†	6.6 ± 1.1
CDAK 1.8†	3.0 ± 0.5
CDAK 2.5†	2.9 ± 0.2
CDAK 4000†	6.6 ± 1.1
TE 15‡	10.5 ± 5.5
Hospal 140§	4.5 ± 0.5

± is Standard Deviation

*Travenol Laboratory, Deerfield, IL
†Cordis Dow, Miami, FL
‡Terumo, Piscataway, NJ
§Hospal, East Brunswick, NJ
Dialyzers were rinsed with saline, water, and hydrogen peroxide and stored in 1 percent formaldehyde. Dialyzer is discarded when fiber volume decreases below 80 percent of original volume.

Dialyzer Configuration

There are three dialyzer configurations in current use (Fig. 5-1):
1. coil dialyzers
2. flat plate dialyzers
3. hollow fiber dialyzers

Although at present there appears to be no clear cut superiority of one dialyzer design over the others, there are some definite advantages and disadvantages of each.

Coil Dialyzers

As discussed in Chapter 4 coil dialyzers were used in the original dialysis experiments of Kolff in 1956. Coil dialyzers consist of fairly large diameter cellophane tubing wrapped around a cylinder. In the original "rotating drum" dialyzer, the cylinder was several feet in diameter and was rotated in a large tub containing dialysate. The cylinder in the coils in current use is 4–6 inches in diameter and remains stationary while the dialysate is pumped over the tubing. Because of the relative inefficiency of this design, it is necessary to circulate the dialysate through the coil at rapid flow rates. In order not to use excessive amounts of dialysate, coil dialyzers are usually used with equipment which recirculates the dialysate over the coil at high flow rates. The recirculating dialysate is kept in a reservoir and is changed at a lower rate of flow.

The main advantage of coil dialyzers is that of cost. They generally cost significantly less than the other types of disposable dialyzers. The disadvantages of coil dialyzers are that they have relatively low solute clearance and ultrafiltration rates, require rather large extracorporeal blood volumes, and have large compliances.

Plate Dialyzers

Flat plate dialyzers are made of a series of rectangular-shaped membranes which are laid on top of each other. These dialyzers are designed so that blood and dialysate flow between alternating sheets of membrane. On each dialysate side of the membrane there is a support structure to give strength and maintain the geometry of the dialyzer.

Plate dialyzers have several advantages over coil dialyzers. They have a higher surface area for the amount of extracorporeal blood volume and therefore higher solute clearance and ultrafiltration rates. Most plate dialyzers have relatively low residual blood volumes and compliances that are less than most coil dialyzers. One problem that occurs with some plate dialyzers is that the solute clearance is markedly decreased at high transmembrane pressures. This is probably

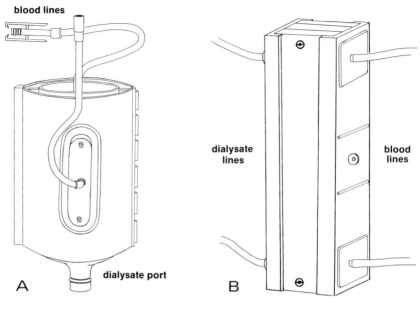
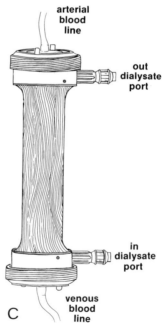

Figure 5-1. Coil dialyzer (A), flat-plate dialyzer (B), capillary fiber dialyzer (C).

the result of masking of the dialyzer membrane by the support structures.

Hollow Fiber Capillary Dialyzer

Hollow fiber capillary dialyzers are made of thousands of small cellulose capillaries which are tightly bound in a bundle. The dialyzer is designed so that the blood flows through the fibers and the dialysate flows in the opposite direction around the outside of the fibers.

Hollow fiber dialyzers have several advantages. In both a theoretical and actual basis they have the highest surface area for the amount of extracorporeal blood volume. The capillary fibers are supported only at their ends and there is no support structure in the dialysate compartment to mask the membrane. Whether compared on the basis of membrane surface area or extracorporeal blood volume, capillary fiber dialyzers have the highest clearance and ultrafiltration rates. Of available dialyzers, capillary fiber dialyzers have the lowest compliance with extracorporeal blood volume changing very little as transmembrane pressure increases.

The major disadvantge of the hollow fiber dialyzer is that they tend to have higher residual blood volumes, which can aggravate the anemia present in patients with chronic renal failure. They also are technically more difficult to manufacture, which results in somewhat higher costs.

DIALYSIS MACHINES

There are two general types of dialysis machines in use: (1) recirculating, single-pass (RSP) machines and (2) parallel flow machines.

The RSP dialysis machine made by Travenol Laboratories (Deerfield, IL) was first introduced into the market in 1967, rapidly became the standard dialysis machine, and was used for most hemodialysis treatments in the early 1970s. It is still used in a significant number of dialysis centers worldwide. With the RSP machine, the entire amount of dialysate to be used is made in a batch by mixing 3.4 liters of dialysate concentrate with 120 liters of water. The RSP machines use exclusively coil dialyzers. The coil dialyzer is placed in a small 10-liter reservoir in the upper portion of the machine which is filled with dialysate. The dialysate in this reservoir is rapidly pumped through the coil dialyzer at a rate of 60 liters/min by a recirculating pump; hence the term recirculating. The dialysate in the reservoir is then changed at a slower dialysate flow rate of approximately 500 ml/min. The RSP machine has the advantage of being very economical with a price significantly lower than any other dialysis machine, is easy to operate, and because of the lack of complexity has low maintenance costs. It, however, lacks many of the features of the newer dialysis machines and because coil dialyzers are less efficient, longer dialysis times are required.

Single-pass, negative pressure dialysis machines are used in most modern hemodialysis centers. There are two basic types in use: those which use a central delivery system for the preparation of the dialysate and those in which the individual patient machine prepares the dialysate.

With a central delivery system the dialysate for the entire dialysis unit is made by a central unit and piped through the walls or floor to each individual patient station. The main advantage of a central dialysate unit is economic. For a dialysis unit of 10 or more stations, the initial set-up cost using a central unit is significantly less than using individual patient units even when a backup central unit is installed. There are also some operational savings in that concentrate does not need to be transported to each individual station.

The main advantage of individual patient units is that it allows the physician to change the constitutents of the dialysate on a patient to patient basis. The importance of this is becoming increasingly recognized as time goes by. An additional advantage of individual patient units is that if the machine malfunctions only one patient is affected and the malfunctioning machine can be easily replaced with a backup machine.

Functions of the Single-Pass, Negative Pressure, Individualized Dialysis Machine

The primary functions of the dialysis machine are the preparation and delivery of dialysate and monitoring the dialysis system. Dialysate is sold in a liquid concentrate containing the constituents at a concentration 35 times that of the final dialysate. The dialysate machine takes 1 part of this concentrate and mixes it with 34 parts of water to prepare the dialysate. There are two basic methods which dialysis machines use to prepare the dialysate. The first method, typified by the Drake Willock® (B.D. Drake Willock, Portland OR) dialysis machine, is the fixed proportioning method. In these machines dialysate concentrate and water are drawn into separate cylindrical chambers by pistons and then expelled into the dialysate system. The volume of the water chamber is 34 times that of the concentrate chamber before creating the

34:1 ratio. The advantage of this system is that it does not depend on any electronic systems to maintain the 34:1 proportions and consequently it is very unlikely that improperly diluted dialysate will be prepared.

The second method of dialysate preparation is typified by the Cordis Dow® dialysis machine. In this machine, water is pumped by a centrifugal pump at a fixed rate and the dialysate concentrate is added with a similar, second, smaller pump. The rate of this second pump is determined by a servomechanism that measures the conductivity of the final dialysate and adjusts the rate so the conductivity falls into a predetermined range. Since the dialysate conductivity is dependent on the dissolved ions, the final dialysate composition is controlled. The advantage of this second method is that, within limits, the concentrations of the final dialysate can be varied away from the 35:1 ratio by changing setting of the servomechanism.

An important aspect of single-pass dialysis machines is the creation of negative pressure in the dialysate compartment of the dialyzer. Dialysate negative pressure is used to remove fluid from the patient during the dialysis procedure and the pressure must be adjustable so that the amount of fluid removal can be controlled. It is created by an additional pump on the dialysate outlet side of the dialyzer. The negative pressure is then adjusted either by changing the speed of this pump or more commonly by changing the size of an orifice through which the dialysate passes on the inlet side of the dialyzer. The amount of fluid removed during dialysis is determined not solely by the dialysate negative pressure but by the total transmembrane pressure, which includes both the pressures in the blood compartment and the dialysate compartment. The rate of fluid removal is independent of the rate of blood flow through the dialyzer. Most dialysis machines measure both the dialysate compartment pressure and the blood compartment pressure. In some machines these two pressures are electronically added and the resultant fed into a meter which then indicates total transmembrane pressure. Some of the newer machines will adjust the negative pressure of the dialysate compartment on the basis of changes in pressures in the blood compartment so as to maintain the transmembrane pressure constant.

Monitoring

A very important function of modern dialysis machines is that of monitoring. Usually blood and dialysate compartment pressures, dialysate temperature, dialysate conductivity, and the presence of air in the blood compartment or blood in the dialysate compartment are monitored.

In order to prevent the patient from being treated with improperly prepared dialysate, it is mandatory that the solute concentration of the dialysate be monitored. This is done by monitoring the dialysate conductivity. Conductivity is a measurement of the ability of the dialysate to conduct an electrical current. The conductivity of a solution is a complex function of the concentration of the various electrically charged solutes in the fluid. The dialysate conductivity varies most closely with the concentration of chloride. In all the currently available single-pass machines the conductivity of the dialysate is continually monitored. If the conductivity does not fall within a fixed range an alarm is activated and the machine is automatically put into a bypass mode so no further dialysate is delivered to the dialyzer until the conductivity is corrected. Many dialysis machines actually have two conductivity monitors, one which can be adjusted into a rather narrow range by the dialysis technician and a further backup conductivity monitor which cannot be adjusted and which automatically puts the machine in bypass mode if the conductivity falls below a certain value.

It is mandatory that dialysis machines have a dialysate temperature monitor. In order to prevent excessive heat loss from the patient, the dialysate is heated to near body temperature. If, however, the thermostat fails and the temperature goes above 44°C hemolysis will occur. Dialysis machines are equipped with a temperature monitor which alarms and places the machine in bypass mode if the dialysis goes above 40°C.

The final dialysate monitor present in the dialysis machine is a blood leak detector which continuously monitors the dialysate outflow from the dialyzer with a photometer. If a break occurs in the dialyzer membrane and blood leaks into the dialysate, the increased optical density of the dialysate is detected and an alarm is activated.

In addition to monitoring the dialysate, most dialysis machines also monitor certain aspects of the blood side of the dialyzer. By convention the blood line leading from the patient to the dialyzer is referred to as the arterial blood line and that which leads from the dialyzer to the patient is referred to as the venous line, even though neither line is usually attached to the arterial blood system of the patient. All currently available dialysis machines monitor the pressure in the venous line and most machines also have an arterial line pressure monitor. The upper and lower pressure limits of these monitors are adjustable and if a pressure limit is set by the dialysis personnel is transgressed, an alarm is sounded and the blood pump is automatically stopped.

Another important monitor present on some, but not all dialysis machines is a detector for the presence of air in the returning blood. This is an important safety device and should be present on all dialysis equipment. Although under ideal conditions air embolism should be exceedingly rare, the presence of a properly functioning air detector on the venous line should completely eliminate this potentially fatal complication. For those dialysis machines which do not have an air detector incorporated into them, separate units can be purchased and used.

There are two basic types of air detectors: photoelectric and sonic. Photoelectric air detectors pass a beam of light across the venous line into a photoelectric cell. If the amount of light reaching the cell increases suddenly, indicating air, the device trips an alarm clamping the venous line and turning off the blood pump. There are two problems with photoelectric air detectors.

1. They are not sensitive enough to pick up the tiny air bubbles (foam) which sometime are drawn into the blood lines from a loose connection.
2. The administration of large amounts of saline will decrease the optical density of the blood and cause the device to set off the alarm.

A better method of air detection is that of the sonic detector. Short pulses of high-frequency sound are transmitted across the blood stream and any significant amounts of air, whether in large bubbles or small bubbles (foam) will be detected and sound the alarm. Sonic detectors are not affected by saline administration.

Another important part of the dialysis equipment is the blood pump. In many systems the blood pump is an integral part of the dialysis machine whereas with other systems it must be purchased separately. All of the dialysis blood pumps in current use are double-headed roller pumps in which the blood is propelled through the blood tubing by compression of the tubing with the roller head against a flat surface (Fig. 5-2). This produces minimal trauma to the blood and results in essentially no hemolysis. It is important that the occlusion of the roller pumps be checked routinely and that the blood flow of the pump be measured periodically to assure that the proper blood flow is obtained during the dialysis procedure.

SINGLE-NEEDLE DIALYSIS

Most hemodialysis treatments are performed using two needles. One needle for removal of the blood and a second separate needle for

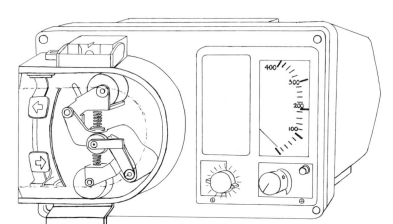

Figure 5-2. A hemodialysis double-headed roller blood pump.

blood return. There have been several systems developed which allow the dialysis procedure to be performed using a single-needle insertion. Proponents of single-needle dialysis allude to several possible advantages. The first and possibly major advantage of single-needle dialysis is the prevention of the further discomfort of a second needle puncture for the patient. It has also been claimed that single-needle dialysis prolongs fistula life by decreasing the number of punctures into the fistula by half. There are, however, no studies which prove this point and it is at least theoretically possible that the increased flow and turbulance that occurs with the higher flow rates and intermittent change in flow direction which occurs through the single needle may in fact decrease fistula life span. The disadvantage of single-needle dialysis is that even under the best of circumstances it is less efficient than double-needle dialysis.

Single-needle dialysis usually involves the use of a device which intermittently clamps the venous and arterial blood lines allowing blood flow through only one of these lines at a time. There are currently two single-needle devices available in the US: (1) the Vital Assists® SND (Hospal, Littleton, CO) and (2) Drake Willock® SND. These units use different methods for determining the length of time that the arterial and venous lines are open.

A schematic of the Vital Assists® single-needle system is shown in Figure 5-3. The clamp system pad is a double solenoid which alternately clamps either the arterial line or the venous line. In the beginning of the cycle the venous return line is closed and the arterial

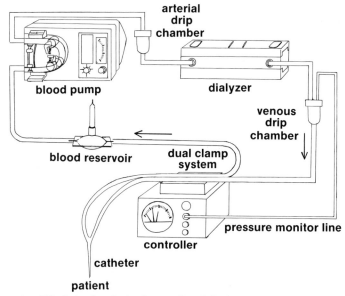

Figure 5-3. Vital Assists® single-needle dialysis system (Hospal Littleton, CO).

line is open. Blood is pumped through the arterial line into the dialyzer system until the pressure in the venous drip chamber reaches a preselected value. At this time the venous clamp is released and the arterial line clamped. During the venous phase, blood is allowed to return to the patient through the venous line. The length of the venous return time varies from 0.5–1.5 seconds and is determined by the dialysis staff. During the venous phase the blood pump delivers blood from the arterial line between the arterial clamp and the blood pump into the dialyzer.

A schematic drawing of the Drake Willock® single-needle device is shown in Figure 5-4. This system involves the use of a single venous line clamp. Similar to the Vital Assist® unit, during the beginning of the cycle with this system the venous line is clamped and the blood pump delivers blood into the dialyzer until the pressure in the venous drip chamber reaches a preselected value. At this time the clamp is removed from the venous line and the blood pump is turned off. Blood is allowed to return through the venous line into the patient until the pressure in the venous chamber falls to a preselected value. At this time the venous clamp is again activated and the cycle begins again.

Keshaviah and co-workers have performed extensive in vitro and in vivo comparisons of these two single-needle systems with routine

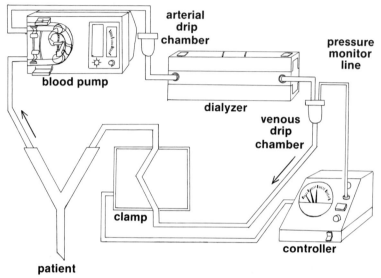

Figure 5-4. Drake Willock® single-needle system (Drake Willock, Portland, OR).

double-needle dialysis.[30] The in vivo results of their studies are summarized in Table 5-6. Both urea and creatinine removal were significantly lower with either single-needle system than with the double-needle system. The urea removal with the Vital Assists® system was significantly better than that with the Drake Willock® system. This is probably due to the fact that the Vital Assists® system blood pump runs throughout the cycle whereas the Drake Willock® system blood pump is shut off between 40 and 60 percent of the total dialysis time.

A major problem with single-needle dialysis is the recirculation of blood from the venous line to the arterial line. Keshaviah et al. found in their in vivo studies that recirculation was similar with both devices (Table 5-6). The amount of recirculation which occurs during dialysis is

Table 5-6
In Vivo Performance of Vital Assist® and Drake Willock Single-Needle Dialysis Devices

	Percentage Urea Removed	Percentage Creatinine Removed	Percentage Recirculation
Vital Assists	58 ± 4	48 ± 5	17 ± 1
Drake Willock	39 ± 4	34 ± 2	9 ± 6
Double needle	70 ± 3	60 ± 2	3 ± 1

inversely related, however, to the blood flow through the fistula, and if fistula flow is less than 300 ml/min, recirculation increases. Keshaviah et al. studied the effect of decreasing fistula flow on both these systems in an in vitro experiment. They found that the Vital Assists® system is more susceptible to decreased fistula flow than the Drake Willock® system (Fig. 5-4). It is important to remember that with decreased fistula flow, recirculation can also occur with the usual double-needle dialysis by blood flowing from the venous return needle back through the vein to the arterial needle.

Thus it apperars that single-needle dialysis is associated with some decrease in small molecular weight clearance. This reduction in clearance is related to both recirculation and decreased total blood flow. Large molecular weight clearances are much less affected by these changes than small molecular weight changes and ultrafiltration rates are essentially unchanged. Whether the increased patient comfort afforded by lack of a second venopuncture is worth the decrease in small molecular clearance is conjectural.

The above results were obtained at pressure and flow rates which were selected to maximize clearances during single-needle dialysis. It must be pointed out that if careful attention is not given to these settings the amount of recirculation can greatly increase and therefore reduce small molecular weight clearances. Decreased fistula flow during double-needle dialysis is usually accompanied by line jumping, bubble formation, and collapse of the arterial line so as to give warning of inadequate flow, whereas decreased fistula flow with single-needle dialysis mainly results in increased recirculation and may go unnoticed unless special procedures to determine the percent of recirculation are performed. One visual indication of very large amounts of recirculation with either single-needle or double-needle dialysis is the visual darkening of the blood (black blood syndrome) caused by the deoxygenation of hemoglobin.

Double-lumen fistula catheters are also available for single-needle dialysis. These are small Teflon catheters that are placed into the fistula and contain two concentric lumens. The outer lumen, which contains side holes, is used to draw blood out of the vessel into the dialyzer circuit and blood is returned through the inner lumen, which discharges blood through the end of the catheter. The total diameter of this device is somewhat larger than the normal dialysis needles and it sometimes is associated with increased bleeding after dialysis. The close proximity of the inflow and outflow ports also may cause recirculation to be higher than with two needles placed farther apart. Similar, longer double-lumen catheters for subclavian vein or femoral vein use are also available.

REFERENCES

1. Easterling RE: Standards for hemodialysis systems (draft). Arlington, Association for the Advancement of Medical Instrumentation, 1901 N. Ft. Myer Dr., Arlington, VA
2. Kjellstrand CM, Eaton JW, Yawata Y, et al: Hemolysis in dialyzed patients caused by chloramines. Nephron 13:427–433, 1974
3. Matter BJ, Pederson J, Psimenos G, Lindermon RD: Lethal copper intoxication in hemodialysis. Trans Am Soc Artif Intern Organs 15:309–315, 1969
4. Berkes SL, Kahn SI, Chazan JA, Garella S: Prolonged hemolysis from overheated dialysate. Ann Intern Med 83:363–364, 1975
5. Van Stone JC, Bauer J, Carey J: The effect of dialysate sodium concentration on body fluid compartment volume, plasma renin activity and plasma aldosterone concentration in chronic hemodialysis patients. Am J Kidney Dis 2:58–64, 1982
6. Gotch FA, Lam MA, Prowitt M, Keen M: Preliminary clinical results with sodium-volume modeling of hemodialysis therapy. Proc Clin Dial Transplant Forum 10:12–16, 1980
7. Ogden DA: A double blind crossover comparison of high and low sodium dialysis. Proc Dialysis Transplant Forum 8:157–164, 1978
8. Robson M, Oren A, Ravid M: Dialysate sodium concentration, hypertension and pulmonary edema in hemodialysis patients. Dial Transplant 6:678–679, 1978
9. Dumler F, Grondin G, Levin NW: Sequential high/low sodium hemodialysis: An alternative to ultrafiltration. Trans Am Soc Artif Intern Organs 25:351–353, 1979
10. Oh MS, Levison SP, Carroll HJ: Content and distribution of water and electrolytes in maintenance hemodialysis. Nephron 14:421–433, 1975
11. Johny KV, Lawrence JR, O'Halloran MW, Wellby ML, Worthley BW: Studies on total body, serum and erythrocyte potassium in patients on maintenance hemodialysis. The value of erythrocyte potassium as a measure of body potassium. Nephron 7:320–240, 1970
12. Goldsmith RS, Furszyfer J, Johnson WT et al: Control of secondary hyperparathyroidism during long-term hemodialysis. Am J Med 50:692–699, 1971
13. Rivera-Vazquez AB, Noriega-Sanchez A, Rammirez-Gonzalez R, Martinez-Maldonado M: Acute hypercalcemia in hemodialysis patients: Distinction from 'dialysis dementia.' Nephron 25:243–246, 1980
14. Hecerli C, Hill AUL: The relationship between the magnesium concentration in the dialysis fluid used and in the plasma and erythrocytes of patients with chronic renal failure treated by regular haemodialysis. Clin Sci 43:779, 1972
15. Pletka P, Bernstein DS, Hampers CL, Merrill JP, Sherwood LM: Effects of magnesium on parathyroid hormone secretion during hemodialysis. Lancet 2:462–463, 1971

16. Fleming LW, Levman JAR, Stewart WK: Effect of magnesium on nerve conduction velocity during regular dialysis treatment. J Neurol Neurosurg Psychiatry 35:342–355, 1972
17. Mion CM, Hegstrom RM, Boen ST, Scribner BH: Substitution of acetate for sodium bicarbonate in the bath fluid for hemodialysis. Trans Am Soc Artif Intern Organs 10:110–113, 1969
18. Graefe V, Milutinovich J, Follette WC, et al: Less dialysis-induced morbidity and vascular instability with bicarbonate in dialysate. Ann Intern Med 88:332–336, 1978
19. Vreman HJ, Assomull VM, Kaiser BA, Blaschke TF, Weiner MW: Acetate metabolism and acid–base homeostasis during hemodialysate. Influence of dialyzer efficiency and rate of acetate metabolism. Kidney Int 18 (Suppl 10):562–574, 1980
20. Kirkendol PL, Devia CJ, Bower JD, Holbert RD: A comparison of the cardiovascular effects of sodium acetate, sodium bicarbonate and other potential sources of fixed base in hemodialysis solutions. Trans Am Soc Artif Intern Organs 23:399–403, 1977
21. Novello A, Kelsch RC, Easterling RE: Acetate intolerance during hemodialysis. Clin Nephrol 5:29–32, 1976
22. Van Stone JC, Cook J: The effect of bicarbonate dialysate in stable chronic hemodialysis patients. Dial Transplant 8:703–709, 1979
23. Sargent JA, Gotch FA: Bicarbonate and carbon dioxide transport during hemodialysis. ASAIO 2:61–72, 1979
24. Ibels LS, Simons LA, King JO, et al: Studies on the nature and causes of hyperlipidemia in uremia, maintenance dialysis and renal transplantation. Quart J Med 44:601–610, 1975
25. Savdie E, Mahony JF, Steward JH: Effect of acetate on serum lipids in maintenance hemodialysis. Trans Am Soc Artif Intern Organs 23:385–391, 1977
26. Wathen R, Keshaviah P, Hammeyer P, Cadwell K, Comty C: Role of glucose in preventing gluconeogenesis during hemodialysis. Trans Am Soc Artif Intern Organs 23:393–397, 1977
27. Gotch FA, Borah M, Keen M et al: The solute kinetics of intermittent dialysis therapy, in: Annual Contractors Report of Artificial Kidney Programs of NIAMDD. DHEW Pub #(NIH) 77-1442, 1977, pp 106–107
28. Swamy AP, Cestero RVM, Campbell RG, Freeman RB: Long-term effect of dialysate glucose on the lipid levels of maintenance hemodialysis patients. Trans Am Soc Artif Intern Organs 22:54–58, 1976
29. Hubner W, Sieberch HG, Dremer A, Finke K, Prange E: Effect of regular haemodialysis with glucose and glucose free dialysate on hyperlipidemia. Proc Eur Dial Transplant Assoc 8:174–178, 1971
30. Keshaviah P, Carlson G, Wathen R: In vitro and clinical evaluation of single needle dialysis. Trans Am Soc Artif Intern Organs 22:367–375, 1976

John C. Van Stone

6
Hemodialysis Prescription

Hemodialysis treatments are complex and contain many variables that can change on an individual patient-to-patient basis. At the present time there, unfortunately, are little objective data available to guide in making appropriate choices on many of these variables. It is undoubtedly true, however, that proper adjustments of these parameters can improve overall patient well-being and decrease the number of untoward reactions during dialysis. These parameters of the hemodialysis treatments are referred to as the dialysis prescription and this chapter offers some guidelines in their determination.

DETERMINING THE AMOUNT OF TOTAL DIALYSIS NEEDED

The total amount of dialysis treatment a patient receives is primarily a function of the size of the dialyzer, the number of hours of dialysis, and the blood flow through the dialyzer. Determining the total amount of dialysis treatment that a patient with chronic renal insufficiency needs is an important but very difficult task. The primary purposes of the dialysis treatments are to remove the toxins which are normally eliminated by the kidney and to maintain mineral and water homeostasis. There are a large number of substances which accumulate during renal failure and which of these are most important to remove is not known at this time. It is generally agreed that the commonly measured substances, i.e., urea, creatinine, and uric acid, have minimal if any toxicities at concentrations present in chronic renal failure. In the past there was a large search for the "uremic toxin" but now it appears evident that the uremic syndrome is probably not caused by the accumulation of a single toxic substance, but is most likely the result of the presence of a number of toxic agents.

While it is not necessary to know the exact composition of these toxic substances in determining the dialysis parameters, it would be helpful to at least know their molecular weight. There are currently two views: Babb and Schribner at the University of Washington feel that the most important uremic toxins have a molecular weight in the range of 1000–2000 daltons, so-called "middle molecules,"[1] while many others feel that the major toxins are much smaller, being in the range of urea (100–200 daltons).

In the early 1970s Babb and co-workers developed what they termed the square meter–hour hypothesis.[1] This theory is based on the supposition that the limiting factor in determining the minimal amount of dialysis needed is middle molecule removal. It states that the removal of molecules in this range is relatively independent of dialyzer blood flow and is related mainly to the available surface area of the dialyzer and the total dialysis time. It also recognizes that the amount of residual renal function of the patient's own kidneys has a much larger impact on the total removal of middle molecular substances than it does on the removal of small molecular weight substances. They developed a dialysis index which is the total weekly clearance of substances of a molecular weight of 1500 daltons.[2] The dialysis index (D_I) is calculated by the formula in Figure 6-1.

An estimate of the residual GFR can be obtained by averaging the patient's urea and creatinine clearance. They suggest a minimum dialysis index of 1.0 which converts to 17 liters/week of middle molecular clearance for each square meter of body surface area or 29 liters/week for the "normal" 1.73-m² patient.

$$D_I = (3.5 \times 10^{-3})(K_D t_D + 168 K_K)/S$$

where

K_D = dialyzer clearance of 1500 molecular weight at the mean ultrafiltration rate used for the patient (ml/min)

t_D = weekly dialysis time (hours)

K_K = residual glomerular filtration rate (ml/min)

S = body surface area (m²)

Figure 6-1. Calculations of the dialysis index.

Interdialysis weight gains have significant effects on total middle molecular clearance. All interdialysis fluid gains must be removed by ultrafiltration during the dialysis treatment. For every liter of fluid removed there is a liter of middle molecular clearance (see Chapter 5). A patient who gains an average of 3 kg between each treatment therefore will have 7.5 liters more middle molecular weight clearance each week than a patient who gains only 0.5 kg between each treatment if the same dialyzer is used for the same number of hours. This may make a 30 percent or greater difference in total weekly middle molecular clearance.

The square meter hypothesis has been studied by several different protocols by varying dialyzer size, total dialysis time, dialysate flow, or blood flow. Some of these studies suggest that if the dialysis index is below one, patients develop peripheral neuropathy, whereas neuropathy does not develop if the index dialysis is greater than one. In none of the available studies, unfortunately, was it possible to change middle molecular clearance without some changes in small molecular clearances. Although there is sugestive evidence that middle molecular clearances are important, it remains to be unequivocally proven. Until the question is settled it is probably wise to attempt to maintain a D_1 of at least one.

Many feel that an important factor in determining the total amount of dialysis needed is the removal of smaller molecular weight substances. In contrast to middle molecular weight substances, where removal is dependent mainly on dialyzer surface area and dialysis time, removal of smaller molecular weight substances are more dependent on total blood flow during dialysis. At present there are no well-established guidelines for the total small molecular weight clearances needed.

Gotch suggests using the serum urea concentration as a guide to small molecular weight clearance.[3] Serum urea levels are dependent not only on total urea clearance but also upon urea generation. Urea generation is a function of the total protein catabolic rate which, in the stable hemodialysis patient, is predominantly a function of protein intake. If serum urea nitrogen concentrations are used as an indication of the adequacy of dialysis, then it is important to determine the protein catabolic rate to make sure that the dietary protein intake is adequate.

The results of a large national cooperative study of the adequacy of dialysis suggests that the BUN concentration has an effect on patient morbidity.[4] This controlled study separated the effects of blood urea nitrogen concentrations and the dialysis treatment times. High BUN concentrations were associated with increased hospitalizations whereas the total number of hours each week on dialysis had no effect on morbidity.

Inadequate dialysis itself can cause inadequate protein intake. Studies demonstrate that patients spontaneously reduce protein intake when the total amount of dialysis is reduced.[5] It is possible that some of the protein catabolic products cause a relative anorexia. A reduction in protein intake can cause protein malnutrition and it is preferable that dialysis patients maintain a protein intake of 0.8–1.0 g/k body weight.

Sargent and co-workers have demonstrated that an estimate of the protein catabolic rate of hemodialysis patients can be obtained from urea kinetics.[6] Total urea generation is determined by adding the amount of urea which accumulates in the body between two dialysis treatments to the amount of urea which is excreted by the kidneys during this time and the protein catabolic rate (PCR) calculated from the amount of urea generated.

For determination of urea generation it is only necessary to measure the serum urea nitrogen concentration at the end of one dialysis treatment and the beginning of the next and to collect and measure the urea in the urine excreted between the treatments. Since urea is distributed in total body water, urea accumulation is calculated by multiplying the increase in serum urea concentration by the postdialysis total body water volume. Since the increase in body weight which occurs between dialysis is predominantly with urea-free water which is then filled with urea, an adjustment is made by multiplying the increase in body weight by the predialysis serum urea concentration. Urea excretion is determined by multiplying urine urea concentration by urine volume. The protein catabolic rate is then calculated from the urea generation rate by a formula which was developed empirically.

An important value in the calculation of urea generation is the estimated total body water. Sargent determines the total body water by dividing the amount of urea removed during dialysis by the intradialysis change in blood urea nitrogen concentration. The total urea removed during dialysis is calculated from the dialyzer clearance and the time on dialysis. An alternate way to determine total body water is to assume that total body water is equal to 56 percent of body weight at the end of dialysis. This assumption appears valid if the patient is clinically in good water balance at the end of treatment. At the University of Missouri total body water was determined with tritiated water in 10 dialysis patients and found that total body water did not vary from 56 percent of body weight by more than 10 percent. Given the variation which exists between dialyzers it is doubtful that dialyzer clearance can estimate total body water more accurately than this and it is certainly much easier and less expensive to use this alternate method.

The Gotch and Sargeant method of determining protein catabolic rate is commercially available through Quantitative Medical Systems, 1710 59th St., Emeryville, CA 64608. (The cost of this service is dependent on the total number of patients and currently ranges between $2.00 and $5.00 for each determination.)

Urea generation and protein catabolic rate can also be determined easily using a small hand-held programmable calculator with the formulas in Figure 6-2. (A program using these formulas for a Texas Instrument 59® programmable calculator has been developed and is available without charge by writing to John Van Stone, M.D., c/o Department of Medicine, University of Missouri–Medical Center.)

Gotch and co-workers suggest that small molecular weight clearances should be sufficient to keep the predialysis serum urea nitrogen level below 80 mg/dl, when measured predialysis after the longest interdialysis interval and when the patient is eating at least 1 g/kg of protein each day.[3] This cannot be converted directly into total urea clearance per week because of the different effects that dialysis and residual renal failure have on the predialysis serum urea level. If one assumes, however, that serum urea levels typically fall to 40 percent of

$$UNG = \frac{(SUN_{PRE} - SUN_{POST}) BW \times 0.56 + SUN_{PRE} \times \Delta BW + UUN \times V}{0.417 \times time}$$

$$PCR = \frac{UNG + 1.7}{0.154}$$

where

UNG	= Urea nitrogen generation (g/24 h)
SUN_{PRE}	= Predialysis serum urea nitrogen concentration (mg/dl)
SUN_{POST}	= Postdialysis serum urea nitrogen concentration (mg/dl)
BW	= Post dialysis body weight (kg)
ΔBW	= Weight gained between dialysis (kg)
UUN	= Urine urea nitrogen concentration (mg/dl)
V	= Urine volume between dialysis (liters)
Time	= Time between dialysis (hours)
PCR	= Protein catabolic rate (g/24 h)

Figure 6-2. Calculation of urea generation and protein catabolic rate.

predialysis levels by the end of the last dialysis of the week, this would equate to a mean serum urea nitrogen level throughout the week of approximately 55 mg/dl. The weekly urea clearance needed to maintain a mean SUN of 55 can be calculated from the protein catabolic rate. One gram of protein each day will produce approximately 130 mg of urea nitrogen each day or 910 mg each week. To clear 910 mg of urea nitrogen/kg each week with a mean serum urea nitrogen of 55 mg/dl, a weekly clearance of 1.7 liters/kg is needed. A 70-kg patient eating 1 g/kg of protein therefore will need 120 liters of urea clearance each week.

DIALYZERS

There are currently an abundant number of dialyzers available in many sizes and configurations. The advantages and disadvantages of the different available configurations are discussed in Chapter 5 and my personal preference leans toward the hollow fiber kidney, although it does not have overwhelming advantages over plate dialyzers. The most important parameters when choosing a dialyzer for a patient are the clearances, both small and middle molecular weight, and the ultrafiltration rate. It seems intuitively apparent that a 220-pound muscular man should be treated with a larger dialyzer than that used for a 100-pound woman. Clinical experience demonstrates that when large-sized dialyzers are used on small patients there is an increased incidence of untoward reactions such as hypotension, vomiting, and muscle cramps. Conversely, if the dialyzer is excessively small in comparison to patient size, either there will be inadequate dialysis or the treatment time will need to be unduly long.

One method of choosing a dialyzer is to first determine the amount of middle molecule clearance needed on the basis of patient size and residual renal function. Then determine the amount of small molecular clearance needed on the basis of protein catabolic rate and residual renal function, and finally determine the amount of ultrafiltration needed on the basis of average interdialysis weight gain. Using these figures and the approximate number of hours each week of dialysis, an appropriate dialyzer can be chosen. The clearances and ultrafiltration rates of many of the dialyzers presently available are listed in Table 6-1.

An alternate method of choosing a dialyzer is to empirically start all patients on a medium-sized dialyzer and change the dialyzer if clinically indicated. Although this method is not as scientific, it is done in many centers with apparently good results.

Table 6-1
Characteristics of Currently Available Parallel Flow Dialyzers

Manufacturer	Model	Type	Material	Wall Thickness	Surface Area	Priming Volume	UFR	Clearance (ml/min)*			
								Urea	Cr	PO_4	Vitamin B_{12}
Cobe (Lakewood, CO)	HF 130	Capillary	Cuprophan	19	1.3	150	2.7	145	125	—	33
	HF 150	Capillary	Cuprophan	16	1.5	170	3.6	156	140	—	41
	PPD 1.3	Plate	Cuprophan	13.5	1.3	77–180	3.4	136	118	—	29
	PPD 1.6	Plate	Cuprophan	11.5	1.6	89–190	4.1	151	131	—	36
	HF 70	Capillary	Cuprophan	—	.7	65	2.8	142	144	—	23
	HF 100	Capillary	Cuprophan	—	1.0	90	4.2	165	132	—	33
	Lento	Capillary	Cuprophan	11	.7	65	2.6	142	114	—	23
	Andante	Capillary	Cuprophan	11	1.0	90	3.8	165	132	—	33
	Allegro	Capillary	Cuprophan	11	1.4	105	5.0	181	145	—	39
Cordis Dow (Miami, FL)	0.6	Capillary	RC	30	0.6	53	1.1	118	90	55	—
	1.3 D	Capillary	RC	30	1.3	100	1.9	160	133	85	23
	1.8 D	Capillary	RC	30	1.8	135	2.3 (2.3)	172 (167)	150 (102)	125	28
	2.5 D	Capillary	RC	30	2.5	180	3.6 (3.6)	184 (190)	154 (165)	140 (144)	40
	3500	Capillary	CA	40	0.9	75	3.2 (5.3)	130 (128)	105 (102)	70 (83)	34
	4000	Capillary	CA	40	1.4	109	4.3	161	129	105	45
	90 SCE	Capillary	Soponified cellulose ester	30	1.1	85	2.2	160	135	109	36

Table 6-1 (Cont.)

Manufacturer	Model	Type	Material	Wall Thickness	Surface Area	Priming Volume	UFR	Clearance (ml/min)*			Vitamin B_{12}
								Urea	Cr	PO_4	
(Cordis Dow, cont.)	135 SCE	Capillary	Soponified cellulose ester	30	1.35	101	3.0	173	147	121	43
Erika (Rockleigh, NJ)	HPF 100	Capillary	Cuprophan	11	0.8	67	3.3 (3.1)	160 (119)	133 (106)	— (81)	57
	HPF 200	Capillary	Cuprophan	11	1.0	78	3.7 (2.9)	170 (150)	142 (123)	— (103)	61
	HPF 300	Capillary	Cuprophan	11	1.3	95	4.6 (3.7)	181 (165)	156 (139)	— (112)	73
Extracorporeal (King of Prussia, PA)	TriEx 1	Capillary	Cuprophan	11	1.0	86	3.2 (3.2)	150 (157)	125 (131)	— (108)	30
	TriEx 3	Capillary	Cuprophan	11	1.6	138	5.5 (4.5)	160 (167)	148 (135)	— (113)	45
Gambro (Barrington, IL)	GLP 11.5	Plate	Cuprophan	11.5	1.0	75	3.4	159	128	86	36
	GLP 17.0	Plate	Cuprophan	17	1.0	62	1.8	142	111	63	22
	GLM 11.5	Plate	Cuprophan	11.5	1.7	103	4.5	170	145	93	46
	GLM 17.0	Plate	Cuprophan	17	1.7	93	1.8	161	130	81	30
	GLP 0.41	Plate	Cuprophan	13.5	0.41	33	1.4	100	73	—	17
	120 L	Capillary	Cuprophan	16	1.1	80	2.0	160	130	90	26
	120 M	Capillary	Cuprophan	11	1.2	80	3.0	170	140	106	38
	120 H	Capillary	Cuprophan	8	1.2	80	4.6	175	152	115	48

Manufacturer	Model	Configuration	Membrane							
Hospal (Littleton, CO)	080	Capillary	Cuprophan	11	.8	2.5	150	130	100	28
	110	Capillary	Cuprophan	11	1.1	3.5	168	140	115	38
	140	Capillary	Cuprophan	11	1.4	4.8	183	160	137	48
	RP-610	Plate	Acrilonitrile	30	1.0	20	150	128	—	60
	RP-607	Plate	Acrilonitrile		.67	14	130	110	—	42
	H 12-10	Plate	Acrilonitrile	30	1.0	20	160	—	—	55
Terumo (Compton, CA)	TH1000	Capillary	Cuprophan	16	1.0	3.2 (3.2)	130 (115)	105 (96)	(77)	32
	TH 1300	Capillary	Cuprophan	16	1.3	4.0 (4.1)	150 (152)	120 (132)	—	35
	TH 1500	Capillary	Cuprophan	16	1.5	5.6 (4.9)	155 (148)	125 (121)	(104)	40
	TE-07	Capillary	Cuprophan	11	.7	2.8	140	118	(109)	30
	TE-10	Capillary	Cuprophan	11	1.0	3.7 (2.7)	155 (154)	130 (130)	—	40
	TE-15	Capillary	Cuprophan	11	1.5	5.2 (5.1)	170 (175)	150 (147)	(73)	50
Travenol (Deerfield, IL)	12.11	Capillary	Cuprophan	11	.8	— (2.6)	162	120	(152)	34
	15.11	Capillary	Cuprophan	11	1.1	— (3.7)	173 (163)	142 (141)	56	34
	23.08	Capillary	Cuprophan	11	1.25	— (3.4)	180 (168)	152 (141)	(63)	47
	CD-1400	Coil	—		1.3	—	135	113	(126)	34
									68	

Abbreviations: RC = regenerated cellulose, CA = cellulose acetate, UFR = ultrafiltration rate.

*Values in parentheses were obtained from in vivo studies conducted at the University of Missouri. Clearances are based on blood flow, 220 ml/min; dialysate flow, 500 ml/min; transmembrane pressure (TMP), 100 mm Hg. Ultrafiltration rates were determined at TMPs of 100, 200, 350, and 500 mm Hg and averaged.

Performance data not in parentheses were obtained from the manufacturer. Typical blood flow was 200 ml/min; dialysate flow, 500 ml/min; TMP 0 mm Hg.

DIALYSIS DURATION AND FREQUENCY

The total number of hours of dialysis which a patient needs is dependent on the total weekly clearance of both small and large molecules needed and the clearance of the dialyzer chosen. A dialyzer generally can be used which is large enough so as to permit the total number of hours of dialysis each week to be 12 hours or less. This provides three, 4-hour treatments each week, which is the most common schedule in our clinics. Another important factor in determining the length of dialysis treatments, in addition to the amount of clearance needed, is the amount of fluid which needs to be removed during the treatment. If the patient gains large amounts of fluid then it may be necessary for the treatment time to be lengthened in order to remove the fluid without the development of hypotension or severe symptoms.

After the dialyzer and total number of hours of dialysis each week is determined, it is necessary to determine the duration of each dialysis treatment and the number of dialysis treatments each week. Patients usually do best by splitting their total dialysis time each week into three treatments. In my opinion, it is mandatory for patients whose residual glomerular filtration rate is less than 1 ml/min to have three treatments each week. Some patients with a residual GFR greater than 1 ml/minute do well with two dialysis treatments each week. It is important, however, for the patient who receives only two treatments each week to restrict fluid intake to a sufficient degree that weight gains are not excessive between treatments. A further problem with placing patients on a twice weekly dialysis schedule is that if their renal function deteriorates to a level that thrice weekly treatments are indicated, as it usually does, it is frequently very difficult to convince them of this fact. For this reason, it is my preference to place most patients on three dialysis treatments each week from the beginning. Mitigating factors, however, such as long travel time to treatments or the attempts to maintain full employment need to be taken into consideration.

DIALYSATE

A thorough discussion of the constituents of the dialysate is found in Chapter 5. If the dialysis unit does not use a central delivery system, then the dialysate can be tailored for individual patients. The most common constituents of the dialysate which are changed are the potassium concentration, calcium concentration, and the base.

Potassium

The majority of patients do well using a dialysate which contains 2 mEq/liter of potassium. This can be reduced, however, to 1 mEq/liter or potassium-free dialysate can be used if the predialysis serum potassium concentrations are high. Although serum potassiums between 5.5 and 6.0 mEq/liter are above the "normal range" they are well tolerated by patients and do not have any obvious harmful effects. The dialysate potassium need not be reduced unless the serum concentration is above 6 mEq/liter. High serum potassiums can also be treated by stricter dietary restriction. It is my personal philosophy that frequently it is better to reduce the dialysate potassium concentration than to decrease the dietary intake. The use of lower dialysate potassium concentrations are associated, however, with an increased incidence of cardiac arrythmias during dialysis. This is particularly true in patients receiving digitalis preparations. In these patients it is better to use a stricter dietary restriction and dialysate potassium concentration of 2–3 mEq/liter. Potassium concentrations below 2 mEq/liter should be used with caution in patients receiving digitalis.

Approximately 10 percent of the patients starting dialysis will have a low serum potassium (less than 4 mEq/liter) when they start their treatments. The low serum potassium in these patients usually is due to a combined effect of diuretics and anorexia from their uremia. In these patients a dialysate potassium of 4 mEq/liter should be used. Diuretics are discontinued at the start of the dialysis treatments and after several weeks of dialysis treatments potassium intake usually increases because of decreased anorexia. As this happens the serum potassium rises and the dialysate potassium concentration must be reduced. There occasionally are patients, however, who need treatments with these higher dialysate potassium concentrations for prolonged periods of time. These patients usually either have high urine outputs and/or are very anabolic, replacing muscle mass which was lost in the catabolic predialysis period.

Calcium

Because of the decreased calcium absorption seen in chronic renal failure (Chapter 1) it is desirable in most patients to have a net positive calcium influx during dialysis. A dialysate calcium concentration of 3.0 to 3.5 mEq/liter will generally accomplish this without causing excessive postdialysis hypercalcemia. Patients with severe hypocalcemia can be treated with dialysate containing 4 mEq/liter but they need careful, frequent monitoring of postdialysis serum calcium. Patients with persistent hyperphosphatemia should not be treated with high calcium dialysate because of the possibility of causing soft tissue and vascular calcification.

Hypercalcemia is not rare in chronic dialysis patients. Its etiology frequently is unclear but at least some of the time it appears to be related to an overshoot of secondary hyperparathyroidism. Hypercalcemia can be treated by decreasing the calcium concentration of the dialysate. In cases of severe hypercalcemia, calcium-free dialysate can be used to rapidly reduce serum calcium concentration. In milder hypercalcemia a dialysate calcium concentration of 2.5 mEq/liter will be sufficient to normalize calcium concentration.

Dialysate Base

Two different bases are currently used in dialysate for hemodialysis, acetate and bicarbonate. Acetate has the advantage of being compatible with the other dialysate constituents in highly concentrated solution and is the base used for most hemodialysis treatments. Bicarbonate has the advantage of being associated with increased cardiovascular stability and less adverse symptoms during dialysis but requires special dialysis machines which use two separate concentrates (see Chapter 5). Because of the additional expense and difficulty of using bicarbonate dialysate, acetate dialysate is used initially in most patients. Those patients who have excessive problems with hypotension or untoward symptoms during dialysis can be given a trial of bicarbonate dialysis to see if this will decrease these problems.

The concentration of acetate generally used in the dialysate varies from 35–40 mEq/liter and is usually not adjusted on an individual patient basis. Because of this the correction of acidosis varies considerably with predialysis serum bicarbonate typically ranging from 15–25 mEq/liter. Many patients have a persistent mild metabolic acidosis. Whether this acidosis has any significant harmful effects on patients is not known at present but it would appear wise to attempt to maintain as near normal acid–base balance as possible. Patients with persistently low serum bicarbonate can be treated several ways. First, the amount of acetate in the dialysate can be increased. This, however, may increase vascular instability in some patients. Second, the patients can receive oral base therapy with sodium bicarbonate or Scholls solution (see Chapter 2). Finally, the patient can be switched from acetate to bicarbonate dialysate and the concentration of bicarbonate in the dialysate increased if necessary without causing vascular instability. With the use of bicarbonate dialysate, however, excessive metabolic alkalosis must be watched for, especially immediately after dialysis and postdialysis serum bicarbonate should be monitored. With the switch from acetate to bicarbonate dialysate there may be a slow, gradual increase in serum bicarbonate concentration over many weeks, probably as the acid sink which accumulated during acetate dialysis is titrated. If the predialysis serum bicarbonate increases above 25 mEq/liter or the postdialysis serum bicarbonate above 30 mEq/liter the dialysate bicarbonate concentration should be reduced.

ANTICOAGULATION DURING HEMODIALYSIS

Hemodialysis treatments require the use of an anticoagulant to prevent clotting of the dialyzer and blood tubing. Heparin is usually used as the anticoagulant. This produces a risk of hemorrhage during or immediately after the dialysis treatments. In order to minimize this risk it is desirable that the heparin dosage be adjusted so that the anticoagulation is sufficient to prevent clotting of the dialyzers but is not excessive.

Heparin is a mucopolysaccharide prepared from various animal tissues, most commonly the lung. It renders the blood incoagulable by interfering with the formation of thromboplastin and inhibiting the action of thrombin. Heparin elimination is a first-order reaction with a relatively short half-life of approximately 1 hour in both normal and uremic subjects. In individual patients, the anticoagulation response to heparin is linearly related to the dose given. There is, unfortunately, marked variability among patients in both the sensitivity, or anticoagulation response to heparin, and in the rate of heparin elimination. The heparin dosage therefore has to be adjusted for each patient.

The anticoagulation response to heparin needs to be quantified in order to adjust the dosage. There are many different methods available for determining the anticoagulation effect of heparin. A simple method is the Lee White clotting time in which 1 ml blood is placed into a test tube, the tube inverted every 30 seconds until the blood clots, and the amount of time required for the blood to clot measured. Usually for hemodialysis, the normal clotting time of 10 minutes should be prolonged to 30 minutes. Although heparin dosage can be adjusted on the basis of Lee White clotting times, the test is time-consuming and the end point tends to be imprecise.

Another method of monitoring the anticoagulation is the activated partial thromboplastin time (APTT). This method has the advantage of reproducibility and a rapid end point (less than 5 minutes) but since it is done on plasma, specimens must be transported to the laboratory for centrifugation before performing the test. There is also considerable amount of scatter at higher heparin levels.

The activated whole blood coagulation time (ACT) appears to be the best test for monitoring heparin administration during hemodialysis. The ACT is performed by adding whole blood to a test tube containing a substance which activates the clotting system and measuring the time it takes for the blood to clot. The substance used to provoke clotting may either be a thromboplastin material prepared from animal tissue or siliceous earth. Evacuated test tubes containing this material are commercially available at a reasonable price. The test may be performed either at room temperature or for slightly more reproducible results, the tubes may be heated to 37°C. The normal ACT time is approximately 90 seconds at 37°C and 110 seconds at room temperature. The increase in the ACT time is linearly related to the plasma heparin concentration.

To properly adjust the heparin dosage, two variables must be determined (Fig. 6-3).[7] The first is *heparin sensitivity (S)*, which is the increase in ACT time produced by each unit of heparin. This determines the initial amount of heparin needed to produce the proper level of anticoagulation. The second variable is the *heparin elimination constant (E)*, which determines the rate at which heparin must be replaced in order to maintain the anticoagulation.

To determine these constants, first the base line ACT time (BL) is measured before the administration of heparin, then a bolus 1000 units of heparin is given and the ACT is repeated (R_1). The heparin sensitivity is equal to the difference in the ACT times (R_1-BL) divided by 1000. The heparin elimination rate is then determined by the repeat determination of ACT 1 hour after the heparin administration (R_2). The elimination constant is then equal to the original increase in ACT time (R_1-BL) divided by the final increase in ACT time (R_2-BL), all divided by the time (T) between the last two ACT determinations, in this case 1 hour.

After the sensitivity and elimination rates are determined, the amount of heparin needed at the beginning of dialysis (loading dose) and the amount that needs to be replaced can easily be determined. The loading dose is calculated by dividing the number of seconds of increase in ACT required by the heparin sensitive constant. The number of seconds increased in ACT time required is equal to the desired therapeutic ACT time minus the patient's base line ACT.

Heparin can be replaced during the dialysis procedure either as a constant infusion with the use of a heparin pump or by giving intermittent bolus of heparin. For patients who have an increased risk

$$S = \frac{R_1 - BL}{1000}$$

$$E = \frac{R_2 - BL}{R_1 - BL}$$

$$LD = \frac{ACT_T - BL}{S}$$

$$RD_1 = LD \times E$$

$$RD_2 = LD \times E + LD \times E^2$$

where

- BL = base line ACT time (seconds)
- R_1 = ACT time immediately after 1000 units of heparin (seconds)
- R_2 = ACT time 1 hour after 1000 units of heparin (seconds)
- ACT_T = desired therapeutic ACT time (seconds)
- S = heparin sensitivity constant (seconds/unit)
- E = elimination constant (%/hour)
- LD = loading dose (units)
- RD_1 = hourly replacement dose (units/hour)
- RD_2 = replacement dose if heparin is administered every 2 hours

Figure 6-3. Calculation of heparin doses.

for hemorrhage, the heparin replacement should be given either as small frequent boluses or with an infusion using an infusion pump. For routine dialysis, heparin can be given, however, as a single dose and a bolus for replacement halfway through the dialysis procedure. If a constant infusion is used, the hourly rate of infusion is calculated by multiplying the loading dose by the elimination constant. If the replacement heparin is going to be administered as a bolus 2 hours after starting dialysis, the dose is determined by multiplying the loading dose by the elimination constant for the first hour and the square of the elimination constant for the second hour.

We have two heparin regimens in our dialysis program. During routine dialysis the patients are given a loading dose and an additional replacement dose at 2 hours. The loading dose is adjusted so as to give an ACT time between 180 and 200 seconds 2 hours starting dialysis, and the second dose is adjusted so as to have the ACT time at the end of dialysis between 150 and 180 seconds.

In the immediate postoperative patient, pericarditis patient, patient with GI bleeding, and other patients predisposed to hemorrhage, we use a low-dose heparin regimen. In these patients an amount of initial heparin is given to prolong the ACT to between 150 and 180 seconds and sufficient replacement heparin is given hourly to keep the ACT in this range, either as hourly boluses or as a constant infusion.

Another heparin regimen used in some dialysis centers is that of regional heparinization. With this technique, no loading dose of heparin is given and heparin is infused into the dialyzer arterial line at a constant rate sufficient to anticoagulate the blood entering the dialyzer. The anticoagulant effect of heparin is then reversed after the blood leaves the dialyzer by a constant infusion of protamine sulfate into the venous line. This technique has the theoretical advantage of having the blood anticoagulated in the dialyzer and not anticoagulated in the patient. While this technique would appear to be ideal for the patient predisposed to hemorrhage, it has several serious drawbacks. Because of varying heparin potencies, each preparation of heparin must be titrated against protamine to determine the relative rates of infusion. Even with this titration it is frequently difficult to adjust the infusion rates so that the kidney remains adequately anticoagulated without any anticoagulation effect in the patient. The total amount of heparin administered during the dialysis procedure is also greater using regional heparinization than during a routine hemodialysis treatment. An additional problem is that protamine is usually metabolized faster than heparin. The higher rate of metabolism of protamine leaves unreversed heparin which causes a rebound anticoagulation in the patient several hours after the termination of dialysis. For this reason, if regional heparinization is used, it is necessary to check the patient's ACT time 3 to 4 hours after the end of dialysis and administer additional protamine sulfate if it is prolonged. Because of these problems many dialysis programs have abandoned the use of regional heparinization in favor of the use of a low-dose heparin regime.

DETERMINING THE TARGET WEIGHT

The majority of patients gain body fluid between each treatment and this fluid needs to be removed. One of the most difficult aspects of the dialysis prescription is the determination of the amount of fluid which needs to be removed during the dialysis procedure.

The best estimate of the fluid balance is the physical examination of the patient. Excessive fluid is manifested by peripheral edema, inspiratory rales in the lung bases, and/or hypertension. The earliest signs of fluid depletion are an increase in pulse rate and decrease in blood pressure when changing from the supine or sitting position to the upright position. Fluid balance, unfortunately, usually must deviate by greater than 5 percent from normal before it can be reliably detected by these parameters and none of these signs are specific for fluid imbalance. It is desirable to control the patients total body fluid with a greater sensitivity than 5 percent as it is very probable that fluid depletion less than that which causes postural changes in the pulse or blood pressure can cause unpleasant symptoms in patients and the long-term consequences of mild chronic fluid overload are unknown.

Fluid balance during dialysis is managed by the development of a target weight for the end of the procedure. The target weight is an estimation of the weight at which the patient is in ideal fluid balance. Fluid is then removed during the dialysis procedure at a rate so that the patient is at his target weight at the end of the treatment. Changes in dry body weight (total body weight − total body water) cause changes in the target weight, so that it needs to be reevaluated frequently.

In order to determine a target weight at the initiation of dialysis treatments a complete physical examination and chest x-ray should be performed. If the patient has no peripheral edema, is normotensive, and the chest x-ray does not indicate cardiomegaly or pulmonary vascular congestion then the present weight of the patient is an appropriate target weight. Most often, however, at the start of dialysis treatment the patient has either peripheral edema, pulmonary vascular congestion, and/or is hypertensive. In this case then it is likely that the patient needs to have fluid removed during the dialysis procedure and his target weight is below his current weight. If the patient is not dyspneic and the blood pressure is not severely elevated, it is best that the excessive body fluids be removed during several of the dialysis treatments rather than attempting to remove all the excess body fluid during the first dialysis treatment. The patient's target weight should be reduced by 0.5−1 kg during each dialysis treatment until the excess fluid is eliminated.

Control of Hypertension

Fluid overload is the most common cause of hypertension in the chronic dialysis patient. About 80 percent of dialysis patients will have their blood pressure controlled without the use of antihypertensive medication by controlling their total body fluids. The remaining 20 percent of patients will need some type of hypertensive medication in addition to fluid control by dialysis. It is frequently difficult to determine whether or not the blood pressure can be controlled by fluid removal alone. It is unfortunately necessary to remove excessive fluid before it can be ascertained that the blood pressure cannot be controlled by fluid removal alone.

One method of determining whether the blood pressure can be controlled without medications is to reduce the target weight by 0.5–1 kg during each successive dialysis treatment until the patient is either normotensive or is having severe hypotension during the dialysis procedure, indicating excessive fluid removal. If the patient is hypertensive before the dialysis procedure but the blood pressure markedly decreases during dialysis when fluid removal is attempted, then it is likely that antihypertensive medication will be required to control the blood pressure. There are two exceptions, however, to this premise. The first is the patient who has gained excessive amounts between dialysis treatments. If the fluid gained between treatments is greater than 4 percent of the total body weight then the hypotension during the dialysis may be related to the necessary rapid rate of fluid removal rather than to the fact that the patient is actually being taken below the actual dry body weight. The second exception occurs in patients who are taking antihypertensive medicines. Even moderate rates of fluid removal during dialysis decreases cardiac output which requires an increase in peripheral vascular resistance to maintain blood pressure. Interference with this increase in vascular resistance by antihypertensive medications may cause hypotension during the dialysis procedure in the absence of actual fluid depletion.

The administration of antihypertensive medications is discussed in Chapter 2.

SYMPTOMS DURING DIALYSIS

Patients unfortunately experience unpleasant symptoms during many of the hemodialysis treatments. Between 15 and 45 percent of treatments are associated with untoward symptoms such as hypotension, malaise, dizziness, muscle cramps, nausea, vomiting, or headaches. The etiology of these symptoms is largely unknown, but they occur much more commonly at high rates of ultrafiltration. Although at present these symptoms cannot be completely prevented, the incidence and severity can be reduced by the proper management of the dialysis prescription.

Hypotension

During the vast majority of dialysis treatments there is a significant fall in both systolic and diastolic blood pressures. Approximately 25 percent of dialysis treatments are associated with symptomatic hypotension. The cause of the decreased blood pressure during dialysis is multifactorial. Depletion of the vascular volume plays a major role. In the beginning of dialysis there is an immediate phlebotomy of between 100 and 300 ml into the extracorporeal blood circuit. During the usual hemodialysis treatment between 1000 and 4000 ml of fluid which has accumulated between dialysis treatments must be removed. This fluid is removed initially from the plasma volume and is then replaced by the movement of fluid from the interstitial space into the plasma volume. There is a limit in the rate at which fluid can move from the interstitial space into the vascular system and plasma volume may be as much as 25–30 percent below normal during dialysis. In addition, if the dialysate sodium concentration is less than plasma, there is a shift of fluid from the extravascular space into the intracellular compartment (see Chapter 5) which can further decrease plasma volume. The decrease in plasma volume reduces blood return to the heart with a resultant reduction in cardiac output. Normally blood pressure is maintained in face of a decrease in cardiac output by an increase in peripheral vascular resistance. By some as yet unknown mechanism, there is a relative inability to increase peripheral vascular resistance during hemodialysis treatments. Several studies have compared the hemodynamic effects of fluid removal during hemodialysis to fluid removal either during isolated ultrafiltration or hemofiltration. These studies indicate that, while reductions in plasma volume and cardiac output are similar, there is a greater fall in blood pressure during hemodialysis compared to either ultrafiltration or hemofiltration, indicating a significant difference in peripheral vascular resistance. The elegant studies of Shaldon and co-workers indicate that the difference in peripheral resistance does not appear to be secondary to changes in osmolality, efficiency of solute removal, or acetate.[8-10]

Acetate plays a significant role in the generation of hypotension during hemodialysis (Chapter 5). Several studies have indicated a significantly greater reduction in blood pressure during hemodialysis with an acetate dialysate compared to bicarbonate dialysate. This appears to be especially true in patients who have a high frequency of hypotension during dialysis and patients undergoing high efficiency, short duration treatments.

There are several ways to minimize hypotension during hemodialysis. Probably the most important is to keep the interdialysis weight gain low. If the weight gain is below 3 percent of the body weight, then the incidence of hypotension is relatively low while the majority of patients will become hypotensive when fluid volumes greater than 5 percent of body weight are removed during a 4-hour hemodialysis treatment. The most important factor in reducing intradialysis weight gain is limitation of sodium intake (see Chapter 15). Many patients are unfortunately unable to limit their weight gain to this degree.

Dialysate sodium concentration also has a definite effect on blood pressure changes during dialysis. Having the dialysate sodium concentration equal to or greater than serum sodium concentration prevents the shift of water from the extracellular compartment to the intracellular compartment and helps maintain intravascular volume. Many patients who have frequent symptomatic hypotension with low or moderate ultrafiltration rates will also benefit from using a bicarbonate-based dialysate.

There are several methods for treating hypotension during dialysis once it develops. Usually the rapid administration of 100 to 200 ml of normal saline and reducing the rate of fluid removal by decreasing the transmembrane pressure will increase the blood pressure. This of course has the problem of decreasing the rate fluid removal. The intravenous administration of mannitol may also help. Mannitol, an extracellular solute (similar to sodium), probably increases blood pressure by causing a shift of fluid from the intracellular compartment to the extracellular compartment. Mannitol is normally metabolized by excretion through the kidneys and patients with chronic renal insufficiency will unfortunately accumulate mannitol to high concentrations if it is administered during each dialysis. Mannitol should therefore not be given during more than one treatment each week. The mannitol administered during one treatment is removed during the following treatment and this removal probably causes a shift of fluid from the extracellular back into the intracellular space and may increase the incidence of symptomatic hypotension during these treatments. The administration of 10–20 ml of 3 percent of NaCl has an effect similar to that of mannitol. It is likely that both mannitol and hypertonic saline cause an increase in thirst and result in increased weight gain.

The administration of 12.5–25 g of human serum albumin draws fluid from the interstitial space into the plasma space and is usually very effective in treating hypotension. It is unfortunately also very expensive.

Some chronic hemodialysis patients have an automatic insufficiency which causes the hypotension.[11] Vasopressors such as norepinephrine, dopamine, ephedrine, or phenylephrine may be effective in increasing blood pressure in these patients. Many of these patients, however, are asymptomatic in spite of severely low blood pressures and do not necessarily need treatment.

Muscle Cramps

Muscle cramps, caused by the involuntary contraction of skeletal muscles, are frequent during hemodialysis treatments. They most commonly involve the calf, abdominal, or back muscles and occur in between 10 and 50 percent of treatments. They are also not rare during the interdialysis period, usually occurring at night. The etiology of muscle cramps is not entirely clear. Intravascular and extracellular volume depletion appears to play a major role and muscle cramps are much more common at high ultrafiltration rates and toward the end of the dialysis treatment when the patient is close to his target weight. Intracellular overhydration from the use of hyponatremic dialysate may also contribute. In isolated muscle preparation, hypotonicity enhances and hypertonicity suppresses the tension and muscle activity of skeletal muscle.[12] This is felt to be due to a direct influence of tonicity on the contractile elements themselves, since little change in membrane excitability can be demonstrated. The incidence of muscle cramps during dialysis can be reduced by increasing the dialysate sodium concentration. Stewart and co-workers demonstrated that the incidence of muscle cramps was reduced from 49-23 percent of treatments by increasing the dialysate sodium concentration from 132-145 mEq/l.[13] A similar but less dramatic effect occurs if sodium is given orally during the treatment.

The prophylactic administration of quinine sulfate during dialysis will also reduce the incidence of muscle cramps. Panadero and co-workers demonstrated in a double-blind study that the administration of 300 mg of quinine sulfate at the beginning of dialysis significantly reduced the incidence of muscle cramps without any secondary problems.[14] Quinine at bedtime is also effective in preventing nocturnal cramps.

Once cramps occur during dialysis there are several effective methods of treating them. The most common method is to clamp the arterial line and administer between 100 and 500 ml of saline. This is usually effective in stopping the cramp within 5-10 minutes. The cramps can also be relieved by the rapid administration of 40-50 mEq of sodium chloride in the form of hypertonic saline or the administration of 12.5–25 g of mannitol. Both of these are usually effective in stopping the cramp within 1 minute of administration. Milutinovich and co-workers have demonstrated that reducing the rate of ultrafiltration and the administration 50 ml of 50 percent glucose over a 5-minute period of time will relieve cramps in the majority of cases.[15] This has the advantage that it avoids loading the patient with sodium or mannitol. Glucose probably should not be used in diabetic patients but in the nondiabetic it causes only a mild transient hyperglycemia with blood glucoses not exceeding 450 mg/dl.

STARTING PATIENTS ON CHRONIC HEMODIALYSIS TREATMENTS

It is important when starting hemodialysis treatments in a patient with chronic renal insufficiency that the first treatments be managed so as to minimize untoward effects during the treatments. Rosa and co-workers have shown that it takes up to 6 weeks for the patient to optimally adapt to the hemodialysis treatments.[16] For reasons that are not entirely clear, patients have many more symptoms during the initial hemodialysis treatments than they do later on during the course of their treatment. This is especially true if the BUN is excessively high (greater than 120 mg/dl) but also occurs at lower BUN concentrations. These untoward effects can be decreased but not completely prevented by careful management of the initial dialysis prescription.

If the patient is very uremic at the beginning of dialysis treatments with excessively high blood urea nitrogen levels, the BUN should be reduced slowly with several daily short hemodialysis treatments. It is also helpful to use a small-sized dialyzer and to keep the blood flow rate low (100–150 ml/min). Unless the patient is severely symptomatic from fluid overload, fluid removal during these initial treatments should be kept to a minimum. It is usually possible to decrease the blood urea level down to reasonable values in two to four short, daily dialyses without precipitating severe symptomotology during these treatments.

Most patients who have been under good medical management prior to starting dialysis will have a blood urea nitrogen concentration below 100 mg/dl at the initiation of dialysis. While these patients do not need daily dialysis at the beginning of their therapy, it is still helpful to use small-sized dialyzers with reduced blood flows during their initial treatments. We generally start with a 2-hour treatment for the first treatment, increase to 3 hours for the second treatment, and then use the normal 4-hour duration for subsequent treatments. Blood flow during the initial week of dialysis is kept below 150 ml/min and a small dialyzer is used for the first few weeks of treatment.

REFERENCES

1. Babb AL, Popovich RP, Christopher TG, Schribner BH: The genesis of the square meter-hour hypothesis. Trans Am Soc Artif Int Organs 17:81–91, 1971
2. Milutinovich J, Strand M, Casaretto A, et al: Clinical impact of residual glomerulofiltration rate on dialysis time. Trans Am Soc Artif Int Organs 20:410–416, 1974
3. Gotch FA, Sargent JA, Keen M, et al: Clinical results of intermittant dialysis therapy guided by ongoing kinetic analysis of urea metabolism. Trans Am Soc Artif Int Organs 22:175–189, 1976
4. Lowrie EG, Laird NM, Parker TF, Sargent JA: Effect of the hemodialysis prescription on patient morbidity. N Eng J Med 305:1176–1181, 1981
5. Lowrie EG, Steinberg SM, Galen MA, et al: Factors in the dialysis regimen which contribute to alterations in the abnormalities of uremia. Kidney Int 10:404–422, 1976
6. Sargent J, Gotch F, Borah M, et al: Urea kinetics: A guide in nutritional management of renal failure. Am J Clin Nutr 31:1696–1702, 1978
7. Farrell PC, Ward RA, Schindhelm K, Gotch FA: Precise anticoagulation for routine hemodialysis. J Lab Clin Med 92:164–176, 1978
8. Shaldon S, Deschodt G, Beau MC, et al: Vascular resistance and stability during high flux haemofiltration compared to haemodialysis. Abst Am Soc Nephrol 12:129A, 1979
9. Shaldon S, Beau MC, Deschodt G, Ramperey P, Mion C: Vascular stability during hemofiltration. Trans Am Soc Artif Organs 26:391–393, 1980
10. Baldamus CA, Ernst W, Lysoyht M, Shaldon S, Koch: Is hemodynamic stability during hemofiltration a sodium balance related phenomenon. Proc Clin Dial Transplant Forum (in press)
11. Kersh ES, Kronfield SJ, Unger A, et al: Autonomic insufficiency in uremia as a cause of hemodialysis induced hypotension. N Eng J Med 290:650–653, 1974
12. Gordon AM, Godt RE: Some effects of hypertonic solutions on contraction and excitation–contraction coupling in frog skeletal muscles. J Gen Physiol 55:254–275, 1970
13. Stewardt WK, Fleming LW, Manael MA: Muscle cramps during maintenance haemodialysis. Lancet 1:1049–1050, 1972

14. Panadero SJ, Perez CA: Action of quinine sulphate on the incidence of muscle cramps during hemodialysis. Med Clin (Barc) 75:247–249, 1980
15. Milutinovich J, Graefe V, Follette WC, Scribner BH: Effect of hypertonic glucose on the muscle cramps of hemodialysis. Ann Intern Med 90:926–928, 1979
16. Rosa AA, Fryd DS, Kjellstrand CM: Dialysis symptoms and stabilization on chronic hemodialysis. Arch Intern Med 140:804–807, 1980

W. Kirt Nichols

7
Vascular Access

Vascular access is a very important aspect of chronic hemodialysis. Chronic hemodialysis treatments require the easy availability of 200–300 ml/min of blood flow and nowhere in the normal body can this amount of blood flow be repeatedly obtained over long periods of time. In the 30 years that hemodialysis has been performed there have been many methods developed to facilitate blood access. None of the methods, however, are yet ideal and many problems remain. Difficulties with vascular access account for more days in the hospital than any other single problem in chronic hemodialysis patients. A study by Mandel et al. revealed that patients require an average of 19 days each year in the hospital as a direct result of problems arising from vascular access.[1]

Vascular access was initially obtained for hemodialysis by cutting down on major arteries and placing stiff cannulas into them which were removed at the end of each treatment. Each vessel could only be used for a very limited number of times, thus restricting the total number of dialysis treatments which could be performed. This prevented patients from being kept alive long periods of time using chronic hemodialysis. The development of an external arteriovenous shunt, using Silastic® tubing and a Teflon® tip, by Quinton, Dillard, and Scribner in 1960 opened the way for the development of chronic hemodialysis.[2] With this technique cannulas were placed in adjacent arteries and veins for blood access. Between uses, the two Silastic® tubes were connected by a short Teflon® connector. Blood continuously flowed through the shunt to prevent clotting. Although this was a major advance over previous approaches, in the best of hands, problems with clotting and infection restricted the average life span of these arteriovenous shunts from 6-9 months.

In 1966 Brescia and Cimino described the creation of an internal arteriovenous fistula for hemodialysis access.[3] With this technique an arteriovenous fistula is surgically constructed by the direct connection of an adjacent artery and vein. The increased blood flow and pressure in the vein results in a gradual increase in caliber of the lumen and a thickening or arterialization of the vein wall.

Although the internal arteriovenous fistula remains the best available access for chronic hemodialysis, in many patients there is insufficient development of the venous system. In these patients an internal arteriovenous shunt can be created by implanting a conduit made either from a autogenous saphenous vein, bovine carotid artery, or a synthetic material such as expanded polytetrafluoroethylene (Gore-Tex,® Impra®). These grafts are tunneled subcutaneously beneath the skin and connected between an artery and a vein. They provide blood access by easy transcutaneous puncture.

TYPES OF CHRONIC HEMODIALYSIS ACCESS

External Silastic®-Teflon® Shunt

A typical external shunt is shown in Figure 7-1. It consists of two small Teflon® or Silastic® tips connected to segments of Silastic® tubing which are surgically implanted into an adjacent vein and artery. The Silastic® tubing from the venous and arterial limbs are brought separately through the skin and are directly connected to the hemodialysis tubing during the treatments. Between treatments the venous and arterial limbs are connected to each other by a short piece

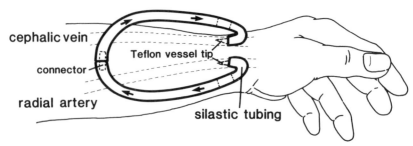

Figure 7-1. A forearm Quinton-Scribner Silastic® shunt from radial artery to cephalic vein.

of Teflon® tubing. The continuous flow of blood through this artificial fistula prevents clotting.

These shunts can be placed at many locations in the body. A convenient place is the ankle between the posterial tibial artery and the greater saphenous vein. Placement here avoids the use of the upper extremity vessels so that these can be saved for a more permanent type of access if necessary. If unable to use the ankle, the Silastic® shunt can be placed in the groin between the greater saphenous vein and the superficial femoral or profunda femoris arteries. In the upper extremities, a shunt can be placed at the wrist between either the radial or the ulnar artery and an appropriate adjacent vein or inserted in the upper arm between the brachial artery and the cephalic vein.

Since distal flow in the artery used for the arteriovenous shunt is stopped, it is important that the tissue supplied by that artery has adequate collateral flow. Unless good radial and ulnar pulses are thus both present at the wrist, the wrist should not be used for an arteriovenous shunt. It is helpful to perform an Allen test preoperatively to check for the patency of the radial and ulnar arteries before creating an arteriovenous fistula or placing an external shunt.

Because of the short life span of the shunts and other complications seen with external arteriovenous shunts, they are seldom used today for chronic hemodialysis. Their primary role at present is for temporary blood access in acute renal failure or for chronic renal failure while a more permanent type of access is maturing. Many dialysis programs now rarely use the Silastic® shunt even for temporary access and use instead subclavian, femoral or jugular vein catherization. (See below.)

Appropriate surgical technique is an important determinant in the longevity of arteriovenous shunts. Although it is beyond the scope of this book to completely describe the surgical technique of arteriovenous shunt implantation, a few salient points should be mentioned. Meticulous attention to detail when placing an arteriovenous shunt will be rewarded by an increased survival time of the shunt. It is important that the endothelial lining of the vessels be traumatized as little as possible during the insertion of the cannula. It is also important that the size of the cannula tip be appropriate for the vessel size; if the tip is either too small or too large for the vessel problems may arise. Particular care must be taken to avoid bending or kinking of the vessel as turbulence at these bends promote the development of thrombosis.

There are several modifications of the basic Scribner shunt available. The Ramirez shunt (Fig. 7-2) has wing tips attached to each limb which help anchor the tubing and prevent torsion on the vessels.

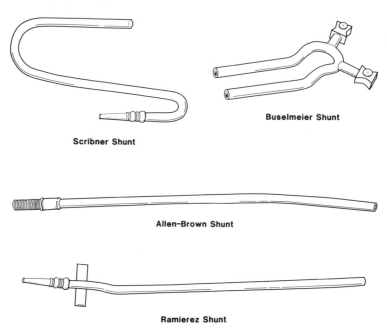

Figure 7-2. Four types of external arteriovenous shunts.

The removal of these shunts is somewhat more difficult. Another shunt in use is the Buselmeier shunt (Fig. 7-2). This shunt consists of a U-shaped continuous Silastic® tubing which is connected to two Teflon® tips. The Silastic® tubing has two side ports on it for the direct connection to the hemodialysis tubing. The entire Buselmeier shunt is placed subcutaneously with only the two side ports exiting from the skin. During the hemodialysis treatments the plugs are removed from the side ports and the hemodialysis tubing directly connected to the ports. The Buselmeier shunt has the theoretical advantage that less pull and torsion is transmitted through the tubing to the vessels.[4] Although increased survival time for this shunt has been claimed, there have been no well-controlled studies and it has not gained wide acceptance.

The Thomas shunt and the Allen–Brown shunt (Fig. 7-2) are usually only used as an access of last resort.[5] It is seldom necessary to use one of these shunts. These two shunts are quite similar and consist of Silastic® tubing attached to a knitted Dacron® prosthesis. The prosthesis is directly sutured end to side to a major vessel, such as the femoral or brachial artery. These shunts provide excellent blood flow, but have the problem that if they become infected, which is not uncommon, suture line hemorrhage may result requiring vessel ligation and the potential loss of an extremity.

The major problem with any external shunt is thrombosis. If the clot is noticed soon after it occurs, the shunt usually can be reopened and may remain patent for long periods of time. It is important that part of the external portion of the shunt be left uncovered so that it can be observed continuously. When a shunt clots, the blood in the tubing rapidly separates into a cellular clot and a plasma component. Patients need to be instructed to watch for this and to seek medical attention immediately if it occurs.

Declotting of a shunt must, of course, be performed under strict aseptic techniques. Occasionally it is possible to open a clotted shunt by syringe aspiration of the venous and arterial limbs. If this is not successful then a small polyethylene tube can be passed through the shunt up into the vessels and normal saline injected in an attempt to loosen and wash out the clot. If the shunt still remains clotted the small polyethylene tube can be removed and small amounts of saline forcibly injected into each limb of the shunt. It is important that no more than 2–4 ml of fluid be injected into the arterial limb of an arm shunt to prevent the possibility of the retrograde movement of the clot back up the artery into the cerebral circulation.[6] This rapid injection will frequently loosen the clot and in the arterial limb it can usually then be withdrawn into the injecting syringe. In the venous limb the clot generally continues up the vein causing a small and harmless pulmonary embolus.

If none of the above procedures are finally successful in declotting the shunt, then removal of the clot with a Fogarty catheter can be attempted. The Fogarty catheter is a long catheter with a small balloon on the tip (Fig. 7-3). To remove a clot, it is inserted 10–30 cm into the vessel, the balloon is inflated with 0.2–0.4 ml of saline and the catheter slowly withdrawn. This will frequently loosen and remove the clot.

After a shunt is successfully declotted it is helpful to temporarily place the patient on heparin to prevent reclotting. A small Teflon® "T" tube can be inserted between the arterial and venous limbs in place of the usual straight Teflon® shunt connector. This provides an injection port through which the heparin can be administered, either by continuous infusion or intermittent injection. If necessary patients can inject heparin through this port on an outpatient basis.

Removal of an arteriovenous shunt after it is no longer needed is usually a simple procedure. The shunt should be clotted for at least 24 and preferably 48 hours before its removal. This is accomplished by

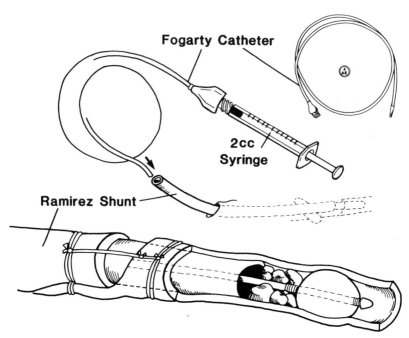

Figure 7-3. Clot removal from a Ramirez shunt with a Fogarty catheter.

simply placing an occluding clamp on the Silastic® tubing. The shunt then can be removed by gentle traction on each of the shunt limbs; usually the shunt will come out with minimal bleeding. It may occasionally be necessary to make a small incision over the shunt insertion site to remove the retaining ligatures: however, this is seldom necessary. Small skin incisions are needed to remove the wing tips of the Ramirez shunt. The Thomas and Allen–Brown shunts need to be removed in an operating room, preferably by a vascular surgeon, so that the artery can be repaired.

It is possible to convert an external arteriovenous shunt into an internal arteriovenous fistula at the time of shunt removal.[7] This is done by surgically removing the Silastic® shunt from the artery and anastomosing the artery to a nearby vein. If the hemodialysis treatments need to be continued urgently, some other type of temporary access must be provided since the new arteriovenous fistula cannot be used until the veins dilate and thicken. If the vessels of an arteriovenous shunt are to be converted to an arteriovenous fistula, it is important that it be done at the time of the shunt removal. If the shunt is clotted prior to its removal, the vessels can never be used for the production of an internal arteriovenous fistula.

Internal Arterial Venous Fistula

An internal arteriovenous fistula is without question the best available vascular access for chronic hemodialysis. If properly constructed and cared for, it can provide good blood flow indefinitely in many patients. Unfortunately there are many patients with chronic end-stage renal disease in whom the venous system of both upper extremities will not develop sufficient dilatation to be used for blood access. This is frequently the result of damage to the superficial veins of the upper extremities by repeated use for intravenous infusion or repetitive venipuncture for laboratory studies. It is helpful to identify potential chronic hemodialysis patients early in the course of their illness and attempt to preserve the superficial venous system of one upper extremity. It is generally advisable to use the nondominant upper extremity for the fistula so that the dominant arm can be free during the hemodialysis treatments.

The most frequent site for placement of an arteriovenous fistula is in the radial artery at the wrist. The ulnar artery at the wrist can also be used, however, if the veins in this area appear better, or an upper arm fistula can be created using the brachial artery. Arteriovenous fistulas are not generally placed in the leg because of the possibility of producing severe varicose veins. Prior to choosing the site for an arteriovenous fistula, it is helpful to place a tourniquet on both upper extremities and observe the superficial venous pattern and select a suitable vein in close proximity to an arterial trunk.

The success of the arteriovenous fistula is dependent on the skill and patience of the surgeon. The arteriovenous fistula is created by making a 5- to 8-mm connection between the artery and vein. A running nonabsorbable suture should be used for the anastomosis to prevent future enlargement of the fistula opening. The anastomosis can be made as either a side to side, end to side (artery to vein), side to end (artery to vein), or end to end. (Fig. 7-4). Although there is no common agreement it is theoretically better to use the end of the artery rather than the side. If the side of the artery is used rather than the end, patients may develop a steal syndrome. Blood from the ulnar artery may be shunted through the palmer arch to the fistula and ischemic symptoms may develop in the hand. If this occurs it can be corrected by ligation of the radial artery distal to the fistula. This additional

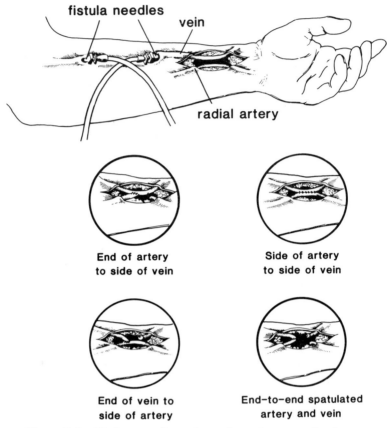

Figure 7-4. Various configurations of arteriovenous fistulae.

surgical procedure is not needed if the end of the artery is used initially. If, for technical reasons, the surgeon is more comfortable making a side to side anastomosis (which is technically easier and has higher flow rates) this can be done and a functional end to side fistula created by ligating the distal radial artery at the time of the original operation.

Surgeons do not agree about whether or not it is best to use the end or the side of the vein in an arteriovenous fistula. With an anastomosis in the side of a vein, retrograde flow of blood into the hand with enlargement of the veins of the hand is common. The veins in the hand are seldom usable for vascular access because they are tortuous and it is difficult to immobilize the hand for the 4-hour dialysis procedure.

The blood that runs through these hand veins frequently returns through the deep venous system of the forearm, thus making it unavailable in the forearm for vascular access. For the above reasons it is usually desirable to prevent the retrograde blood flow through the venous system either by ligating the vein distal to the anastomosis if the side of the vein is used or by using the end of the vein for the anastomosis. The venous anastomosis, however, must be individualized on the basis of the venous pattern in the patient's arm. My preference at present is an end vein to side artery fistula. "Steal" symptoms have been infrequent.

Although it is sometimes possible to use an internal arterial venous fistula immediately after its production, it is generally not best to do so. After creation of an arteriovenous fistula there are gradual changes in the vein wall occurring over several weeks. The increased pressure and flow caused by the shunting of arterial blood causes a gradual thickening or arterialization of the venous walls. This wall thickening aids in the sealing of the puncture wound after the dialysis needle is withdrawn. If the access is used before adequate time has been allowed for the wall to thicken, the increased pressure and flow in the vein may permit a leak and result in a large hematoma. Compression produced by the hematoma may block blood flow through the fistula and result in loss of a previously good arteriovenous fistula. It is therefore wise to allow an arteriovenous fistula to develop for a minimum of 4-6 weeks prior to use as a hemodialysis access site even if it appears to be adequate for use prior to this time. It is also important not to use an arteriovenous fistula for routine phlebotomy or intravenous fluid administration. Blood pressures should not be taken in the extremity with the arteriovenous fistula unless absolutely necessary.

Internal Arteriovenous Shunts

If the venous system of the arm does not develop to sufficient caliber or have sufficient flow for use as a hemodialysis access, then a conduit can be placed subcutaneously between an artery and a vein for use as a vascular access. Many different types of material can be used for subcutaneous arteriovenous shunts. The most commonly used at present are autogenous saphenous veins, bovine carotid arteries, tanned, reinforced human umbilical arteries, and expanded polytetrafluoroethylene (PTFE) (Gore-Tex,® Impra®) grafts.

There are numerous locations in the body where these internal arteriovenous shunts can be placed. One of the best locations is in the forearm with a straight graft between the radial artery and an antecubital vein. If the wrist arteries are unsuitable for access, the forearm still can be used by anastomosing the graft to either the proximal radial or ulnar artery or directly to the brachial artery. The straight graft then can be anastomosed to a vein at the wrist or if there are no usable veins at the wrist, then the graft can be looped through the forearm and anastomosed to a vein in the antecubital fossa or above (Fig. 7-5). The anterior upper thigh is also a good place for an internal arteriovenous shunt. If the saphaneous vein is used, it can be ligated and transected immediately above the knee, dissected free and tunneled subcutaneously in a loop with the distal end anastomosed to the profunda femoris or the superficial femoral artery in the groin. Other variations of internal arteriovenous shunts can also be used in the thigh, either as a straight graft going from one of the arteries in the groin down to the saphenous vein above the knee or as a loop graft going from either the superficial or profunda femoris artery in the groin to the saphenous

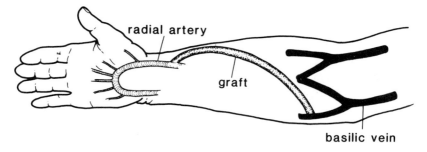

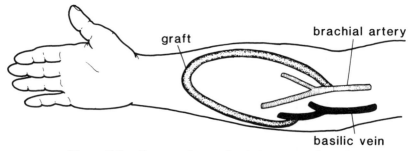

Figure 7-5. Forearm internal arteriovenous shunts.

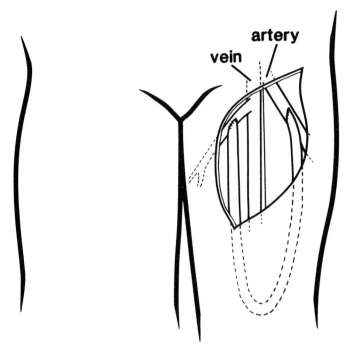

Figure 7-6. Thigh loop internal arteriovenous shunt.

vein at the fossa ovalis (Fig. 7-6). There are many other alternate locations for internal arteriovenous shunts, such as the axillary–axillary shunt in which the graft is anastomosed to the axillary artery on one side and the axillary vein on the other side and tunneled subcutaneously across the anterior chest.

There is no universal agreement as to what material makes the best internal arteriovenous shunt. Each of the various materials have their proponents. Although there are numerous studies in the literature detailing experiences using the various types of grafts, these are invariably retrospective reports describing an individual experience and prospective controlled studies comparing the various materials are not available.[8-10] The three most commonly used materials are autogenous saphenous vein grafts, bovine carotid artery grafts, and the expanded PTFE grafts. Most surgeons now feel that the saphenous vein graft does not appear to offer any advantage over the bovine xenograft or PTFE and since it requires a more extended surgical procedure, saphaneous veins are not used as frequently as in the past.

Bovine carotid arteries are removed from calves or adult cattle at the time of slaughter and digested with ficin which removes the elastin and muscular material and leaves behind a collagenous tube. Subsequent tanning is accomplished by immersing the tube in 1.3 percent dialdehyde solution thereby providing a nonanergic graft.

PTFE is a man-made material which is very nonreactive in the human body. It provides an internal arteriovenous shunt comparable to bovine xenograft and because PTFE comes in many different sizes, is readily available, and costs less, it appears to be the material of choice at this time. There is a suggestion that prolonged bleeding from puncture sites may be a greater problem with PTFE, whereas aneurysm formation and hemorrhage, if infection occurs, appear to be a more frequent complication with bovine xenografts.

Internal shunts can also be placed as an arterial to arterial graft rather than as an arterial to venous bridge graft. This may be helpful in patients with severe vascular disease in whom shunting of blood from the arterial system may result in ischemic symptoms. It also is occasionally necessary to use an arterial-to-arterial shunt because of the lack of a suitable vein for an anastomosis. These patients, however, are exceedingly rare. A major problem with the arterial-to-arterial shunt is the possibility of distal arterial emboli arising from a thrombus in the graft.

Although it is possible to use any of these subcutaneous arteriovenous shunts immediately after surgery for vascular access, it is best not to do so. With time a pseudointima forms in the foreign conduit by the migration of cells from the host vessels. It takes approximately 2 weeks for the internal surface of the conduit to develop an pseudointimal lining and for some tissue ingrowth into the graft to occur. This lining helps to seal the puncture site after the withdrawal of the dialysis needle. If the conduit is used before adequate time has been allowed for the pseudointimal lining to form there is an increased risk of hematoma formation at the puncture site with the possibility of compression and occlusion of the internal arteriovenous shunt. Infection may also develop in the hematoma. An internal arteriovenous shunt should therefore not be used for the first 2 weeks after its placement unless absolutely necessary.

IMMEDIATE BLOOD ACCESS FOR HEMODIALYSIS

If blood access is needed for hemodialysis immediately and the patient does not have a mature access, a fresh internal arteriovenous fistula or shunt should not be used. Although an external Silastic® shunt can be inserted for temporary access, it has several drawbacks. First, it should be inserted in an operating room by an experienced surgeon, which requires the scheduling of the room and surgeon. Second, it usually results in the eventual loss of a peripheral artery which may be needed for more permanent hemodialysis access at a later time. Third, it is not always possible in patients whose access sites have already been lost by previous operations, venopuncture, or arterial puncture. For these reasons external arteriovenous shunts are very seldom used for hemodialysis access in our program. We prefer instead to use cannulation of the large central veins via the femoral, subclavian, or external jugular veins for immediate, temporary hemodialysis access.

Femoral Vein Cannulation

Cannulation of the femoral vein for hemodialysis access is usually an easy, quick, and safe procedure. In our program, at the University of Missouri, this procedure is done by physicians or specially trained registered nurses. Femoral vein cannulation has one major disadvantage in that the cannula cannot be left in place between dialysis treatments without immobilization of the patient. Although hematoma formation around the femoral vein may make repeated use of the vein difficult or impossible, in most instances the femoral vein can be used many times for hemodialysis access. We have had patients who have had hemodialysis performed by repeated femoral vein cannulation 3 times each week for over 6 weeks without difficulty.

Cannulation of the femoral vein for hemodialysis by the Seldinger technique was first introduced by Shaldon in 1961.[11] The groin area is shaved, prepped with an antiseptic solution, and a sterile field is then produced by the appropriate placement of sterile drapes. Sterile gloves are worn; the femoral vein is located by palpating of the femoral artery and a 16-gauge angiocath is inserted medial to the medial edge of the artery with the tip of the angiocath needle pointed slightly cephalad. The angiocath is attached to a syringe and slight negative pressure is kept on the syringe during the insertion so that as soon as the femoral vein is entered, blood will "flash" into the syringe. It is a common technique when using the femoral vein as a source for a blood specimen to place the needle completely through the vein and locate the vein by the slow withdrawal of the needle. This is not desirable during placement of a catheter for hemodialysis access because of the production of an extra puncture wound in the back of the vein. As soon as the angiocath enters the vein, the metal needle is withdrawn slightly from the catheter which is then further advanced into the vein. The needle is then completely removed from the angiocath and a 0.89mm guidewire introduced through the angiocath into the vein. The guidewire is advanced into the femoral vein and the angiocath is removed. The dialysis catheter is then inserted over the guidewire into the femoral vein and the guidewire removed. If the femoral vein is to be used with a single-needle device then a catheter with an appropriate "Y" piece such as that made by Sorenson Research Company must be used. Unless the patient is to be kept at bed rest, the catheter is removed at the end of the procedure and pressure is applied over the venous puncture wound. It is important that pressure be held over the femoral vein for a minimum of 20–30 minutes after removal of the catheter and that the patient be observed for an additional 30 minutes for the development of a hematoma.

Subclavian Vein Cannulation for Temporary Hemodialysis Access

The use of the subclavian vein for hemodialysis access was largely developed and perfected by Uldall.[12] It has an advantage over femoral vein cannulation in that the catheter can be left in place for long periods of time without restriction of the patient's mobility. It has a disadvantage in that it is a technically more difficult procedure to perform and should be performed only by physicians who are experienced in the technique. Although controlled comparative studies are not available, subclavian vein catheterization likely has a greater complication rate than femoral vein catheterization.

Subclavian cannula insertion can be done in the dialysis unit or in the patient's hospital bed. The patient should be placed in the supine position with the head turned to the side opposite of the site of insertion. The skin above and below the clavicle is prepared with an antiseptic solution and a sterile field created with sterile drapes. Local anesthesia is infiltrated into the insertion site, which is immediately above and lateral to the junction of the clavicle with the first rib (Fig. 7-7). A small stab incision is made with a scalpel blade at the insertion site. Using a hemostat a subcutaneous tunnel is then made from this incision to a point 5 cm outward and downward for the subcutaneous tunneling of the catheter. A 16-gauge angiocath is then inserted into the subclavian vein through the incision and a 0.89mm guidewire introduced into the subclavian vein through the angiocath. The guidewire is then advanced into the superior vena cava. It is important that the length of guidewire advanced into the patient is greater than the total

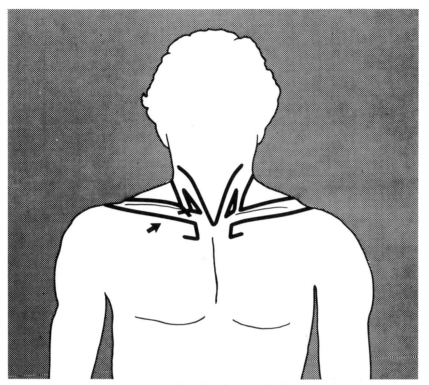

Figure 7-7. Insertion site for subclavian cannula.

length of the subclavian catheter. The currently available subclavian dialysis catheters are stiff and if advanced into the superior cava beyond the guidewire tip can puncture the wall of the superior vena cava. After passing the guidewire into the superior vena cava the proximal end of the guidewire is passed out through the previously prepared subcutaneous tunnel. It is pulled straight to eliminate the kinking which invariably occurs; the subclavian cannula is passed over the guidewire through the subcutaneous tunnel and down into the subclavian vein. The catheter is filled with heparinized saline and the incision is closed with one or two sutures. The cannula is then held in place by two (10 × 14 cm) sterile transparent dressings, the first applied below and reflected back under the cannula and the second applied above and on top of the cannula so that it covers the insertion site. The Silastic® extension is thus completely enclosed in the two layers of sterile adhesive dressing. This arrangement has the effect of anchoring the cannula and avoids any need for sutures to hold it in place. It is our practice to check the placement of the cannula with a chest x-ray prior to its use.

At the end of the dialysis, one limb of the Y tubing is capped and the other limb is flushed with heparinized saline and either attached to a continuous intravenous infusion, if the patient is hospitalized and requires intravenous therapy, or connected to a small intravenous extension tube with a rubber diaphram on the end. If there is no intravenous infusion through the catheter, it is filled with 1 ml of 5000 units/ml heparin. Patients are allowed to go home and the subclavian catheters are used on an outpatient basis.

In some centers the catheters are routinely changed on a weekly basis in attempt to prevent infection. In our center, the catheters are only changed if clotting occurs. Changing is easily accomplished by the passage of a guidewire through the existing cannula which is then withdrawn over the guidewire and a fresh cannula inserted. It has been our practice only to place or change catheters in a hospital setting. In order to minimize complications such as pneumothorax, hemothorax, and infection, it is important that the subclavian catheters be placed or changed only by experienced physicians who have been specially trained in the proper technique.

VASCULAR ACCESS COMPLICATIONS

The major complications which can occur with any type vascular access include thrombosis, infection, aneurysm formation, stenosis, and high-output cardiac failure.

Thrombosis of the vascular access is the most frequent complication. It can and does occur with all types of vascular access. Some patients appear to be much more prone to thrombosis of their vascular access than other patients. Although at present it is not possible to separate out these patients by routine laboratory testing, it appears that these patients may be more "hypercoagulable." It may be that some of these hypercoagulable patients in reality are more like the normal population and patients who do not have trouble with vascular access clotting may benefit from some of the coagulation abnormalities common to renal insufficiency. Attempts to create arteriovenous fistulas in patients without renal failure for purposes other than hemodialysis have been plagued with recurrent thrombosis. It is also very common for thrombosis of the vascular access to occur after successful renal transplantation.

There are several modes of therapy which can be used to treat this group of hypercoagulable patients. We have administered warfarin to several of these patients with seemingly very good results. It is likely, however, that hemodialysis patients given chronic anticoagulants have an increased risk of major and minor hemorrhagic complications.

Since part of the problem with access thrombosis appears to be related to platelet aggregation, platelet inhibitors such as aspirin and dipyridamole have been used. Harter and co-workers have demonstrated that aspirin will prolong the life of external arteriovenous shunts.[13] We are currently involved in a double-blind study evaluating the effect of dipyridamole administration to patients with internal arteriovenous shunts. The results of this study are not available at this time. Although both aspirin and dipyridamole are effective in inhibiting platelet aggregation, dipyridamole has the advantage of not causing gastric irritation or gastrointestinal bleeding. It is, however, rather expensive.

Kauffman and co-workers feel that many patients who experience repeated access clotting have specific, treatable coagulation abnormalities.[14] In an uncontrolled series, they found that 45 percent of patients with spontaneous thrombosis of a technically adequate internal arteriovenous shunt had either antithrombin III deficiency or increased spontaneous platelet aggregation. These investigators suggest treatment of the antithrombin III deficiency with fresh, frozen plasma which is started before access surgery and continued for 3–5 days after surgery and treatment of platelet hyperaggregation by giving aspirin and dipyridamole. They feel that these treatments were successful, in that all of their 13 patients so treated had successful arteriovenous grafts which had remained patent for the follow-up period of 8–36 months. Larger controlled studies are needed before treatment can be universally recommended.

Bedside Treatment of a Clotted Internal AV Fistula

Techniques for declotting of external arteriovenous shunts are described above. If clotting occurs in an arteriovenous fistula or an internal arteriovenous shunt, it is sometimes possible to declot the access without surgical intervention.[15] The declotting is most likely to be successful if clotting has occurred suddenly in a previously well-functioning access as often occurs after severe hypotensive episodes, surgical procedures, or cardiorespiratory resuscitation.

The first step in the bedside declotting of an internal arteriovenous fistula is to place a tight venous tourniquet around the upper arm. The majority of sudden fistula occlusions occur at the site of vascular anastomosis. This maneuver distends the veins with liquid blood immediately adjacent to the area of the clot, either through antegrade flow via the still patent distal veins or by persistent, albeit feeble arterial flow across the anastomosis. If an acutely clotted arteriovenous fistula can be distended down to the vascular anastomosis by this maneuver the chances of reopening it are extremely good, and in fact the venous distention in and of itself may on occasion reestablish flow.

The second step in declotting procedure is to smartly flick the skin directly over the vascular anastomosis. This is a painful procedure and the patient should be forewarned. The purpose of this is to break up the thrombus and dislodge it into the vein. The next step is to knead the area of anastomosis for approximately 10 seconds using a rocking motion with the ball of the thumb in an effort to milk the fractured clot from the area of anastomosis into the venous limb of the fistula. The venous tourniquet is then removed and the fistula inspected for return or improvement of the thrill and bruit. The entire procedure may be repeated several times if necessary.

Zimmerman found this procedure to be successful in 85 percent of acutely clotted Brescia arteriovenous fistulas, but only in 1 out of 5 cases of internal arteriovenous shunts.[15]

Stenosis

A frequent problem of internal arteriovenous fistulas and shunts is the development of progressive stenosis near an anastomotic site. The stenosis is believed to be caused by histologic changes resulting from turbulent blood flow across the anastomosis. Turbulent flow causes endothelial injury which leads to platelet and fibrin deposition on luminal surface which leads to progressive myointimal proliferation. If the stenotic area is at the arterial anastomosis it is usually first manifested by an inability to obtain adequate blood flow for dialysis. If the stenosis is at the venous anastomosis, high pressures will be noted in the graft during dialysis and there will be difficulty in stopping the bleeding from the puncture site after dialysis. If stenotic areas are not corrected, they will ultimately lead to complete thrombosis and loss of the vascular access. Generally the stenotic areas can be corrected by surgically opening the vessel and doing a patch graft angioplasty at the stenotic area.

Infection of Internal Hemodialysis Accesses

Between 50 and 70 percent of all infections in chronic hemodialysis patients involve the vascular access. With bacteremia, which is not rare, the mortality may be as high as 20 percent.

Staphylococcus aureus causes 70 percent of vascular access infections, which implies that most are the result of access puncture for dialysis.[16]

The nasal carrier rate for *S. aureus* in hemodialysis patients is 62 percent compared to 10 percent in the normal population.[17] The use of phage typing has demonstrated that most access infections are due to autoinfection by organisms which colonize the patients skin and nasal cavity. It is impossible to completely prevent these infections but their incidence can be kept to a minimum by proper medical management. It is important that meticulous care be given to prepping of the skin over the access site prior to needle insertion.

The infection rate of the various types of access are different. The highest infection rate occurs in the external arteriovenous shunt and the lowest rate is in the internal Brescia–Cimino fistula, with the infection rate of internal arteriovenous shunts being in between. There is some evidence that PTFE internal shunts may have a slightly lower infection rate than the Bovine hetrograft, but the difference, if real, is minimal.

Experimental work in dogs indicate that newly implanted grafts are more susceptible to infection than grafts which have been in place for at least 2 or 3 weeks. This is an additional reason not to use the internal arteriovenous grafts for 2–3 weeks after surgical implantation.

Aneurysm

Another complication of arteriovenous access is aneurysm formation. Aneurysms may form in the Brescia–Cimino arteriovenous fistula or with any of the internal arteriovenous shunts. The aneurysm in the Brescia arteriovenous fistula is usually a true aneurysm with the wall being formed from expansion of the vein wall. The aneurysm associated with internal arteriovenous shunts are usually anastomotic aneurysms caused by a defect at the anastomosis site. Pseudo-aneurysms may also occur due to loss of integrity of the graft wall. It has been postulated, in either case, that a part of the etiology of aneurysm formation is related to multiple needle sticks in a small area and the incidence of aneurysm formation probably can be decreased by rotating the puncture sites.

Many of the aneurysms do not need surgical intervention. The incidence of rupture or other complications such a emboli appears to be quite low. Large aneurysms and those which appear to be enlarging rapidly, however, should be surgically repaired. The portion of the vein or internal shunt with the aneurysm usually must be resected and a bypass graft, using a small piece of PTFE graft or other suitable material, inserted.

High-Output Cardiac Failure

The shunting of blood directly from the arterial system into the venous system which occurs with all types of arteriovenous vascular access produces the potential for high-output cardiac failure. This complication, however, is rare. The blood flow of a properly constructed arteriovenous fistula or internal shunt is between 300 and 1000 ml/min. If the arteriovenous anastomosis is too large, larger flows of 2000 ml/min or greater may occur and precipitate congestive heart failure. Cardiac failure is most likely to occur in the patient who is severely anemic or has some underlying cardiac disease.

Determining the contribution of an arteriovenous fistula to cardiac failure in the hemodialysis patient is a difficult task. While a significant decrease in pulse rate with occlusion of the fistula (Branham's sign) is very suggestive that the fistula flow may be excessive, the absence of this finding does not eliminate this possibility. An estimate of blood flow through the fistula can be made by several different methods. A common technique is the use of Doppler ultrasonic flow meter.[18] The doppler technique measures the velocity of blood flow through the vessels and an estimate of the of the vessel diameter must be made in order to calculate volume flow rate. Errors in the diameter estimate decrease the accuracy of this method markedly. Flow through the brachial artery above the fistula can be measured by the Doppler technique both before and after fistula occlusion and fistula flow estimated by the difference between the two values.

Blood flow through internal arteriovenous shunts may be determined by isotope dilution.[19] With this technique a solution containing a known amount of radioactivity is injected at a fixed rate into the proximal end of the arteriovenous shunt and blood is withdrawn downstream from the shunt. Flow through the internal arteriovenous shunt is calculated by the dilution principle. Blood flow is equal to the infusion rate of the isotope solution times radioactivity of this solution divided by the radioactivity of the collected blood. Blood flow through a Brescia arteriovenous fistula can be measured by this method, but may grossly underestimate flow if there are multiple venous channels present for the blood to return to the heart.

Cardiac output can be measured by thermal dilution, dye dilution, or impedance cardiography before and after occlusion of the fistula. With a normal functioning fistula there is usually a significant decrease in cardiac output with occlusion with the fistula. The drop in cardiac output with fistula occlusion is usually less than the actual flow through the fistula, probably because of increased blood flow to areas which were underperfused while the fistula was functioning.[20]

If there is excessive flow through the fistula, flow can be decreased by banding the vein or synthetic graft or by decreasing the diameter of the arteriovenous anastomosis.

ANGIOGRAPHIC FISTULA EVALUATION

When technical problems such as decreased arterial blood flow, increased venous resistance, difficult needle cannulation, or suspected clot formation arise with arteriovenous fistulas and internal arteriovenous shunts, it is helpful to evaluate the access by venous angiography. Anderson and co-workers have developed a method which does not require arterial puncture and visualizes the veins, the graft if present, the arteriovenous anastomosis, and the immediate adjacent arterial segment.[21] With this method a 19-gauge scalp vein needle is inserted into the proximal venous limb so that the tip of the needle lies 1 cm away from and points toward the arteriovenous fistula. A blood pressure cuff is placed around the upper arm and inflated above systolic pressure. A 20-ml bolus of x-ray contrast material is manually injected over 4 seconds while an assistant controls the bulb of the blood pressure cuff. Radiography is begun ½ second before the end of injection and the pressure in the cuff is released 1 second later. Rapid serial films are taken at 2/second for 4 seconds. To obtain optimum information it is best if x-rays are taken in two projections at right angles to each other. This procedure is very helpful in demonstrating the anatomy of the vessels and can show significant vascular stenoses, thrombus formation in the vessels, aneurysmal dilatation, excessive flow rates, and steal phenomena. Complications from this procedure are exceedingly unusual.

REFERENCES

1. Mandel SR, Martin PL, Blumoff RL, et al: Vascular access in a university transplant and dialysis program. Arch Surg 1122:1375–1380, 1977
2. Quinton W, Dillard D, Scribner BH: Cannulation of blood vessels for prolonged hemodialysis. Trans Am Soc Artif Intern Orgaans 6:104–113, 1960
3. Brescia MJ, Cimino JE, Appel K, Hurwich BJ: Chronic hemodialysis using venipuncture and surgically created arteriovenous fistula. N Eng J Med 275:1084–1094, 1966
4. Buselmeier TJ, Kjellstrand CM, Quinton WE, et al: The Buselmeier shunt, specific method of surgical placement. Dial Transplant 3:30–35, 1974

5. Thomas GI: A large vessel applique A-V shunt for hemodialysis. Trans Am Soc Artif Intern Organs 15:288–292, 1969
6. Lowenstein E, Little III JW, Lo HH: Prevention of cerebral embolization from flushing radial artery cannulas. N Eng J Med 285:1414–15, 1971
7. Schwartz AD, Declement FA, Bowen R, et al: Conversion of external arteriovenous hemodialysis shunt to internal fistula. JAMA 239:1788–1783, 1978
8. Sabanayagam P, Schwartz AB, Soricelli RR, et al: A comparative study of 402 bovine heterografts and 225 reinforced expanded PTFE grafts as AVF in ESRD patients. Trans Am Soc Artif Intern Organs 26:88–92, 1980
9. Haimov M, Burrows L, Schanzer H, et al: Experience with arterial substitutes in the construction of vascular access for hemodialysis. J Cardiovasc Surg (Torino) 21:149–154, 1980
10. May J, Harris J, Patrick W: Polytetrafluoroethylene (PTFE) grafts for hemodialysis: Patency and complications compared with those of saphenous vein grafts. Aust NZ J Surg 49:639–642, 1979
11. Shaldon S, Chiandussi L, Higgs B: Haemodialysis by percutaneous catheterization of the femoral artery and vein with regional heparinization. Lancet 2:857, 1961
12. Uldall PR, Woods F, Bird M, Byck R: Subclavian cannula for temporary hemodialysis. Proc Dialysis Transplant Forum 9:268–272, 1974
13. Harter HR, Burch JW, Majerus PW, et al: Prevention of thrombosis in patients on hemodialysis by low dose aspirin. N Eng J Med 301:557–559, 1979
14. Kaufman HM, Ekbon GA, Adams MB, Hussey CV: Hypercoagulation-A cause of vascular access failure. Proc Dialysis Transplant Forum 9:28–30, 1979
15. Zimmerman, CE: Bedside manipulation of the clotted arteriovenous fistula. Dial Transplant 10:837, 1981
16. Dobkin JF, Miller MH, Steigbigel NH: Septicemia in patients on chronic hemodialysis. Ann Intern Med 88:28–33, 1978
17. Kirmani N, Truazon U, Murray HW, Parrish AE, Sheagren JN: *Staphylococcus aureus* carriage rate of patient receiving long term hemodialysis. Arch Intern Med 138:1657–1659, 1978
18. Kasulke RJ, Lichti D, Kapsch E, Silver D: Transcutaneous quantitation of arterial blood flow with the dopper ultrasonic flowmeter. Surg Forum 31:325, 1980
19. Kaye M, Lemaitre P, O'Regan S: A new technique for measuring blood flow in polytetrafluoroethylene grafts for hemodialysis. Clin Nephrol 8:533–534, 1977
20. VanderWerf BA, Kuman SS, Pennell P, Gotliek S: Cardiac failure from bovine graft arteriovenous fistulas: Diagnosis and management. Trans Am Soc Artif Intern Organs 24:474–475, 1978
21. Anderson CB, Gilula LA, Harter HR, et al: Venous angiography and the surgical management of subcutaneous hemodialysis fistula. Ann Surg 187:194–204, 1978

Michael I. Sorkin

8
Peritoneal Physiology

ANATOMY AND HISTOLOGY

The peritoneal dialysis system is composed of three parts: first, the blood which is supplied to the dialyzing membrane by the peritoneal blood vessels, second, the peritoneal membrane which the solutes must cross, and third, dialysis fluid which is instilled into the peritoneal cavity and becomes dialysate when components of the blood are transferred into it across the peritoneal membrane.

The peritoneal blood supply (Fig. 8-1) is made up of branching arteries which become progressively smaller until the muscle layer is gone and they become true capillaries. The capillaries merge to form venules and then veins that carry blood away from the peritoneal membrane back to the systemic circulation. Blood flow to these capillary beds is governed by the action of muscular elements located in the arterioles just before the vessels break up into the capillary bed.[1] These muscular sphincters are known as precapillary sphincters. Apparently some control of outflow resistance is provided by an additional set of muscular sphincters at the venular end of the capillary arcade—these are known as postcapillary sphincters.

The peritoneal capillaries are not entirely analagous to glomerular capillaries since they do have fenestrae in the endothelial cell bodies. They do have, however, a basement membrane which acts as a component of the filtration barrier after the endothelial cytoplasm. Molecules may traverse the capillary wall through the endothelial cytoplasm but most likely the major molecular transfer occurs through the spaces between the endothelial cells known as intercellular gaps.[2]

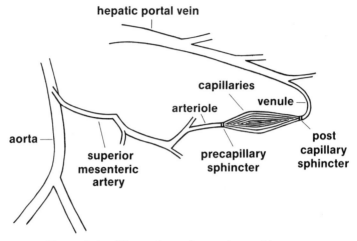

Figure 8-1. The peritoneal vascular architecture.

These gaps probably make up about 0.2 percent of the surface area of the capillary wall. Adjacent to the basement membrane is a layer of loose connective tissue which averages approximately 100 μ from blood vessel to mesothelium. This interstitial matrix is covered by a single layer of mesothelial cells. The whole package from capillary lumen to mesothelial cells is the dialyzing segment of the peritoneal membrane.

The peritoneal membrane is divided into visceral and parietal components. The visceral peritoneum covers all those organs which are anatomically adjacent to the peritoneal cavity. The parietal peritoneum lines the abdominal wall. Some differences have been demonstrated between the control of circulation to the parietal and visceral peritoneum in animals but anatomically and histologically they appear much the same. There is an important difference in venous drainage. The visceral peritoneal circulation drains into the portal system while the parietal veins drain into the inferior vena cava. This means that at least part of solutes absorbed from dialysis fluid goes to the liver before entering the general circulation.

Under normal circumstances there is no "peritoneal cavity." The peritoneal dialysis system takes advantage of the fact that the smooth, glistening peritoneal membrane forms a continuous structure which covers the intraabdominal contents thus forming a potential cavity which can be filled with fluid much like a balloon is expanded by air. The size of this cavity is limited by the elasticity of the abdominal wall, the size of the intraabdominal organs, the encroachment upon the cavity by extraperitoneal structures (including the kidneys or other masses), and disruption of the smoother peritoneal membrane by adhesions.

FACTORS CONTROLLING PERITONEAL DIALYSIS

The movement of the solvent and solute across the peritoneal membrane depends on the same factors that govern the movement of solvent and solute across any dialysis membrane (Chapter 5). Blood must reach the dialyzing surface and be carried away. Membrane characteristics, especially surface area and permeability, are important; dialysis fluid must reach the peritoneal membrane and be carried away. Unlike "dead" cellophane membranes, the "living" peritoneal membrane characteristics are potentially continuously variable, depending on the hormonal factors that influence blood supply and blood vessel permeability, connective tissue matrix, and cellular composition. Other modifying factors include vagaries of dialysate distribution, influence of dialysate composition, and filtration pressure. The net result of all these factors is not always predictable. A careful review of the available information is helpful, however, in understanding the clinical implications and limitations of peritoneal dialysis.

Blood Flow

In order to cross the dialyzing membrane, molecules must come in contact with it. Blood flow to the peritoneal membrane is thus the first factor controlling peritoneal dialysis. Blood flow depends on: (1) systemic blood pressure to provide the force that moves the blood, (2) pre- and postcapillary sphincters that regulate blood flow, and (3) filtration pressure at the capillary wall. Blood flow is a more important limiting factor for small molecules which cross the peritoneal membrane easily since they equilibrate more quickly than larger molecules that cross the peritoneal membrane slowly. Existing evidence suggests that blood flow to the peritoneal membrane is approximately 100 ml/min in man.

Two pieces of evidence suggest that blood flow is not a significant limiting factor for peritoneal dialysis in man or animals. First, the best urea clearance obtainable is in the range of 30 ml/min.[3] Urea is the smallest (60 daltons) commonly measured molecule, is uncharged, and passes across most biological membranes with ease. If peritoneal blood flow were an important limiting factor, the clearance of urea should therefore equal or nearly equal the rate at which it is delivered to the dialyzing membrane—approximately 100 ml/min. Second, peritoneal dialysis of urea is affected relatively little by severe decreases in systemic blood pressure.[4] Reducing a dog's mean arterial pressure to 25 percent of normal reduces the urea clearance to only 75 percent of normal. Assuming that blood flow decreases parallel systemic pressure and the fact that filtration pressure at the capillary must certainly fall as systemic pressure falls, indicates that there are other more important limiting factors than blood pressure and blood flow. These other factors are inherent in the two other parts of the dialysis system—the peritoneal membrane and dialysis fluid.

The Membrane

The peritoneal membrane may be thought of as a group of resistances in series as illustrated in Figure 8-2. The first resistance is caused by the fluid film in the capillary. Solute must diffuse through the plasma to reach the second resistance—the capillary endothelium. The endothelial cell may in fact provide such a high resistance that most of the movement of solute and solvent occurs through the gaps between cells. This reduces the effective area available for dialysis to about 0.2 percent of the capillary surface area. These gaps are probably big

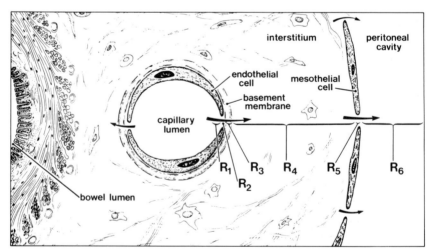

Figure 8-2. The resistances through which solute must pass during peritoneal dialysis. Reprinted with permission from Nolph KD, Miller F, Rubin J, Popovich R: New directions in peritoneal dialysis concepts and applications. Kidney Int 18 (Suppl 10):S111–S116, 1980.

enough so that they do not limit the size of molecules that reach the next resistance. The third resistance is the capillary basement membrane. This is a relatively homogenous structure that does provide the first size discrimination by the characteristics of its matrix. It may also provide some charge discrimination since some basement membranes, such as glomerular capillaries, have been shown to contain charged molecules that may enhance or retard the movement of charged molecules present in the blood. The fourth resistance is the layer of connective tissue extending from the capillary basement membrane to the mesothelial cells forming the surface of the peritoneal membrane. Although this is loose connective tissue, the distance from blood vessel to mesothelium is relatively large. This distance and the tissue permeability characteristics probably provide a significant barrier even to relatively small molecules. The fifth resistance lies in the mesothelial cell layer itself. Little is known about the characteristics of this resistance. Molecules may pass between the cell bodies to reach dialysate or they may pass through the cells. The contribution of each of these is yet to be determined. Most authorities suggest, however, that this mesothelial cell layer is a relatively minor resistance. The sixth resistance is the dialysate. This is the fluid film that solute must diffuse through analagous to the first resistance caused by capillary fluid films.

Dialysate Flow

Molecules move across the peritoneal membrane until their concentration in the dialysate equals their concentration in the blood. The smaller the molecule the sooner this equilibration generally occurs. Larger molecules cross the peritoneal membrane considerably slower than smaller molecules and their concentration in the dialysate increases more linearly than small molecules. This means that small molecule removal tends to increase with higher dialysate flow rates whereas the clearance of larger molecules is less affected by dialysate flow.

In older dialysis systems (hemodialysis and intermittent peritoneal dialysis) dialysate flow rates are high enough (500 and 65 ml/min, respectively) that dialysate flow rate is not a major factor limiting dialysis efficiency. In the continuous anbulatory peritoneal dialysis (CAPD) system, dialysate flow rate is relatively low (6–7 ml/min) and is the limiting factor for small molecule clearances. This is because clearances achievable with high dialysate flow rates approach 30 ml/min for urea clearance and 20 ml/min for creatinine clearance. If the dialysis fluid flow is only 6 ml/min, the clearance must be limited to 6 ml/min regardless of what clearances the system is capable of achieving under ideal conditions.

FACTORS AFFECTING PERITONEAL DIALYSIS EFFICIENCY

Diffusion

Most mass transfer across the peritoneal membrane occurs by the simple process of diffusion. The most important driving force for diffusion is concentration. Molecules diffuse from an area of higher concentration to an area of lower concentration. The role of electrical forces in the control of diffusion in the peritoneal dialysis system has not been explored.

Convection

Convection is the process by which molecules are swept along with the solvent, usually water, through the dialyzing membrane in the process of forming ultrafiltrate. Increasing the ultrafiltration rate during peritoneal dialysis may be used to increase solute removal through this convection transfer phenomenon.

Permeability

Permeability is the property of the membrane that determines the rate at which a solute passes through that membrane. In the peritoneal dialysis system this may be influenced by local factors in the dialysate, including pH, osmolality, and type of buffers. The permeability may also be altered by presence of endogenous factors in blood or dialysate including histamine, bradykinin, prostaglandin, parathormone, catecholmines, and others. Permeability should also decrease as the thickness of the membrane increases.

Surface Area

The area available for dialysis is another factor that determines the rate at which molecules cross from blood to dialysate. The area of the blood side of the membrane (capillary surface area) and the dialysate side of the membrane (usually called the peritoneal membrane) are very important. Increasing the surface area of the membrane generally increases the rate that solutes and water are transferred from blood to dialysis fluid.

Net Filtration Pressure

Movement of water across biological membranes (osmosis) is driven primarily by pressure. The pressures acting on the dialysis system include (1) hydraulic pressure (peritoneal capillary blood pressure), (2) intracapillary oncotic pressure generated by plasma proteins, (3) interstitial oncotic pressure generated by connective tissue proteins, (4) peritoneal cavity hydrostatic pressure, and (5) peritoneal dialysis fluid osmotic pressure generated by the glucose concentration. The algebraic sum of these pressures is net filtration pressure.

Ultrafiltrate

The water and solutes driven across a membrane by net filtration pressure are called ultrafiltrate. The membrane limits the passage of cells and protein molecules but permits the passage of electrolytes and small- and middle-sized molecules. In the peritoneal dialysis system the ultrafiltrate is hypotonic because of the peculiarities of the membrane and the dialysate. The net result is the loss of fluid with a sodium concentration of about 70 mEq/liter. Of course solutes others than NaCl are present, especially urea.

MEASUREMENTS OF PERITONEAL DIALYSIS EFFICIENCY

Clearance

It is frequently useful to think of solute removal in terms of the volume of blood cleared of that solute each minute. Clearance (C) in the peritoneal dialysis system is calculated exactly the same as clearance in renal physiology. It is the concentration of a solute in the dialysate (Ds) divided by plasma or serum concentration of the same solute (Ps) times dialysate flow (in ml/min)(Vo):
$C = (Ds/Ps) \, Vo.$
The time interval used for this calculation begins with the start of dialysis fluid inflow and terminates at the end of outflow. The flow rate is the total volume drained out divided by the time interval.

Mass Transfer Area Coefficient

The term mass transfer simply refers to the movement of molecules from blood to dialysate or from dialysate to blood. It makes no implications about how molecular transfer occurs—it is simply the amount of solute transferred across the membrane. The amount of solute transferred across the peritoneal membrane is the sum of the amounts moving by diffusion and the amounts moving by convection. The amount of solute moving by diffusion is dependent on the permeability of the membrane and its surface area. Since both the dialyzing area and the permeability of an individual peritoneal membrane are difficult to measure, a composite term has been used to describe the rate at which an individual molecular species is transported across the peritoneal membrane. This composite term has been called mass transfer area coefficient (MTAC).[5] The peritoneal membrane permeability may be characterized by its MTAC. This is calculated by measuring the clearance of the specific solute at multiple points in time, subtracting convective transfer, and then extrapolating the diffusive clearance back to 0 time—the time at which the instantaneous clearance should be the greatest since the gradient is the largest. MTAC (expressed in ml/min) is the theoretical maximum dialyzing capability of the peritoneal dialysis system for the molecule in question. The calculation measurements required to determine MTAC are complicated and are not routinely used to assess peritoneal function. Clearance mesurements are instead usually relied upon clinically.

DYNAMICS OF PERITONEAL DIALYSIS

The only pressure that is readily controlled in the peritoneal system is the dialysis fluid osmotic pressure. By increasing the osmotic agent (commonly glucose) the movement of water and most solutes can be enhanced. The osmotic pressure exerted by the glucose is reduced by dilution as ultrafiltrate is added to the dialysis fluid and is also reduced by the absorption of glucose across the peritoneal membrane into the blood stream. Dialysate glucose concentration and, therefore, the osmotic gradient diminishes rapidly so that ultrafiltration rate is maximum at 10–20 minutes and is falling rapidly by 20–30 minutes.[6]

In spite of this rapid diminution in glucose concentration and osmotic gradient, a positive net ultrafiltration can be achieved during long dwell exchanges (Fig. 8-3).[7] While drainage volume is maximum at

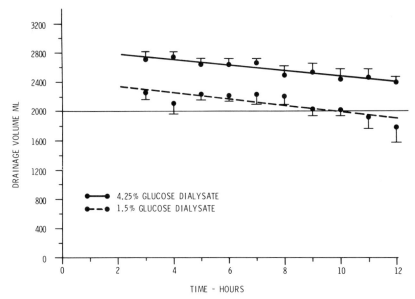

Figure 8-3. The change in drainage volume during long dwell peritoneal dialysis with 4.25 percent glucose and 1.5 percent glucose dialysate. Reprinted with permission from Rubin J, Nolph KD, Popovich RP, Moncrief JW, Prowant B: Drainage volumes during continuous ambulatory peritoneal dialysis. ASAIO 2:54–60, 1979.

2–3 hours after instillation of dialysis fluid, more dialysate is drained than instilled in the average patient as long as 6–8 hours after instillation with a dialysis fluid 1.5 percent glucose concentration. Volume "breaks even" at about 14–18 hours with dialysis fluid glucose concentration of 4.25 percent. It is thus possible to achieve adequate volume removal even with long dwell exchanges by selecting osmotic concentration based on individual patient requirements.

Solute transfer from blood to dialysis fluid is a function of time as well as membrane permeability, net filtration pressure, and membrane surface area. The largest concentration gradients exist during the first few minutes of dialysis but urea concentration in dialysate has not reached 75 percent of plasma concentration until more than 100 minutes have elapsed.[8] Although most efficient solute removal is obtained during short duration exchanges, solute removal continues during long dwell exchanges until equilibrium is reached (Fig. 8-4). For urea (60 daltons), D/P is only about 55 percent at 1.5 hours and is just approaching 100 percent at 5 hours, creatinine D/P is about 75 percent

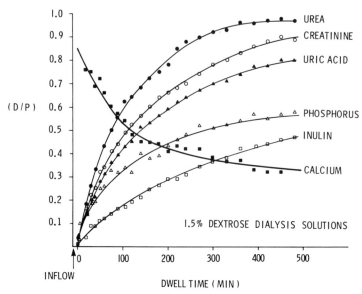

Figure 8-4. The change in dialysate to plasma concentration ratio of different molecular weight solutes during long dwell peritoneal dialysis. (D/P = dialysate/plasma concentrations. N = 4.) Reprinted with permission from Nolph KD, Twardowski ZJ, Popovich RP, Rubin J: Equilibrium of peritoneal dialysis solutions during long-dwell exchanges. J Lab Clin Med 93:246–256, 1979.

at 4 hours. Larger molecules equilibrate much more slowly so that the increase in dialysate solute concentration is almost linear as size approaches 5200 daltons (inulin). For long dwell exchanges, drainage volume is thus the most important determinant of small molecule removal and dialysis time is the most important factor in large molecule removal. These properties have been beautifully exploited in the CAPD system.

ALTERATION OF PERITONEAL PHYSIOLOGY BY EXOGENOUS AGENTS

Local conditions and circulating factors modulate peritoneal physiology under normal conditions. Exercise reduces splanchnic blood flow, histamine increases mesenteric vessel permeability, and peritonitis causes marked protein exudation and increases solute transfer. Certainly the addition of exogenous agents should have some effect on the peritoneum. In this section, several agents will be discussed because they have potential clinical significance.

Dialysis Solutions

The peritoneal dialysis fluid itself has large effects on the peritoneum. The major effect of the application of dialysis solution to the peritoneum is vasodilatation although the parietal peritoneum does undergo a brief period of vasoconstriction as illustrated in Figure 8-5.[1,9] This vasodilatation seems largely due to a combination of hyperosmolality plus the acetate or lactate used as the bicarbonate substitute. The vasodilatation should ensure that peritoneal blood flow is near maximal during uncomplicated peritoneal dialysis.

Although there are differences between peritoneal dialysis solutions marketed by different manufacturers, they all currently have equivalent effects on the peritoneal membrane and equivalent clear-

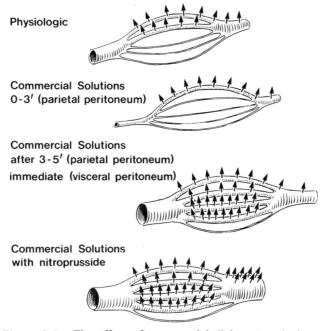

Figure 8-5. The effect of commercial dialysate and nitroprusside on peritoneal vasoconstriction and permeability. (Density of arrows indicates permeability.) Reprinted with permission from Nolph KD, Miller F, Rubin J, et al: New directions in peritoneal dialysis concepts and applications. Kidney Int 18 (Suppl. 10): S111–S116, 1980.

ances for all substances tested thus far. The major differences between manufacturers and between solutions made by the same manufacturer lie in the buffer composition. Lactate or acetate are both used. Some solutions may also differ in the concentration of magnesium.

The pH of peritoneal dialysis solutions generally is adjusted to about 5.5 by the manufacturer. This is done to prevent glucose from caramelizing during the sterilization process. The low pH apparently has no adverse effects on the peritoneal membrane or its function. Serial pH measurements demonstrate that the pH is adjusted to physiological pH within minutes after the fluid is instilled.

Dialysis fluid temperature also effects mass transfer. As expected, the higher the temperature the greater the diffusive mass transfer. Fluid temperatures are therefore usually raised to near body temperature before instillation. This is more important for the short dwell exchanges than long dwell exchanges. In long dwell exchanges, the dialysis fluid is warmed quickly enough so that dialysis solution instilled at ambient temperature has little effect on clearance.

Increasing dialysis fluid osmolality has a twofold effect. First, ultrafiltration rate and drainage volume are increased. Convective mass transfer is thus increased and removal of all solutes will be enhanced. Second, exposure of the membrane to hyperosomotic solutions by itself apparently increases the clearance of solutes. These effects may be used clinically to augment clearances with the proviso that the patient must be carefully observed to prevent volume depletion or hypernatremia.

Vasodilators

Sodium nitroprusside is the most commonly mentioned vasodilator used in conjunction with peritoneal dialysis. Sodium nitroprusside dilates peritoneal vessels just as it does other systemic vessels. Although it has no appreciable effect on ultrafiltration, nitroprusside does increase the MTAC of urea, creatinine, and inulin. This increase in MTAC is greatest for the larger inulin molecule. Most of the increase in MTAC is probably due to increased permeability rather than increased blood flow since blood flow is already increased by the dialysis solution alone. Nitroprusside seems to have its most important clinical effect at the venular end of the capillary arcade as indicated in Figure 8-5. Venular diameter is increased and venular permeability may be selectively increased.

The ability of nitroprusside to increase MTAC has been used as a tool to evaluate peritoneal function.[10] It offers only a relatively small gain in clearances in the clinical setting when balanced against the additional risk of accumulation of toxic metabolites, systemic blood pressure effects, and the risk of contaminating the sterile system when adding the drug. It is not currently used in the treatment of patients.

The list of other agents that have been tested and found to have some effect on peritoneal physiology is quite long. All the compounds tested thus far have only theoretical advantages and are not used clinically.

CLINICAL APPLICATIONS

Improving Dialysis

The "best" dialysis schedule for intermittent peritoneal dialysis is a composite of: (1) the time over which maximum ultrafiltration occurs, (2) the dialysate flow rate that maintains the largest solute gradient, and (3) the practical aspects of performing the exchange (operator time, machine requirement, and cost). Analysis and application of these factors have led to the current recommendations for 30-minute exchanges of 2 liters each. Shorter exchanges result in a relatively small advantage in ultrafiltration and solute removal but a relatively greater technical and cost problem.

Increasing ultrafiltration may be used to increase solute removal by increasing convective transfer. This is accomplished simply by using a larger number of exchanges containing glucose concentration greater than 1.5 percent.

Limiting Factors

The major clinical problems that limit the use of peritoneal dialysis are factors influencing peritoneal surface area or permeability. The presence of prior abdominal surgery may lead to the development of scars and adhesions. The function of the peritoneal system depends on the ability of the dialysate to circulate within the peritoneal cavity freely so that maximum surface area is used for dialysis. Adhesions may interfere with this and limit surface area thus decreasing the efficiency of the dialysis. Any increase in thickness of the peritoneal membrane as might occur with recurrent peritonitis may decrease permeability significantly and interfere with dialysis.

Permeability clearly changes in the presence of peritonitis. Glucose absorption is enhanced, more protein leaks out of the capillaries into the dialysate and the clearances of most molecules are enhanced. Formation of ultrafiltrate suffers since osmotic forces are rapidly dissipated. Although the ultrafiltration rate may initially be very high, the reabsorption of ultrafiltrate in the face of a rapidly falling pressure for ultrafiltration results in difficulty achieving adequate ultrafiltration. During peritonitis, in other words, solute clearance increases but fluid removal is decreased.[11]

REFERENCES

1. Miller FN, Nolph KD, Harris PD, Rubin J, Wiegman DL, Joshua IG, Twardowski ZJ, Ghods AJ: Microvascular and clinical effects of altered peritoneal dialysis solutions. Kidney Int 15:630–639, 1979
2. Karnovsky MJ: The ultra structural basis of capillary permeability: Studies with peroxides as a tracer. J Cell Biol 35:213–235, 1967
3. Tenckhoff H, Ward G, Boen ST: The influence of dialysate volume and flow rate on peritoneal clearance. Proc Eur Dial Transplant Assoc 2:113, 1965
4. Erbe RW, Green JR, Weller JM: Peritoneal dialysis during hemorrhagic shock. J Appl Phys 22:131, 1967
5. Popovich RP, Pyle WK, Bomar JB, Moncrief JW: Peritoneal dialysis. Am Inst Chem Eng Symp 75:31–45, 1979
6. Popovich RP, Pyle WK, Moncrief JW: Kinetics of peritoneal transport, in Nolph KD (ed): Peritoneal Dialysis. The Hague, Nijhoff, 1981
7. Rubin, J, Nolph KD, Popovich RP, Moncrief JW, Prowant B: Drainage volumes during continuous ambulatory peritoneal dialysis. ASAIO 2:54–60, 1979
8. Nolph KD, Twardowski ZJ, Popovich RP, Rubin J: Equlibration of peritoneal dialysis solutions during long dwell exchanges. J Lab Clin Med 93:246–256, 1979
9. Nolph KD, Miller F, Rubin J, Popovich R: New directions in peritoneal dialysis concepts and applications. Kidney Int 18 (Suppl 10):S111–S116, 1980
10. Rubin J, Nolph KD, Arfania D, Brown P, Prowant B: Follow up clearances in patients undergoing continuous ambulatory peritoneal dialysis. Kidney Int 16:619–623, 1979
11. Rubin J, McFarland S, Hellems EW, Bower JD: Peritoneal dialysis during peritonitis. Kidney Int 19:460–464, 1981

Michael I. Sorkin

9
Clinical Aspects of Peritoneal Dialysis

Peritoneal dialysis has been available for at least as long as hemodialysis. In spite of its longevity, peritoneal dialysis did not come into widespread use until the recent development of continuous ambulatory peritoneal dialysis (CAPD). This lack of popularity is illustrated by the fact that most people even now take the term "dialysis" to be synonymous with hemodialysis. In the past several years both the acute and chronic use of peritoneal dialysis to support patients with end-stage renal disease (ESRD) has increased considerably. In 1977 the number of patients on chronic peritoneal dialysis were numbered in the hundreds. By the time this book goes to press more than 9000 patients will be on peritoneal dialysis in the United States alone. This chapter traces the development of peritoneal dialysis and provides a background for its clinical use intended to be of value to house officers, clinicians, and paramedical personnel.

HISTORY

The first description of peritoneal dialysis with clinical applicability is credited to Ganter in 1923.[1] Widespread clinical use awaited, however, the development of readily available equipment and solutions to support this simple procedure. Although the development of the peritoneal dialysis support system paralleled the development of hemodialysis, the dialysis fluids used in these different types of therapy differ in one very important regard—the peritoneal dialysis fluid must be sterile before it is infused into the peritoneal cavity. Sterile solutions that could be prepared commercially were described by Maxwell et al. in 1959 and eliminated the need to mix and sterilize solutions immediately before use.[2] The most important piece of equipment needed was a device to provide easy access to the peritoneal cavity. A catheter desgined by Westin and Roberts in 1965 provided a simple, inexpensive, effective means of access to the peritoneal cavity and soon was also made commercially available.[3] With dialysis fluid and access devices available, acute peritoneal dialysis was underway. It was difficult to maintain patients on chronic peritoneal dialysis because the catheters available at the time unfortunately usually became infected if left in place for more than 36–48 hours. Although several alternative devices were developed, a catheter that finally made peritoneal dialysis feasible on a chronic basis was reported by Tenckhoff and Schechter in 1968.[4] The catheter is constructed with a Dacron cuff which is placed in the subcutaneous tissue to prevent bacteria from descending into the peritoneal cavity around the outside of the catheter. It has become so well known that in many places all peritoneal access devices are known as Tenckhoff catheters. As you will see in the following pages other devices are now available but the Tenckhoff catheter will continue to be the most popular for some time to come.

At about the same time Tenckhoff was developing the catheter another member of the same group, Boen (pronounced Boon) was developing an automated technique for performing peritoneal dialysis.[5] Much like hemodialysis machines, these peritoneal dialysis machines delivered dialysis fluid to the patient automatically, thus eliminating the need to enter the sterile fluid path periodically to change bottles. This was directly responsible for a significant decrease in the rate of peritonitis. The sterile fluid path had to be interrupted only at the beginning and at the termination of the dialysis treatment. This automated system for mixing solution and timing cycles coupled with the Tenckhoff peritoneal dialysis catheter resulted in a very safe dialysis system.

In spite of its safety and simplicity, peritoneal dialysis was eclipsed by hemodialysis. Two or possibly three problems seem to be responsible. First, the peritoneal dialysis system is considerably less efficient than hemodialysis. The average hemodialysis patient even in the early days was spending less than 20 hours a week "on the machine," and the average peritoneal dialysis patient required at least 30 hours. This discrepancy has become even more marked since the high efficiency hemodialyzers available today allow the average hemodialysis patient in most centers to spend 12 hours each week "on the machine." While the the time requirement for hemodialysis decreased, it has been necessary to increase the dialysis time for most patients on peritoneal dialysis to 40 hours or more each week. Second, many patients and physicians continue to fear peritonitis even though this has not been a significant problem with automated peritoneal dialysis for more than 10 years.[6] Third, there is the feeling that peritoneal dialysis patients "don't do as well" as hemodialysis patients. This may be related to an element of underdialysis. As nephrologists began to extend the time that patients spent on peritoneal dialysis, the patients seemed to "do better" but the time requirement became even more of a deterrent. Another important improvement in the management of peritoneal dialysis patients came with increased emphasis on nutritional factors—especially larger protein intakes.

In 1975 an important change in the peritoneal dialysis technique resulted in the enormous increase in popularity that peritoneal dialysis is experiencing today. Popovich and Moncrief collaborated to solve an individual patient problem.[7] The patient had no vascular access and they had no facilities for chronic peritoneal dialysis. They devised a simple system that allowed the patient to perform his own peritoneal dialysis at home without the aid of complicated equipment or the requirement for a prolonged training course. This technical innovation, now known as CAPD, proved to be a very effective dialysis technique. The multiple daily entries into the sterile fluid path required to change dialysis fluid unfortunately resulted in a marked increase in the rate of peritonitis. Over the succeeding years, technical improvements in the system have again reduced the incidence of peritonitis to acceptable levels.[8]

THE PERITONEAL CATHETER

Acute Peritoneal Dialysis Catheter

In many centers the patient's first acute peritoneal dialysis is performed using a variant of the catheter devised by Westin and Roberts. This catheter consists of a length of rigid plastic tubing containing an end hole and multiple side holes along the intraperitoneal length of the catheter. Before use, a metal stylet is inserted into the plastic catheter so that a few millimeters of the sharpened stylet extends beyond the tip of the plastic catheter. The plastic is constructed so that the intraperitoneal segment curves when the stylet is withdrawn. This curve makes it easier to direct the catheter to the most dependent portion of the peritoneal cavity.

Catheter insertion should be performed using careful aseptic technique by personnel wearing sterile caps, masks, gowns, and gloves. The patient should be supine. The bladder should be empty to reduce the risk of puncture when the peritoneal catheter is inserted. A site is selected in the midline approximately 2 cm below the umbilicus. The skin is prepared with sterile povidone–iodine solution. After a skin wheal is raised with a 25-gauge needle, an 1½" (or longer, if necessary) needle is advanced perpendicular to the skin to infiltrate the subcutaneous tissue, linea alba, and peritoneum with local anesthetic. The next step is designed to minimize the risk of bowel perforation. A 14-gauge needle, or over a needle plastic catheter, is inserted into the peritoneal cavity, 2 liters of dialysis fluid are infused, and the needle or catheter withdrawn before placing the dialysis catheter. Using a No. 11 blade, a stab wound is then made in the skin just large enough to admit the catheter. With the stylet in place, the catheter is placed through the skin incision perpendicular to the skin and advanced into the peritoneal cavity using a twisting motion. It is helpful to have the patient flex his rectus abdominus by lifting his head while the catheter is being advanced. Usually two distinct barriers can be recognized. First, the fascia of the linea alba provides the most resistance and gives away suddenly. Second, the catheter penetrates the peritoneal membrane. As soon as the second "pop" is felt, the stylet is withdrawn several millimeters inside the catheter to avoid lacerating the bowel. If dialysis solution has been infused prior to catheter placement, penetration of the peritoneal cavity is obvious—when the stylet is withdrawn fluid appears in the catheter. The catheter is then angled to the right or left quadrant within the peritoneal cavity, advanced as far as possible, and the stylet entirely withdrawn. The catheter should then be connected to an appropriate sterile tubing system and secured to the abdominal wall with sterile tape alone or a suture placed around the catheter. The patient and the system are now ready for immediate dialysis. This catheter is simple, easy to insert (usually), and it is compatible with either automated or manual peritoneal dialysis techniques. The major diasadvantage of this catheter is that the incidence of peritonitis increases considerably after it is left in place for 36–48 hours. It is therefore usually removed after each treatment and reinserted just before the next.

Since many nephrologists have become more aggressive in using dialysis therapy, most patients will require more than one "acute" dialysis. This increased number of dialyses is in keeping with the philosophy of prophylactic dialysis (Chapter 12). Patients should be dialyzed before they get sick and enough dialysis treatments provided to prevent the patient from becoming sick. To this end, many centers are now inserting "chronic catheters" for acute renal failure.

Chronic Peritoneal Dialysis Catheters

The most popular chronic dialysis catheter is the Tenckhoff peritoneal dialysis catheter. This catheter consists of a length of silicone rubber tubing with end and side holes much like the acute catheter described above (Fig. 9-1). The Silastic material is flexible and does not maintain a curve. It is therefore, usually placed with the help of a stylet. The innovation that made this catheter acceptable for chronic use is the presence of one or two Dacron felt cuffs on the extraperitoneal portion of the catheter. The single-cuff model of this catheter may be inserted by the nephrologist using a specially constructed trocar. Most nephrologists prefer to have the double-cuff model placed surgically. The purpose of the cuff is to provide a matrix for fibroblast ingrowth which in turn provides a reliable bacteria-tight seal. The seal prevents infection of the peritoneum by organisms descending around the catheter from the skin exit site into the peritoneal cavity. The catheter is usually inserted into the peritoneal cavity in the midline just below the umbilicus. A tunnel is then constructed laterally through the subcutaneous tissue and the extraperitoneal end of the catheter is brought out through the second incision in the skin at a site distant from the point where it enters the peritoneal cavity. If the catheter has two cuffs, one is placed just superficial to the peritoneum and the second cuff is buried in the subcutaneous tissue 1.5 or 2 cm deep to the skin exit site. The deep cuff must be entirely outside the peritoneum. Placed intraperitoneally, the Dacron tends to attract omentum and contributes to catheter failure. If the catheter has a single cuff, that cuff is usually placed midway between the peritoneal membrane and the skin or at a point 1.5–2 cm deep to the exit site depending on the preference of the physician. The double-cuff catheter has the theoretical advantage of providing two bacteria-tight seals but many centers use the single-cuff catheter with equal success.

Since the insertion of this catheter requires a larger hole in the peritoneal membrane than the "acute" catheter, more caution must be used in the initial phase of dialysis. A leak may develop around the catheter allowing dialysate to flow to the outside or infiltrate the subcutaneous tissues. The prevention of these leaks provides the rationale for the multiple types of catheter break-in techniques described in Figure 9-2.

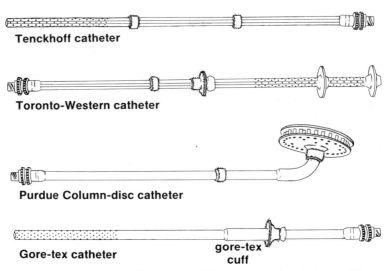

Figure 9-1. The Tenckhoff, Toronto-Western, Purdue-Column Disc, and Gore-Tex permanent peritoneal catheters.

In spite of careful placement techniques, the Tenckhoff catheter may fail to drain properly. Since it tends to float free in the peritoneal cavity, the catheter may be displaced from its dependent position, omentum may invade the catheter and obstruct the holes, or fibrin may encase the catheter and obstruct the holes. To prevent the problems caused by fibrin, heparin is added to the dialysis fluid when the catheter is being broken in, when fibrin is observed in the dialysis fluid, and when the fluid appears bloody or turbid.

Several catheters have been developed to prevent the problem of displacement and plugging by omentum. The Toronto–Western Hospital® peritoneal dialysis catheter (Accurate Surgical Instruments, Toronto, Canada) was designed by Zellerman and Oreopoulos in an effort to correct the problems of displacement, plugging, and leakage encountered with the standard Tenckhoff catheter.[9] The Toronto–Western catheter consists of a silicone rubber tube with end and side holes much like the standard Tenckhoff catheter with the following modification: Two disks spaced near the end of the catheter serve to "anchor" the tip in the desired location as well as to keep omentum and bowel away from the catheter; a Silastic button and a larger deep cuff with an enlarged flange go on either side of the peritoneum to reduce the likelihood of leaking around the catheter (Fig. 9-1). The catheter is placed surgically since the disks at the distal end of the catheter make it difficult to place percutaneously. The surgical inser-

Figure 9-2. Catheter break-in techniques.

Standard Technique
- Begin peritoneal dialysis as soon as possible after insertion of catheter.
- Dialysis to run 48 hours.
- Use 5-minute inflow, 10-minute dwell, and 15-minute outflow (2 cycles each hour).
- Heparin 500 U/liter for entire dialysis.
- Begin with 500-ml exchanges for the first 12 hours — if inadequate drainage is obtained go to 1000 ml.
- If no leak appears at the end of the first 12 hours, advance to 1000 ml (or remain at 1000 ml if starting volume was 1000 ml) for the second 12 hours.
- If no leak at the end of the second 12 hours advance to 1.5 liters.
- At the end of the third 12-hour period advance to 2-liter exchanges.
- Clear liquids for the meal following catheter insertion, then resume previous diet as tolerated.

Dry Method
- At the time of surgery attach 500-ml bag of saline with 500 units of heparin.
- When patient returns to floor flush catheter with 50-ml bolus of heparinized saline from attached bag, then flush with 50 ml of heparinized saline qid until dialysis starts.
- IPD, CAPD, or CCPD may begin 5–7 days post catheter insertion.

Irrigation Method
- At the time of catheter insertion attach bag of 500-ml normal saline with 500 units of heparin.
- Infuse entire 500 ml of heparinized saline and immediately drain.
- Patient to perform these in and out exchanges tid until start of dialysis using the same bag of heparinized saline.
- Bag should be replaced by peritoneal dialysis personnel when the outflow volume is less than 200 ml or is very turbid.
- Begin IPD, CAPD, or CCPD 5–7 days post catheter insertion.

Comment: Catheter break-in techniques are extremely variable from center to center. To a large extent they depend on local surgical techniques, nephrologists' preference, and other intangibles. There is no evidence that one technique is better than the other.

tion technique is similar to the surgical technique used with the Tenckhoff catheter.

The Purdue column-disk catheter (LIFECATH Peritoneal Implant,® Physiocontrol Corp., Redmond, Washington) designed by Ash has a single end hole and is attached to a Silastic disk which is separated from another silicone rubber disk by Silastic columns (Fig. 9-1).[10] The disk that serves as the end of the catheter is placed against the peritoneal membrane in either the midline, right or left lower quadrant below the level of the umbilicus. The outer disk serves to protect the catheter end hole from invasion by omentum and/or plugging by bowel. Since the catheter is located against the peritoneum and does not dangle free in the peritoneal cavity, it cannot be displaced. It is a double-cuff catheter that requires surgical placement because of the 5-cm-diameter disk. Great care must be taken to be sure that no material from the cuff lies intraperitoneally. Even though these catheters do not reach the most dependent part of the peritoneal cavity, they have demonstrated very good drainage characteristics. Apparently catheters do not need to be placed in the most dependent part to drain well.

The Gore-Tex® (W.L. Gore and Associates, Inc., Elkton, Md.) catheter was designed to combat problems of cuff and pericatheter infections. This catheter is a standard Tenckhoff catheter with an expanded polytetrafluoroethylene mesh sleeve and flange. This is, in essence, a single-cuff catheter with a Gore-Tex® sleeve and flange placed under the skin extending straight down toward the peritoneal cavity. This material is designed to allow better epithelialization and fibroblast ingrowth thus preventing the development of a space between two cuffs where fluid can accumulate and provide medium for bacterial growth. This catheter is still in clinical trials and may be available by the time this book is published.

The above catheters (except the column-disk catheter) come with a radiopaque stripe so that they may be visualized on abdominal films. At least two views of the abdomen should be taken when catheter position is to be determined. A catheter loop may appear as a kink or the location may be determined incorrectly unless the catheter is visualized in two planes. Additional aids used to visualize the catheter when malfunction occurs include laparoscopy and/or the pneumoperitoneogram. The laparoscopy, of course, visualizes the end of the catheter directly and may be very helpful in selecting a place for catheter insertion. The pneumoperitoneogram provides contrast to visualize the catheter by injecting air into the peritoneal cavity. This has been particularly helpful with the column-disk catheter since it is not radiopaque. Filling the catheter with radiopaque contrast medium may be helpful in delineating encasement of the catheter tip.

Troubleshooting Catheter Malfunctions

During each dialysis cycle at least the volume of dialysate infused should be returned during the first 20 minutes of starting the drain period. If this volume has not drained, the person performing the dialysis procedure frequently assumes that the small drainage volume has occurred because the outflow is slow and that allowing more time for outflow will increase the drainage volume. This is not usually true. If drainage times longer than 20 minutes are required, outflow should be observed by watching the bag or drip chamber until outflow stops. A better method of measuring the outflow is to place the drainage container on a scale. When the bag weight stops increasing, the outflow phase is clearly ended. Usually there is very little additional drainage after 20 minutes.

Two types of problems may be responsible for incomplete drainage. First, the catheter may be covered by fibrin, omentum, or bowel that acts as a one-way valve allowing normal inflow but limits the outflow. This valve effect usually stops outflow suddenly soon after outflow is initiated. Catheter obstruction usually means the catheter must be replaced. Second, the catheter tip may be out of the pool of peritoneal fluid after part of the fluid has drained. These patients can have normal drainage volumes if they have more than the standard 2-liter peritoneal fluid pool.

A helpful troubleshooting sequence when drainage volumes are low involves adding an additional 1 or 2 liters of dialysis fluid to the peritoneal cavity during the inflow phase and observing for normal drainage volumes of 2 or more liters. The "extra" fluid left in the peritoneal cavity during this one exchange usually will be removed over the duration of the dialysis. Alternatively to adding this extra 1 or 2 liters in the form of an extra inflow volume, the drainage volume may be recorded but the drain time maximum of 20 minutes strictly adhered to so that regardless of the drainage volume at 20 minutes the next inflow of 2 liters is started. Usually this will build up the required "pool" over the next several exchanges and the dialysis will proceed normally thereafter. If this procedure fails to produce normal drainage volumes, the catheter usually must be replaced. Attempts at repositioning or instrumenting peritoneal catheters are usually unsuccessful and may be dangerous unless performed by a person with experience in this area.

As with any troubleshooting procedures, the obvious should not be overlooked. Kinked lines or catheters will prevent inflow and outflow. Anyone can forget to release an inflow or outflow clamp. Some catheters have normal drainage characteristics only when the patient is in a particular position so a variety of positions should be tried before the catheter is changed.

Constipation may interfere with catheter function for unknown reasons. A strong laxative such as castor oil or Dulcolax® (Boehringer Inglheim Ltd, Ridgefield CT) may provide relief for both the constipation and the catheter malfunction. Even if the patient is not constipated, occasionally the catheter can be moved by the use of strong laxatives and frequently this is the first-line therapy for catheter malfunction.

TECHNIQUES FOR EXCHANGING DIALYSIS FLUID

Over the last 10 or 15 years, techniques for performing peritoneal dialysis have become extremely diversified. Some health professionals still consider peritoneal dialysis to be primarily for acute dialysis using hourly exchanges performed by changing glass bottles manually over a total of 36 hours. Although many centers continue to use this technique, much safer techniques are available. Peritoneal dialysis programs can now be custom designed for a particular problem in a particular setting using a variety of automated systems and a variety of exchange times. The following section describes most of the techniques used today and their clinical application. Additional details on "how to do it" can be found in the figures.

Manual Peritoneal Dialysis

Strictly speaking, manual refers to any procedure performed by hand. Manual peritoneal dialysis, however, means changing bottles hourly by hand. A sterile "Y" tubing is attached to the patient's peritoneal catheter. One arm of the "Y" terminates in a "spike" and the other arm is connected to a drainage bag. The spike is inserted through the stopper in the 2-liter glass bottle and dialysis fluid is allowed to flow into the patient by gravity. The inflow rate is controlled by the height of the bottle above the catheter tip and usually takes about 10 minutes. The fluid is allowed to "dwell" in the peritoneal cavity for 30 minutes and then drained by gravity into the drainage bag. Usually 20 minutes are allowed for the drainage or "outflow" phase although the time required is dependent on the height above the bag, catheter position, and structures surrounding the catheter tip. Drainage time should actually be about 10 minutes with the patient 1 m above the bag.

A major problem with the manual technique is the high incidence of peritonitis. Every time an old bottle is removed or a new bottle is "spiked," bacteria may be injected into the peritoneal cavity. Personnel usually treat this bottle change just like an IV bottle change. When this change must be performed hourly through the night for 36 hours or more it is easy to see that busy personnel may become lax in using aseptic technique. Adding potassium, heparin, or medications to the dialysis fluid provides other sources of possible contamination. The incidence of peritonitis is a function of the number of times the sterile system is broken. For this reason, automated systems are desirable if they are available.

CAPD

Continuous ambulatory peritoneal dialysis is a variant of the manual method that is designed primarily for chronic home maintenance dialysis. As the name indicates, the patient is being dialyzed 7 days a week, 24 hours a day, for 168 hours a week. The average patient performs 4 exchanges each day, although a few patients with more residual renal function may use 3 exchanges and a few larger patients may require 5 exchanges each day. (See Fig. 9-3 for routine dialysis orders.)

This new techinique uses dialysis fluid in plastic 2-liter bags. A single transfer set, much like an IV tubing set, connects the catheter to the bag. The patient infuses fluid by gravity, folds the bag, and carries it with him until time to drain. The patient then unfolds the same bag and drains by gravity. When the drainage phase is completed, the full bag of spent dialysate is disconnected and discarded. A fresh 2-liter bag of dialysis fluid is connected and infused.

An average complete exchange requires about 30 minutes. Inflow and outflow time each should be about 10 minutes with the patient to bag distance of 1 m and a catheter that is functioning well. Disconnecting and connecting tubing using appropriate aseptic precautions and antiseptic devices accounts for an additional 10 minutes. The patient is free to perform sedentary tasks like dictating letters or eating during the drain and inflow phases.

This system is simple and allows great flexibility. The timing of exchanges is not critical and can be adjusted to meet the individual

Figure 9-3. Routine dialysis orders—CAPD.

- Three exchanges using 1.5 percent glucose and one exchange with 4.25 percent glucose h.s. for a total of 4 exchanges daily, 7 days a week.
- Exchanges may be performed at the patient's convenience but usually before breakfast, lunch, dinner, and bed.
- Heparin 500 U/liter prn for fibrin or blood—use for 2 or 3 exchanges after last exchange fibrin or blood is observed.
- Potassium O.
- Medication O.
- Laboratory tests to be performed during clinic visits: Monthly—CBC with differential, Na, K, CL, CO_2, glucose, calcium, inorganic phosphorus, albumin, alkaline phosphatase. Before first dialysis and every 3–6 months—SGOT, SGPT, hepatitis B surface antigen.
- ECG before first dialysis, then every 6–12 months.
- X-ray: Chest (PA and lateral); skull, clavicle, and hand films for renal osteodystrophy—before first dialysis and every 6–12 months.

patient's requirements. The independence from machines reduces training time and allows considerable mobility. Companies supplying the solutions usually will ship direct to various locations for business trips or vacations if requests are made far enough in advance.

The risk of peritonitis is minimized by careful adherence to aseptic technique, continuous protection of the spike–bag junction by povodine–iodine-inpregnated wraps, and use of a special titanium connector which prevents bacterial contamination and accidental disconnection. The development of in-line filters and other new devices currently being tested should further reduce the peritonitis risk.

Semi-Automated Devices: The Cycler

This device, in essence, is a switch with a timer. As shown in Figure 9-4, bags of dialysis fluid are attached by means of an 8- or 12-armed transfer set to a single patient inflow line. The cycler then controls the amount of fluid allowed to reach the patient and the outflow time. The cycler, in addition, warms the dialysis fluid and provides information about the amount of drainage volume. It has alarms which indicate when the drainage volume is inadequate or the warming device is inoperative. These are simple, relatively inexpensive devices that can be operated by the patient alone. They have the disadvantage that multiple connections must be made, thus providing

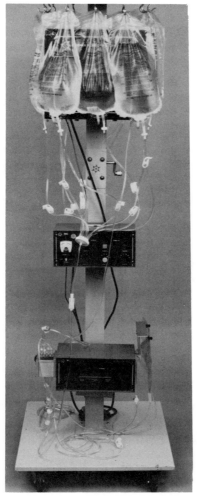

Figure 9-4. A peritoneal dialysis cycler (PDC,® Travenol Laboratory, Inc, Deerfield, IL.)

more chances of contaminating the fluid path than the completely automated technique.

The cycler has found its major use in chronic maintenance home dialysis but also provides a simple system for hospital or center acute or chronic peritoneal dialysis. The average chronic dialysis patient requires 40 hours each week, usually 10–14 hours three or four times each week during the night. Appropriate alarms are provided which wake the patient in the event of a malfunction or inadequate drainage.

It is therefore quite safe for the patient to operate by himself without a helper.

Semiautomated Techniques: CCPD

Continuous cycling peritoneal dialysis (CCPD)—in essence uses the cycler to perform CAPD. The patient is connected to the cycler each evening. The cycler performs three exchanges with 2-liter volumes of approximately 3 hours each over a total of 10 hours through the night. When the patient disconnects in the morning, he leaves an additional 2 liters of dialysis fluid in his peritoneal cavity. This serves as a 14-hour long dwell exchange. In the evening he then connects to the cycler, drains the residual fluid, and starts his nighttime long dwell exchanges. (See Fig. 9-5 for routine dialysis orders.)

CCPD seems to be very comparable to CAPD. The major advantage of CCPD is freedom from doing exchanges through the day. The major disadvantage is the loss of mobility that goes with dependence on the device. Clearance of metabolic wastes are slightly less than with CAPD, but if CCPD is used 7 days a week this difference is probably not significant for the average patient. The risks of peritonitis should be similar to CAPD because bags are used. Initial reports indicate, however, a much lower incidence of peritonitis.

Automated Systems: "The Machine"

Completely automated peritoneal dialysis devices, such as the one in Figure 9-6, are very similar to hemodialysis machines. Tap water is filtered, sterilized, and purified by reverse osmosis. The product water is then mixed with concentrated dialysis fluid by a proportioning pump

Figure 9-5. Routine dialysis orders—CCPD.

- To start dialysis connect patient to cycler using aseptic technique and drain peritoneal fluid present into cycler drain bag.
- Dialysis fluid: Night exchanges—1.5 percent glucose; day exchange—4.25 percent glucose.
- Cycle times: Night—10 minute inflow 2.5-hour dwell 20-minute outflow. When night exchange No. 3 complete, infuse 2 liters 4.25 percent glucose dialysis fluid, disconnect peritoneal catheter from cycler patient tubing, then cap catheter—all procedures with aseptic technique.
- Additives: Heparin 500 U/liter dialysis fluid if fibrin has been observed in drained dialysate. Potassium O.

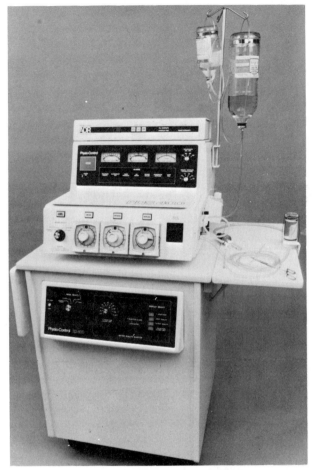

Figure 9-6. A completely automatic peritoneal dialysis machine. (PDS 400®, Physiocontrol, Redmond, Washington.)

to yield the dialysis fluid that is pumped into the patient's peritoneal cavity. The dialysis fluid is continuously monitored by a conductivity sensor with feedback to the proportioning system so that appropriate corrections are made when changes in ionic concentration occur. The fluid is warmed by the machine before entering the patient. Most peritoneal dialysis machines have a system for sounding an alarm if an appropriate volume of dialysate is not drained with each cycle. The dialysis fluid is actively pumped into the peritoneal cavity and this inflow can be controlled for inflow time, inflow rate (in ml/min), and inflow volume. Dwell time and outflow time are set by a timer and switching from inflow to dwell to outflow is accomplished automatically by the machine. Most centers use a cycle of 2 liters every 30 minutes for a total of 4 liters/h. This system is associated with a low incidence of peritonitis since the dialysis fluid path is open only at the beginning when the patient is connected and at the end of the procedure when the patient is disconnected. Since the device operates entirely automatically and has appropriate alarms to warn the patient when inflow, outflow, osmolality, heating, and water purification problems develop, the system can be used by the patient without a helper and while the patient sleeps. A major advantage of peritoneal dialysis over hemodialysis is that no sudden life-threatening events can happen—fluid shifts are relatively slow and no blood leaves the patient. (See Fig. 9-7 for routine dialysis orders.)

The automated system should be the safest and most economical of the various peritoneal dialysis techniques. It is the safest because it has the fewest interruptions in the sterile path. This is reflected in the very low rates of peritonitis reported by most centers using automated systems. It has the lowest maintenance cost since it uses the least amount of disposable items when compared with the cycler, CCPD, or CAPD. The cost of the machine is considerably greater than the cycler, however. Even though it provides more efficient dialysis than any of

Figure 9-7. Routine dialysis orders—automated IPD.

- Dialysis fluid concentrate 30 percent to make 1.5 percent glucose dialysis fluid, potassium 0, heparin 20,000 U/2 liters of concentrate to make 500 U/liter dialysis fluid (Heparin is optional unless fibrin strands are observed in dialysate).
- Two-liter exchanges with a 5-minute inflow, 10-minute dwell, and 15-minute outflow for a total cycle time of 30 minutes.
- Dialysis to run 20 hours. (This time is dictated by the clinical setting. If it is a routine outpatient dialysis standard, options would be 20 hours twice a week or 40 hours once a week—acute peritoneal dialysis would usually be 36–48 hours for the first dialysis.)
- Predialysis lab work: (Weekly for center- or monthly for home-dialysis patients) CBC with differential, BUN, creatinine, Na, K, Cl, CO_2, glucose, calcium, inorganic phosphorus. Monthly—Alkaline phosphatase, total protein, albumin. Before first dialysis then every 3–6 months—SGOT, SGPT, and hepatitis B surface antigen.
- ECG before first dialysis, then every 6–12 months.
- X-ray: Chest (PA and lateral); skull, clavicle, and hand films for renal osteodystrophy—before first dialysis and every 6–12 months.

the other peritoneal dialysis systems it unfortunately provides the least amount of total dialysis because it is only performed 40 hours each week. The time factor more than compensates for the decreased efficiency of the CAPD and CCPD systems. As shown in Table 9-1, the total weekly clearances of CAPD are clearly greatest, followed closely by CCPD. Hemodialysis clearances are included for reference purposes. Clearances will of course vary from patient to patient and the figures in the table represent approximate values calculated using published clearance figures for the various dialysis techniques.

THE DIALYSIS FLUID

The major composition difference between fluid used for peritoneal dialysis and that used for hemodialysis lies in the glucose concentration. The peritoneal dialysis system depends on the generation of osmotic pressure to produce ultrafiltrate whereas the hemodialysis system induces ultrafiltration by increasing hydraulic pressure within the blood path ("positive pressure") or by decreasing the pressure around the blood path in the dialysis fluid ("negative pressure"). Increasing the peritoneal dialysis fluid glucose concentration increases the concentration of osmotically active particles which in turn increases the ultrafiltration rate and volume of ultrafiltrate formed. The manual dialysis systems and the semiautomated systems use fluid prepared in its final form. The glucose concentration is fixed by the manufacturers and in the United States is available as 1.5, 2.5, and 4.25 percent glucose.

Glucose is added to the solution as hydrated glucose. The glucose concentration in the dialysate as measured by current analytical techniques is therefore lower than the concentration indicated on the label. The difference between the hydrated glucose and the anhydrous glucose is so small, however, that it is not clinically important.

To prevent the glucose from carmelizing during sterilization, the pH of the dialysis fluid is usually lowered to about 5.5. This results in a relatively acid solution but the pH is rapidly corrected to physiologic pH within the peritoneal cavity. The low pH has been occasionally associated with discomfort at the beginning of dialysis so that sodium bicarbonate or sodium hydroxide must be added to the dialysis fluid to produce physiologic pH before infusion.

Although some peritoneal dialysis solutions still have a sodium concentration of 140 mEq/liter, for most dialysis procedures the sodium concentration should be between 130 and 132 mEq/liter. The

Table 9-1
Comparative Clearances in Liters/Week

Solute	MW	Human Kidney	HD	IPD	CAPD	CCPD
Urea	60	750	135	60	70	67
Creatinine	113	1200	90	28	60	58
B_{12}	352	1000	30	16	50	45
Insulin	5500	1000	5	12	30	27

MW—molecular weight.
Human kidney—normal clearance with a GFR of 100 ml/min.
HD—hemodialysis (12 hours/week).
IPD—intermittent peritoneal dialysis (40 hours/week, two exchanges/hour).
CAPD—(four 2-liter exchanges each day, average drainage of 2.5 liters).
CCPD—(four 2-liter exchanges each day).

relatively low sodium concentration was formulated because the high glucose in the dialysate generates a hyponatric ultrafiltrate.[11] Removing more water than sodium can produce hypernatremia in the patient and the lower dialysate sodium concentrations offset this problem.

No potassium is added to peritoneal dialysis fluid by the manufacturer. Any potassium must be added prior to infusion and the amount added depends on the clinical situation. Most patients do not need potassium added to the dialysis fluid.

The commonly used calcium concentration of 3.5 mEq/liter in peritoneal dialysis fluid is designed to promote positive calcium balance. This concentration is equal to 7 mg/100 ml and is usually above the ionized calcium concentration in the plasma. The gradient therefore favors calcium diffusion into the patient from the dialysis fluid which is usually desirable (Chapter 1).

The buffer used in the peritoneal dialysis system is either lactate or acetate. As in the hemodialysis system, these molecules are converted to bicarbonate in the liver. Although acetate has been associated with a decrease in myocardial contractility and decreased vascular resistance, the acetate load in peritoneal dialysis is not great enough to cause significant clinical problems. Some patients report diffuse abdominal discomfort with acetate but not lactate dialysis solutions. The concentration of acetate or lactate in dialysis fluid is usually 35 mEq/liter but some patients require more bicarbonate-generating molecules to maintain normal plasma bicarbonate.

The usual concentration of magnesium in peritoneal dialysate is 1.5 mEq/liter. Similar to hemodialysis dialysate this was developed empirically with little investigation into the effects of different magnesium concentrations. Recently CAPD fluid containing magnesium 0.5 mEq/liter and lactate 40 mEq/liter has become available. This magnesium concentration is 1 mEq/liter less than standard solutions. It is designed to be used in patients with high serum magnesium concentrations or patients who do not tolerate aluminum hydroxide as a phosphate binder. With this new solution, patients can be given oral phosphate binders which are a combination of magnesium and aluminum hydroxide. The magnesium that is absorbed from the oral magnesium hydroxide is removed by the low magnesium dialysis fluid. Serum magnesium concentrations should be followed carefully, however, if magnesium-containing compounds are prescribed. The low magnesium solution also has a lactate concentration of 40 mEq/liter. The increased buffer concentration should be used in patients who fail to maintain midrange normal bicarbonate. This theoretically should help maintain normal bone mineralization. In the future dialysis fluid with varying concentrations of the different constituents will become available so that individualized treatment can be prescribed.

For CAPD, bags of dialysis solutions are available in 0.5, 1.0, 1.5, 2.0, and 3.0 liter size. Specifically for the cycler, 2.0, 3.0, and 4.0 liter bags are used. Dialysis fluid is available in a concentrated form for the automated systems. The concentrate is prepared with either 30 or 50 percent dextrose. The proportioning pumps of the machine mix the concentrate with water to supply the patient with a glucose concentration of 1.5 or 2.5 percent, respectively. In most automated peritoneal dialysis systems additional glucose can be added to the concentrate to increase the final glucose concentration up to 5 percent.

No solutes should be added to the dialysis fluid unless prescribed by the physician. If heparin, potassium, or antibiotics are needed they must be added under strict aseptic conditions. Any time the sterile system is violated the danger of inducing peritonitis exists.

Whether the dialysis fluid is contained in bottles or plastic bags, extreme care must be used in connecting the container to the peritoneal dialysis system. The major cause of peritonitis in peritoneal dialysis patients is contamination of the fluid path during the time the containers are changed. If bottle or bag changes are being performed for intermittent dialysis rather than using automated techniques, personnel must be specially trained and special precautions must be used each time a container is connected or disconnected.

THE PATIENT

There is only a single absolute contraindication to peritoneal dialysis—the inability to perform peritoneal dialysis. This rare occurrence is usually caused by the presence of adhesions or intraabdominal surgery that has interrupted the continuity of the peritoneal cavity; i.e., the space available for the instillation of dialysate or the surface area of the peritoneal membrane has been too severely limited to allow instillation of fluid for adequate dialysis. Even more unusual is the formation of peritoneal membrane fibrosis that decreases membrane permeability even though membrane surface may be adequate. For these reasons, a careful history and physical examination of the patient is extremely important. A history of significant abdominal surgical procedures, trauma, or infection may indicate potential problems in peritoneal dialysis. However, in reality, the number of times a patient's peritoneal dialysis career is limited by previous surgery, injury, or infection is very small. In spite of the presence of abdominal scars, most nephrologists will go ahead with a therapeutic trial of peritoneal dialysis.

A simple procedure can be performed to determine whether the patient's peritoneal membrane area and permeability are adequate. Two liters of dialysis solution is infused into the abdominal cavity using a large-gauge needle or intravenous plastic catheter and allowed to dwell for 4 hours. If the patient's peritoneal cavity is capable of holding the 2 liters comfortably, limitation of peritoneal membrane surface area will not be a problem. Permeability should be normal if the dialysate to plasma creatinine ratio at 4 hours is greater than 0.75 and usually patients will be acceptable candidates if the ratio is between 0.50 and 0.75.[12]

Many relative contraindications to peritoneal dialysis exist. These include the presence of recent abdominal surgery with the presence of ostomies (i.e., colostomy, nephrostomy, ureterostomy), the presence of multiple abdominal scars, or the history of significant previous intraabdominal infection. Patients with large muscle mass have been selectively shifted to hemodialysis because most nephrologists feel that the greater efficiency of the procedures offers them better dialysis.

Many patients with these relative contraindications may in fact be successfully dialyzed using peritoneal dialysis. The decision of what mode of dialysis to use frequently rests on the patient's other problems, i.e., cardiovascular, hemodynamic, and the availability of vascular access. It is possible to peritoneally dialyze a patient in spite of the presence of abdominal drains.

Patients with bacterial peritonitis can be started or continued on peritoneal dialysis. At one time peritoneal lavage, which is in essence peritoneal dialysis, was advocated for the treatment of severe peritoneal infection. The infections that generally require catheter removal or preclude catheter placement are fungal peritonitis and tuberculous peritonitis. These patients should be carried on hemodialysis until infections are cleared.

What patients are generally considered primary candidates for peritoneal dialysis? Patients with no vessels available for hemodialysis access, of course, head the list. Next are those patients who are hemodynamically unstable during hemodialysis as indicated by difficulty in controlling hypotension, angina, or other disconcerting symptoms. Specific problems that may become worse with hypotension or heparin, like recent myocardial infarction or stroke, may be an indication for peritoneal dialysis over hemodialysis. Diabetics have been selectively placed in the past on peritoneal dialysis, especially those patients with diabetic retinopathy. The rationale was that patients with a potential for retinal hemorrhage would have fewer problems if they were not treated with systemic heparin. Information available in this literature is conflicting. Several centers performing comparative studies support peritoneal over hemodialysis[13,14] but vision can be preserved in diabetic patients on hemodialysis.[15] The long dwell exchanges in CAPD serve as a good insulin delivery system and some diabetics may go to CAPD as a means of providing good blood glucose control.

Patients must maintain good nutrition since they lose protein and amino acids in the dialysate—a problem not encountered with hemodialysis. Patients with a low protein intake, especially alcoholics, must therefore be watched carefully since they may "fail to thrive" on peritoneal dialysis. Patients with a large muscle mass or those who are hypercatabolic may require hemodialysis, particularly for acute dialysis. These patients have a rapidly rising BUN and creatinine and are frequently hyperkalemic and acidotic. As a rule, patients whose BUN rises more than 50 mg/dl/day or whose creatinine increases more than 5 mg/dl/day should be followed carefully since they may require hemodialysis to keep up with their metabolic requirements. Many "hypercatabolic" patients have been successfully dialyzed, however, using peritoneal dialysis by increasing the frequency and duration of dialysis.[16] Clinical judgment should dictate whether the patient is tried on peritoneal dialysis or goes direct to hemodialysis. The patient who needs emergency treatment for hyperkalemia probably will do better on hemodialysis since it is considerably more efficient for potassium removal. Even considering the relatively low efficiency of potassium removal by peritoneal dialysis, patients whose hyperkalemia can be anticipated may be managed fairly well if peritoneal dialysis is started early. Patients with pulmonary edema or significant volume overload can be managed quite well using peritoneal dialysis.

Patients with marked impairment of pulmonary function in the past have been considered primarily for hemodialysis since theoretically the presence of intraabdominal fluid may compromise respiratory function. Only patients with marked impairment of pulmonary function will in fact have problems with the presence of dialysate in the range of 2–3 liters. This volume produces relatively small change (on the order of a few hundred milliliters) of total lung capacity.[17,18] Even patients with severe pulmonary dysfunction can therefore be managed successfully—even if this means that smaller volumes of dialysis fluid must be used. With modern techniques, small volume and relatively short exchange periods may be used to achieve the same amount of dialysis as more conventional techniques. Some patients with severe lung disease and heart failure may prefer CAPD since the steady-state dialysis may allow greater dietary freedom with better volume control than is possible on hemodialysis.

There is no evidence thus far to indicate that intraabdominal fluid is harmful to patients with serious lower extremity vascular disease. There is very little information, however, in this area and patients with peripheral vascular disease should be observed carefully for the development of decreased blood flow to the lower extremities. These patients, unfortunately, are exactly the ones that are likely to have no vascular access and cannot go to hemodialysis.

The presence of abdominal wall or inguinal hernias should be taken into consideration when arranging for peritoneal dialysis. Although it is doubtful that peritoneal dialysis by itself causes hernias, it certainly will demonstrate the presence of these defects. Hernias should therefore be repaired, if possible, before the patient is placed on peritoneal dialysis. The patient may be dialyzed acutely using peritoneal dialysis and then at a later time have the hernias repaired. Usually this requires that the patient not be dialyzed peritoneally for a period of time that varies from a few days to 3–4 weeks depending on the size and location and the preferences of the surgeon performing the procedure. Hemodialysis via subclavian or femoral vein catheters can be used in most cases to carry the patient until he can return to peritoneal dialysis.

Certain coexisting diseases may cause problems with peritoneal dialysis. Patients with large intraabdominal masses such as large polycystic kidneys occasionally may experience some discomfort during peritoneal dialysis because of the additional volume within the abdomen. Most patients will adjust to the volume without much difficulty and this is an unusual reason for peritoneal dialysis to fail. Patients whose appetites are already impaired may complain of further decrease in appetite because of the full feeling during peritoneal dialysis. Patients with a hiatus hernia may develop symptoms during inflow or when their intraabdominal volume is largest. Patients have solved these problems by eating with their peritoneal cavity empty. Smaller volume exchanges may also alleviate the problem—providing the patient receives adequate dialysis.

The lifestyle of the patient must be considered when selecting peritoneal dialysis. Patients who are swimmers or do vigorous physical activity may wish to try hemodialysis preferentially. The risk of infection may be greater if the patient submerses his peritoneal catheter for any length of time, especially in water that may be contaminated with organisms of uncertain pathogenicity. Some peritoneal dialysis centers, however, have not discouraged patients who want to continue swimming or heavy physical activity. Techniques are available for minimizing the risks of infection during swimming. The simplest of these techniques is to allow the patient to swim without modifying his CAPD procedure until he is out of the water. The assumption is that the spike–bag junction and the catheter-tubing connector are water and bacteria tight. Therefore the patient can enter the water without any special precautions. When he leaves the water he wraps the spike–bag junction with a fresh sterile sponge impregnated with providone–iodine and leaves the wrap in place for 1 hour before changing bags. This should kill bacteria on the spike and spike port that were picked up during the swim. The patient then performs the bag change using standard techniques. A second technique requires that the catheter be disconnected, capped, and secured under an ostomy device so that it is not exposed to water. This requires extensive disconnect and reconnect procedures. A third method consists of wrapping the catheter and bag in a plastic bag then securing the mouth of the bag around the catheter with tape so that it can be submerged without wetting the spike–bag junction. All of these techniques have been used successfully by patients.

Not much information is available about patients who would like to return to heavy manual labor since very few on either hemodialysis or peritoneal dialysis do. Patients may be allowed to carefully increase activity until the desired level is achieved or until definite indications suggest curtailing physical activity.

Patients with major concerns about body image may have some problems with the peritoneal dialysis catheter or the catheter and bag system used for CAPD. Patients who have gone on to try the system have generally discovered that these changes in body image really are not a problem. Many, especially younger patients, will select hemodialysis, however, because of the concern for peritoneal catheter presence in the abdominal wall. Because this is a sensitive subject, great care should be taken to select a catheter site that interferes as little as possible with appearance, clothing, and sexual activity.

NUTRITION

Peritoneal dialysis patients face several problems that are not seen in patients on hemodialysis. Patients on CAPD may in fact require dietary manipulations that seem contrary to standard teaching for the therapy of end-stage renal disease. Patients on peritoneal dialysis lose protein with the dialysate. These losses have been estimated at $6-8$

g/day for CAPD patients and 10–15 g/day for intermittent peritoneal dialysis patients. Most diets are therefore arranged to compensate for these losses by including more protein than is usually recommended for hemodialysis patients. It must be kept in mind, however, that many nephrologists no longer recommend significant protein restriction in hemodialysis. Most patients do tend to "autoregulate" their protein intake depending on "how well dialyzed" they are and other even less well-defined factors. Protein also supplies a large part of the potassium, phosphorus, and hydrogen ion intake and this may be an additional reason for limiting protein intake aside from the obvious increase in BUN seen with a large protein intake. For reasons not fully understood CAPD patients may have low serum potassium concentrations and require potassium supplementation. Peritoneal dialysis patient are subject to a significant glucose load during their dialysis. This may be helpful to those patients who begin with calorie malnutrition but is a serious problem to those patients who already have more than a normal amount of body fat. The glucose provides, in addition, a stimulus for elevation of plasma triglycerides. The long-term significance of hypertriglyceridemia, which is sometimes seen in CAPD patients, remains to be evaluated.

As with hemodialysis, the peritoneal dialysis system is an aqueous medium and water soluble vitamins are removed. Water soluble vitamins must therefore be replaced as well as those vitamins which serve for cofactors in systems that may have reduced activity in uremic patients.

Since the ultimate goal is to provide the patient with the program that will lead him to the best possible state of health, the dietary program must be individualized so that the diet is optimal for each patient. Equally important, the patient must be able to follow the diet—the diet must be realistic. It is usually better to institute dialysis before imposing significant restriction of protein.

In the following discussion, all dietary requirements are expressed in terms of "ideal body weight," which in this context means body weight for an age-, sex-, and height-matched normal individual.[19] If the patient is overweight, his or her dietary requirements therefore will be adjusted to prevent any increase in body weight. If the patient is below the ideal body weight, he or she diet will automatically be corrected to increase his weight.

Calories

During peritoneal dialysis, patients absorb significant amounts of glucose. This will be most important in the CAPD patients because their glucose absorption is continuous. CAPD patients generally require a dietary intake of 25–30 kcal/kg body weight for maintenance and 35–50 kcal/kg to replete the malnourished patients. Recommendations for the IPD patients are 35 kcal/kg body weight for "normals" and 50 kcal/kg for patients who are malnourished. The dialysis program must be arranged so that the patient's glucose absorption is consistent with his energy requirements. Patients who are obese should be cautioned to be careful of their sodium and water intake so that they require fewer exchanges with high glucose concentrations that result in greater glucose absorption. One way of increasing the caloric intake of the patient who is thin is to increase his sodium and water intake so that he requires more exchanges with high glucose concentration thereby increasing his calorie intake.

Protein

Current evidence suggests that peritoneal patients are in nitrogen balance when they take in between 0.8 and 1.2 g of protein/kg body weight each day. A daily protein intake of 1.2 g/kg should therefore maintain nitrogen balance. Protein intake should be increased to 1.4 or 1.5 g/kg each day for those patients who are protein malnourished.

Protein intake may be evaluated using two methods. First, increasing serum albumin will generally reflect positive nitrogen balance while a falling serum albumin indicates negative nitrogen balance. The physician must be careful to consider the presence of other factors when observing serum albumin, such as the presence of peritonitis or other infections that may make the patient abruptly and catastrophically catabolic. In the absence of these mitigating circumstances, the albumin concentrations are useful for follow-up. Second, the serum urea nitrogen may be helpful. Very low BUN concentrations (below 30 or 40 mg/dl) suggest low protein intake. Normal (60–100 mg/dl) or high (greater than 100 mg/dl) serum urea concentrations may indicate adequate protein intake. Marginal protein intake in a patient who is "underdialyzed," may also result in normal or elevated BUN. Those patients "autoregulate" their protein intake to maintain hemeostasis. They may decrease their protein intake due to the underdialysis with the result that their BUN appears normal. Protein intake can be evaluated by urea kinetics, similar to hemodialysis (Chaper 4). In this case, however, the total daily urea removal in the dialysate needs to be added to urinary urine urea excretion.

Vitamins and Minerals

Current evidence indicates that the daily administration of the currently recommended daily allowance of water soluble vitamins to peritoneal dialysis patients will make up for the dialysis losses of these vitamins. These patients also require ascorbic acid 100 mg daily, folic acid 1 mg daily, and pyridoxine 5 or 10 mg daily.

Calcium and Vitamin D

The objectives of calcium and vitamin D therapy are to prevent or treat renal osteodystrophy by promoting bone mineralization and suppressing parathormone release. Patients on intermittent peritoneal dialysis require calcium supplementation even though calcium is present in the dialysis fluid. Current recommendations include at least 1–1.5 g of elemental calcium each day. Many centers suggest prescribing vitamin D in addition to calcium supplementation. This should be in the form of the most active vitamin D metabolite 1, 25-D3 (Calcitriol) starting at 0.25 mcg and increasing gradually while carefully following serum calcium concentrations. An alternative is starting with the vitamin D analog dihydrotachysterol 125 mcg/day and increasing cautiously while following the plasma calcium concentrations until the desired levels of calcium are observed.

Great caution must be used when calcium and vitamin D are employed together. Before using vitamin D, the patient's serum phosphorus concentration should be in the normal range to prevent the metastatic calcification which may be seen with sudden increase in serum calcium. As a rule if the calcium in mg/dl × phosphorus in mg/dl equals or exceeds 70 the risk of metastatic calcification is high.

Calcium and vitamin D supplements in CAPD patients are somewhat controversial. Patients on CAPD are being continuously dialyzed against a calcium concentration of 3.5 mEq/l which should place them in a continuous positive calcium balance. While anecdotal information suggests that standard calcium supplements may cause hypercalcemia in CAPD patients, a recent study indicates that most CAPD patients are in slightly negative calcium balance.[20] Calcium and vitamin D supplementation in CAPD patients must therefore be performed with careful monitoring.

Phosphorus

Hyperphosphatemia causes bone disease by lowering serum-ionized calcium which stimulates parathormone release (Chapter 1). To help maintain normal serum phosphorus, aluminum hydroxide or aluminum carbonate should be used to prevent intestinal phosphorus absorption. This may be given in the form of suspension, capsule or tablet—whichever suits the patient best. The dose is given when the phosphorus load is taken. A standard starting dose might consist of 1 or 2 capsules, 3–4 times daily, taken with meals, snacks, and before bed. If serum phosphorus is high (more than 7–8 mg/dl) weekly follow-up and dose adjustment, as well as dietary counseling, is required. Serum phosphorus should then be followed monthly.

Most centers report that CAPD patients have a decreased requirement for phosphate binding agents and tolerate a more liberal dietary phosphorus intake than intermittent peritoneal or hemodialysis patients. At the beginning of CAPD treatments, however, the patient should be counseled in the use of a low phosphorus (i.e., 800 mg/day) diet and given phosphate binders. This can be liberalized, if appropriate, at a later time. It is much more difficult to persuade the patient to restrict his diet if he starts with no restriction. The average CAPD patient needs phosphate binders.

Potassium

Potassium intake is largely determined by protein intake and it is difficult to reduce potassium intake below 75–90 mEq/day when peritoneal dialysis patients require 1.2 g of protein/kg/day. Serious hyperkalemia is relatively unusual in the chronic peritoneal dialysis patient. It occurs most frequently during seasons when fresh fruits and vegetables high in potassium are available. The patient, with or without the aid of a dietition, can usually identify the indiscretion responsible. Symptoms of weakness or paralysis signal the need for serum potassium measurement.

A small percent of patients will be in negative potassium balance (i.e., they will lose more potassium than they take in). Symptoms are much the same as those caused by hyperkalemia. Hypokalemia is not as life-threatening as hyperkalemia unless the patient is taking a digitalis preparation. This negative potassium balance is much more common in CAPD than in IPD. These patients will probably need potassium supplements. Hypokalemic CAPD patients should receive the potassium in the form of potassium chloride elixir or slow-release wax matrix capsule form. Potassium is usually not added to the CAPD solutions because this requires an extra break in the sterile system that may result in the development of peritonitis. Increasing dietary potassium to increase serum and total body potassium may be difficult and sometimes expensive since the patient must eat quite a few bananas or a significantly larger amount of animal protein. Careful review of the individual's problem by the renal dietitian and the physician will help formulate the most appropriate treatment. IPD patients may have potassium added to the dialysis fluid with little risk of bacterial contamination since this can be done as a single injection at the beginning of the dialysis procedure.

Hyperalimentation

The seriously ill or anorexic patient will require aggressive nutritional therapy to prevent the negative nitrogen balance that rapidly follows decreased protein and calorie intake. Continuous ambulatory peritoneal dialysis is well suited to the management of fluid volumes required to maintain adequate nutrition by either parenteral or enteral hyperalimentation. During intercurrent illness, patients require even more attention to dietary therapy since they may be very catabolic. Protein losses increase dramatically during peritonitis. Although drainage volumes tend to decrease during peritonitis in CAPD and IPD patients, increased nutritional requirements can still be met and adequate ultrafiltration achieved if the program is individualized to the specific patient's changing status.

Miscellaneous

Great care should be taken when selecting vitamin preparations and alternate food sources to ensure that they do not contain substances that are dangerous and not well dialyzed. As an example, many vitamin preparations contain magnesium and other trace metals that may not be good for the dialysis patient.

Insulin

Many centers are now administering insulin intraperitoneally during IPD and CAPD treatments for patients with diabetes mellitus. This generally provides a very convenient and smooth method of controlling blood glucose. There was initial reticence toward adding insulin to peritoneal dialysis solutions because of the risk of causing peritonitis as well as uncertainty about insulin absorption, adsorption by plastic bags, tubing, and the peritoneal membrane. The empiric use of intraperitoneal insulin has led to the clinical assessment that it is a reasonable form of therapy. The incidence of peritonitis in diabetics using intraperitoneal insulin is no greater than incidence in diabetics using subcutaneous insulin or in nondiabetic CAPD patients.[2] Because of insulin losses within the system most patients require two or three times their usual daily insulin dose.

A simple method of calculating the dose of insulin for CAPD is to first average the total daily insulin doses used on the several days preceding conversion to IP insulin. Next multiply the mean dose by three and divide this dose by the number of exchanges each day. The result is an estimate of the number of units of regular insulin to be added to each bag of dialysis fluid. Only regular insulin should be used intraperitoneally. More complicated programs are available for calculating insulin doses.[22,23] As in the management of any insulin program careful monitoring and dose adjustment are required to determine the appropriate dose.

Some clinical observations suggest that the patient will initially need larger amounts of insulin than after he is settled into a stable routine. This may be caused by the presence of insulin receptors on the peritoneal membrane that must be saturated before transperitoneal absorption of insulin is at a steady rate. Since insulin requirements may decrease after the first several days on intraperitoneal insulin, careful monitoring is very important. Patients can be monitored at home using one of the several glucose measuring devices available for home use with blood obtained from a "finger stick." Using intraperitoneal insulin and home glucose measuring devices, blood sugars in diabetic CAPD patients can be maintained with the normal range a large percent of the time.

PROBLEMS

Peritonitis

The major problem with peritoneal dialysis today is still peritonitis. The risk is very low in the intermittent peritoneal dialysis system using a machine. Using the semiautomated devices (cyclers) the risk is greater and in the CAPD system the risk is greatest. There is such a good correlation in fact between the number of times the sterile path is broken and the occurrence of peritonitis that statistics from the National CAPD Registry recently revealed that there is even a difference in incidence of peritonitis among CAPD groups doing three, four and five exchanges daily. Every attempt should therefore be made to maintain the integrity of the sterile pathway. When the sterile path is to be interrupted, the risk of injecting bacteria can be minimized by very careful handling of the components as well as pretreatment of medication ports and spike with betadine. To be effective medication ports must be soaked in povidone–iodine for at least 5 minutes before use. This may be accomplished by simply placing a drop of povidine–iodine on the port and letting it sit for 5 minutes before injecting the medication. The medication bottle must be treated in the same fashion unless the stopper is sterile. A simple wipe with alrohol or povidine–idodine is not acceptable pretreatment. Under certain circumstances povidone–iodine may not be sterile.[24] Careful surveillance of technique and infection statistics is extremely important. Only specially trained personnel should handle sterile components of the dialysis system or the dialysis catheter—this usually excludes physicians.

Organisms

Gram-positive organisms continue to account for about 70 percent of peritoneal infections. Two-thirds of gram-positive peritonitis will be caused by *Staphylococcus epidermidis* and about one-third will be *S. aureus*.[25] About 20 percent of peritonitis will be gram-negative organisms, which include *Pseudomonas, Enterobacteriaceae,* and *Acinetobacter* and less than 5 percent are caused by fungi—the most common of which are *Candida* species.

Catheter

Tunnel and exit infections are usually *S. epidermidis* or *S. aureus*.

Diagnosis

Peritonitis in CAPD patients is associated with (1) cloudy dialysate, (2) greater than 100 white blood cells for each microliter of dialysate, (3) greater than 50 percent of the white blood cells are neutrophils, (4) abdominal discomfort and peritoneal signs, and (5) a "flu-like" syndrome (nausea, vomiting, and fever). Under normal circumstances the patient makes his own diagnosis by observing the cloudy character of the dialysate during the drain period, hopefully, before symptoms or signs develop.

The diagnosis of peritonitis in patients on intermittent peritoneal dialysis is not quite so clear-cut. Cloudy dialysate and appearance of abdominal discomfort up to and including peritoneal signs are helpful.

Because of variable interdialytic periods and intraabdominal fluid volume present, the cell count is not so helpful as in CAPD. Counts of 100 and certainly those greater than 350 cells/μl are suggestive of peritonitis—especially if more than 50 percent are neutrophilis. If the fluid is turbid or any reason exists to suspect peritonitis, a cell count and differential should be performed on a sample of the dialysate. At the same time a sample should be sent for culture and an additional sample spun down for a gram stain.

Since the peritoneal fluid volume is relatively large, the concentration of organisms in bacteria for each milliliter may be relatively small. About 5 percent of uncentrifuged samples of peritoneal fluid from patients with peritonitis reveal organisms whereas the centrifuged sample will disclose organisms over 50 percent of the time. Since the concentration of organisms may be relatively low (i.e., on the order of 10–100 colonies/ml dialysate), large volumes of dialysate should be sampled. This may be done by filtering a large volume, perhaps 100 ml, through a Falcon 7102 Filter® (Becton-Dickinson, Cockeysville, Maryland) or equivalent and planting the filter on blood agar culture medium. This gives a colony count as well as helping in identifying the organism. Alternatively, 5–8 ml of dialysate may be injected into two blood culture bottles. This does not give quantitative results but gives a large enough volume so that organisms are likely to be identified if they are present. Using these large volume culture techniques, the incidence of "sterile peritonitis" has been virtually eliminated.

Treatment

Every effort should be made to diagnose peritonitis and treat the patient as quickly as possible. (See Fig. 9-8 for orders for suspected peritonitis.) For patients on home intermittent peritoneal dialysis or CAPD, the time interval from the onset of symptoms or cloudy dialysate until treatment starts should be no longer than 3–4 hours. If the diagnosis is in question or will be delayed, it is best to treat as though the patient has peritonitis.

For CAPD, tobramycin and cephalosporin may be mixed with heparin in the dialysate even though some pharmacy manuals indicate that these are incompatible. Good studies indicate that with the concentrations used in CAPD, the effectiveness of the individual drugs is not impaired by mixing in standard dialysis fluids.[27] The higher concentrations used when drugs are mixed in dialysis fluid concentrate have not been well studied and should be observed for the formation of precipitate if this method is chosen. Of course, whenever precipitate is

Figure 9-8. Orders for suspected peritonitis.

- Dialysate cell count with differential.
- Dialysate culture for aerobic organisms—"filter culture" with 100 ml of dialysate and/or innoculate two aerobic blood culture bottles with 5–8 ml dialysate in each bottle.
- Gram strain on sediment from centrifuged 10- to 12-ml sample of dialysate.
- If the cell count on uncentrifuged sample is greater than 100 cells/μl with greater than 50 percent neutrophils and no organism seen on gram stain, the following treatment regimen may be used.
  CAPD:
  1. One to three "in and out exchanges" to establish catheter patency and clear fluid, then
  2. Cephalosporin 125 mg/liter (250 ml/2 liter bag) for 4 days then change to cephalosporin 250 mg p.o. qid for 6 days to give a total of 10 days treatment.
  3. Heparin 500 U/liter (1000 U/2-liter bag) until dialysate has been clear for 3 exchanges, then discontinue heparin.
  4. During treatment use patient's usual number of exchanges each day.

  Comment: The patient may go home if he is relatively comfortable and the physician and nurse feel that this is safe. Allowing the patient to return home can only be successful if there is good follow-up. The nurse or the physician should check with the patient in 12–24 hours to determine whether he has improved. Patients who fail to improve in 12–24 hours or who get worse should be admitted to the hospital as soon as possible.

  IPD:
  1. Cephalosporin 250 mg p.o. *qid* or 1 g IM or IV daily for 14 days.
  2. Cephalosporin 50 mg/liter of dialysate during each dialysis.
  3. Heparin 500 U/liter.
  4. Potassium O.
  5. Begin dialysis with 3 in and out exchanges then go to 2-liter exchanges with 10-minute inflow, 30-minute dwell, and 20-minute outflow. *Comment:* Patients should require little or no medication for pain. They usually feel better fairly quickly after the in and out exchanges and rarely are uncomfortable enough to require narcotics.
  6. Continue regular outpatient dialysis schedule unless patient evaluation indicates hospital admission.
- If gram-negative organisms are seen the cephalosporin may be replaced by an IV loading dose of tobramycin 1.7 or 2.0 mg/kg and 5 mg/liter of dialysate.
- If both gram-negative and gram-positive organisms have been seen or there is a high suspicion that this is a mixed infection, cephalosporin and tobramycin may be used together. Tobramycin may be given IM or IV and cephalosporin intraperitoneally.

observed the solution should be discarded and another technique should be used. Aminoglycoside doses should be followed carefully by determining serum concentrations since permanent vestibular and ototoxicity can result from standard doses of these drugs.

Treatment is dictated primarily by the results of the gram stain. if no organisms are seen, statistically the organism will be a gram-positive coccus and treatment is started with one of the cephalosporins. If the patient is on CAPD, 250 mg of cephalosporin for each bag (125 mg/liter) is added to each exchange. Several rapid exchanges without antibiotic should first be performed "in and out" just to ensure that the fluid is not so turbid that it will plug up the catheter. Then the patient goes back to the regular 4 exchanges each day. Heparin 500 U/liter should also be added until the dialysate clears to prevent obstruction of the catheter by fibrin. CAPD patients are usually treated for 4 to 5 days with intraperitoneal antibiotics and then changed to oral cephalosporin 250 mg qid to complete a 10-day course.

The protocol for IPD is somewhat different. The patient is usually given a cephalosporin 250 mg qid by mouth or 1 g IV in addition to cephalosporin 50 mg/liter of dialysis fluid. IPD patients are usually treated for 14–21 days with oral cephalosporin 250 mg qid between dialysis treatments. Both intraperitoneal and oral cephalosporins are used during each treatment period.

If the organism is found to be gram negative, tobramycin, gentamycin, or one of the third-generation cephalosporins such a moxalactam or cephotaxime may be used. Although gentamycin has the advantage of low cost, most centers prefer tobramycin because of its lower oto and vestibular toxicity. Moxolactam is an excellent drug but is quite expensive, especially in the amount that must be used for intraperitoneal treatment.

The patient may receive a standard loading dose of aminoglycosides either IV, IM, or IP. If this loading dose is administered intraperitoneally, it should be given during the first long dwell exchange. Each long dwell exchange should have 5–8 mg/liter of the antibiotic to maintain plasma concentrations of about 4 μg/ml.

Dosage schedules for moxolactam or its analogs are not yet fully developed for dialysis. Current recommendations are, however, a single 1-g IV loading dose followed by 100 mg/liter of dialysis fluid. Third-generation cephalosporins have advantages for patients in unusual locations who have difficulty reaching a lab or a physician. Virtually all the organisms that are serious pathogens are killed by these antibiotics. Most experts still feel, however, that *Pseudomonas* requires more than these cephalosporins and cultures still must be obtained if at all possible.

Peritonitis symptoms and cloudy fluid should resolve rapidly—usually within 12–24 hours. If the fluid does not clear, the infection may be caused by an unusual organism or an organism not sensitive to the antibiotic being used; the antibiotic may be used incorrectly; the patient may have an unusual source of infection such as a nidus within the catheter or tunnel; or the patient may have an intraabdominal abcess or leaking viscus.

Infections that are caused by multiple organisms or that clear and return rapidly after the cessation of treatment suggest perforated bowel. There is no evidence that ruptured diverticuli or other bowel problems are more likely to happen in CAPD or IPD patients. These complications may be more treacherous in the CAPD or IPD patient, however, since the physician may assume that the problem is primarily peritonitis rather than a leak in the bowel. Diverticular disease is not an absolute contraindication to peritoneal dialysis and when a patient with known bowel disease develops peritonitis, diverticulitis or perforation should be suspected. Peritoneal dialysis patients require an aggressive diagnostic and therapeutic approach since these problems carry a high mortality rate.

Herniae

Peritoneal dialysis and CAPD, in particular, seem to be the best provocative test developed for hernia thus far. Patients walking around with 2 liters of fluid in their peritoneal cavity seem to develop hernias more often than intermittent peritoneal dialysis patients. Any variety of abdominal wall hernia may develop and most often these hernias are quite benign.

Hernias, especially inguinal hernias, if they are present should be repaired prior to beginning of dialysis if possible, otherwise at the beginning of therapy. Asymptomatic hernias developing during the CAPD training or outpatient period require careful evaluation and judgment as to whether they need to be repaired immediately or can be repaired electively. Postoperatively these patients may be maintained on hemodialysis or small volume peritoneal exchanges. Usually 1-liter CAPD exchanges will not stress the abdominal wall or suture line and may provide adequate dialysis to tide the patient over until he can return to 2-liter exchanges. This will result in inadequate dialysis if used more than a week and alternate hemodialysis may need to be arranged if an increase in the number of exchanges each day is not possible. For extensive repairs or if any question exists, the patient should wait for 2–4 weeks before starting normal CAPD again. This interval ensures good wound healing and minimizes the chance of leak or wound disruption. IPD patients may get adequate dialysis on 1-liter exchanges performed twice hourly. The optimal program can only be determined by careful collaboration between the surgeon and nephrologist.

Vascular Disease

There is no evidence thus far that the presence of vascular disease in the lower extremities is made worse by the intraabdominal dialysis fluid. Many patients coming to peritoneal dialysis already have far advanced vascular disease which makes hemodialysis technically difficult due to inadequate vascular access, hemodynamic instability, or coronary artery disease. The presence of extensive vascular disease, therefore, is not a contraindication to IPD or CAPD. Even with repair of abdominal aortic aneurysms, most surgeons feel that within 3 months of the surgical procedure the patient should have no ill effects from the dialysis as far as injury or infection of the vascular graft is concerned. Careful evaluation is necessary to determine whether adhesions have formed which could interfere with the efficiency of the dialysis. In most cases this can only be evaluated by a trial of dialysis.

INTEGRATED APPROACH TO THE PATIENT

With the development of CAPD, the improvement in IPD and hemodialysis techniques, and continued success with renal transplantation there is great flexibility in developing treatment programs for the patient with end-stage renal disease. The nephrologist, the transplant surgeon, the patient's referring physician, and the patient should develop a program that fits the patient's lifestyle and requirements. If possible, the patient should be encouraged to return to work and his normal daily activities with relatively little modification.

An integrated approach whereby the patient is introduced to hemodialysis (both center and home), IPD, CAPD, CCPD, and renal transplantation as he approaches the requirement for end-stage renal disease treatment is best. Those patients with obvious contraindications to one or the other modality may be steered gently by indicating the contraindications and the types of treatment available in their location. The renal social worker, dietitian, and nurse should be introduced as early as possible since they will play a major role in the patient's program.

Discussing dialysis and transplantation at the same time with patients eligible for transplantation is perfectly acceptable. The patient will usually need some temporary dialysis support system until transplantation. Evaluation for transplantation should not preclude home-training programs since the patient has no guarantee that the transplant will occur in the near future nor that it will be successful. Virtually anyone with a helper can be trained for home hemodialysis and anyone with reasonable strength and manual dexterity can be trained for CAPD—if they are properly motivated. The patient who has no desire to go to home dialysis will generally make a poor home-training candidate. The patient who is highly motivated to do well at home, however, will usually be able to train for home dialysis and succeed at home.

Some preplanning should go into the placement of vascular access devices and the location of Tenckhoff catheters. This requires some discussion between surgeon, nephrologist, and patient about the appropriate locations for these devices, especially the peritoneal catheter.

Many words have been written about the selection criteria for home dialysis generally and CAPD specifically. There is no evidence thus far that any of the selection criteria have proved to be helpful. In our experience we have not been able to accurately predict whether a patient will or will not make a good CAPD patient. Motivation seems to be the most important factor. The patient and the dialysis team must approach home treatment with the expectation of success but with the realization that if the patient or the training team fail, the patient still has other modes of treatment available.

REFERENCES

1. Ganter G: Uber die Besitigung fiftiger Stoffe aus dem Blute durch Dialyse. Muenchener Medizinische Wochenschrift 70:1478–1480, 1923
2. Maxwell MH, Rockne RE, Kleeman CR, Twiss MR: Peritoneal dialysis. I. Technique and applications. JAMA 170:917–924, 1959
3. Westin RE, Roberts M: Clinical use of stylet catheter for peritoneal dialysis. Arch Intern Med 115:659–662, 1965

4. Tenckhoff H, Schechter H: A bacterialogically safe access device. Trans Am Soc Artif Intern Organs 14:181–187, 1968
5. Boen ST, Mion CM, Curtis FK, Shilipertar G: Periodic peritoneal dialysis using the repeated puncture technique and an automated cycling machine. Trans Am Soc Artif Intern Organs 10:409–414, 1964
6. Gauntner WC, Feldman HA, Puschett JB: Peritonitis in chronic peritoneal dialysis patients. Clin Nephrol 13:255–259, 1980
7. Popovich RP, Moncrief JW, Decherd JF, Bomar JB, Pyle WK: The definition of a novel portable/wearable equilibrium peritoneal dialysis technique (Abstract). Trans Am Soc Artif Intern Organs 5:64A, 1976
8. Nolph KD, Sorkin M, Rubin J, et al: Continuous Ambulatory peritoneal dialysis: Three-year experience at one center. Ann Intern Med 92:246–256, 1980
9. Oreopoulos DB, Izatt S, Zellerman G,, et al: A prospective study of the effectiveness of three permanent peritoneal catheters. Proc Dialysis Transplant Forum 96, 1976
10. Ash SR, Johnson H, Hartman J, et al: The column disc peritoneal catheter: A peritoneal access device with improved drainage. Am Soc Artif Intern Organs 3:109–115, 1980
11. Nolph KD, Hano JE, Teschan PE: Peritoneal sodium transport during hypertonic perittoneal dialysis. Ann Intern Med 70:931, 1969
12. Popovich RP, Pyle WK, Moncrief JW: Kinetics of peritoneal transport, in Nolph KD (ed): Peritoneal Dialysis, The Netherlands, Nijhoff, 1981, pp 104–105
13. Quellhorst E, Schuenemann B, Mietzsch, Jacob I: Haemo- and peritoneal dialysis treatment of patients with diabetic nephropathy—A comparative study. Proc Eur Dial Transplant Assoc 16:205–212, 1979
14. Mitchell JC, Frohnert PP, Kurtz SB, Anderson CF: Chronic peritoneal dialysis in juvenile-onset diabetes mellitus: A comparison with hemodialysis. Mayo Clin Proc 53:775–81, 1978
15. El Shahat Y, Rottembourg J, Bellio P, Guimont MC, Rousselie F, Jacobs C: Visual function can be preserved in insulin-dependent diabetic patients treated by maintenance haemodialysis. Proc Eur Dial Transplant Assoc 17:167–172, 1980
16. Cameron JS, Ogg C, Trounce JR: Peritoneal dialysis in hypercatabolic acute renal failure. Lancet 1:1188–1191, 1967
17. Winchester JF, Da Silva AMT, Davis W, et al: Altered pulmonary function with continuooous ambulatory peritoneal dialysis (CAPD). Proc Int Sym Peritoneal Dialysis 2:329–334, 1981
18. Singh S, Dale A, Morgan B, Sahebjami H: Pulmonary function tests in patients on continuous ambulatory peritoneal dialysis. Proc Int Sym Peritoneal Dialysis 2:356–358, 1981
19. Marks HH: Body weight facts from life insurance records. Hum Biol 28:107, 1956
20. Delmez JA, Slatopolsky E, Martin KJ, Gearing BN: Minerals, vitamin D,

and parathyroid hormone in continuous ambulatory peritoneal dialysis. Kindey Int 21:862–867, 1982
21. Nolph KD, et al: National registry of CAPD patients pilot study. Dial Transplant 10:744–750, 1981
22. Amair P, et al: CAPD in diabetes with end stage renal disease. N Engl J Med 306:625–630, 1980
23. CAPD in diabetes, Peritoneal Dialysis Bulletin, Supplement vol. 2, no. 2, 1982
24. Parrott PL, et al: *Pseudomonas aeruginosa* peritonitis attributed to a contaminated iodophor solution—Georgia. MMWR 31:197–198, 1982
25. Pyle WK, Hiatt MP, Nolph KD: Patient population demographics and selected outcome measures. NIH CAPD Patient Registry Report No 82–3, 1982
26. Rubin J, Rogers WA, Taylor HM, Everett ED, et al: Peritonitis during continuous ambulatory peritoneal dialysis. Ann Intern Med 92:7–13, 1980
27. Koup Jr, Gerbracht L: Combined use of heparin and gentamicin in peritoneal dialysis solutions. Drug Intell Clin Pharm 9:388, 1975

John C. Van Stone

10
Hemofiltration

Hemofiltration is a treatment modality for renal insufficiency that has many similarities to hemodialysis but uses a different physical principle to remove toxins from the bloodstream. Hemofiltration removes large quantities of fluid from the bloodstream through a semipermeable membrane with the majority of the fluid volume being replaced back into the bloodstream in the form of an infusion solution. The removed solution, or ultrafiltrate, contains the toxins and minerals which accumulate in renal insufficiency and the infusion solution replaces the excess salts and fluid which were removed. The composition of the infusion solution is usually very similar to that of the dialysate for hemodialysis.

The primary difference between hemofiltration and hemodialysis is that with hemofiltration all the substances are removed by convective transport whereas the primary method of removal of substances during hemodialysis is by diffusive transport. As discussed in Chapter 5, the amount of a substance removed by convective transport is governed solely by concentration and membrane permeability, whereas, diffusive transport is dependent not only on plasma concentration and membrane permeability, but also on molecular weight. Because of this, hemodialysis removes larger molecular weight substances much less efficiently than smaller molecular weight substances independent of any membrane sieving effects. When the usual hemofiltration procedure is compared to the usual hemodialysis procedure, it is found that small molecular weight substances, such as urea, are removed at a faster rate with hemodialysis whereas substances in the so-called middle molecular weight range (1000–5000 mol wt) are removed much faster with hemofiltration. Large molecules such as proteins are not removed to any significant degree by either procedure.

Hemofiltration was first conceived by Dr. Lee Henderson and his co-workers in 1967.[1] They conjectured that since urine formation begins as an ultrafiltrate of plasma formed through the glomerular capillary wall, it would be more physiologic to remove uremic toxins from the plasma by the process of ultrafiltration rather than the process of diffusion and ultrafiltration should be more efficient in removing large molecular weight toxins. In conjunction with the Amicon Corporation the high-flux membranes needed were developed. Hemofiltration was clinically tested and found to have some apparent advantages over hemodialysis.

There are two problems associated with hemofiltration treatments which are not part of hemodialysis treatments. The first is that the membrane used for hemofiltration must be capable of high rates of ultrafiltration and the second is the requirement for large quantities of sterile, pyrogen-free fluid. High-flux membranes have been developed which in the hemofilters currently used are capable of filtering protein-free fluid at a rate of 2–3 liters/minute at reasonable transmembrane pressures. The major factor which limits the ultrafiltration rate in clinical hemofiltration is the protein content of the blood. Plasma protein concentration increases as fluid is removed during hemofiltration which increases the osmotic pressure and inhibits the further removal of fluid.

Whereas the dialysate for hemodialysis does not need to be sterile or pyrogen-free, the infusion solution for hemofiltration must be both, since it is injected directly into the bloodstream. During most hemofiltration procedures between 20 and 40 liters of fluid are infused. If the liter bottles normally used for intravenous infusion fluids were used, hemofiltration would be prohibitively complex and costly. Hemofiltration infusion fluid was originally prepared and sterilized in large carboys by hospital pharmacies. This, however, is also cumbersome and costly. Recently techniques have been developed where the fluid can be rendered sterile and pyrogen-free by passing it through a membrane filter.[2] This filter can be identical to the hemofilter used to filter the blood in the hemofiltration procedures and can be directly incorporated into the infusion line so that the fluid is filtered on line during the hemofiltration procedure.

Another requirement to make hemofiltration practical is that there must be a method of automatically matching the rate of infusion of fluid to the ultrafiltration rate. Because of the very rapid rate of fluid removal, a small percent difference in the ultrafiltration rate and the infusion rate can rapidly lead to volume depletion or volume overload. For this reason hemofiltration can only be performed if there is a method of accurately monitoring the ultrafiltration rate and adjusting the infusion rate accordingly. The monitoring of the ultrafiltration rate can be done either volumetrically or gravametrically. The infusion rate is generally slightly less than the ultrafiltration rate so that over the course of the treatment the patient will lose the amount of fluid which accumulated between treatments.

POSTDILUTION VERSUS PREDILUTION

There are two different modes of hemofiltration: postdilution and predilution. In the postdilution hemofiltration mode the blood travels through the hemofilter and the fluid removed prior to administration of the infusion solution. In the predilution mode, the infusion fluid is added to the blood before it enters the hemofilter. There are advantages and disadvantages of each of these two modes. In the postdilution mode, the concentration of the toxic solutes in the ultrafiltrate are equal to their plasma water concentration, whereas in the predilution mode the concentration is considerably less since the plasma has been diluted with infusion solution prior to the formation of the ultrafiltrate. The amount of toxins removed for each liter of ultrafiltrate is therefore higher in the postdilution mode. Since the rate of formation of ultrafiltrate varies inversely with the plasma protein concentration, however, the ultrafiltration rate in the predilution mode is greater than with the postdilution mode. These two factors thus, tend to cancel each other out so that in the postdilution mode we have ultrafiltrate being formed at a relatively low rate with high concentrations of toxic solutes and in the predilution mode we have relatively low solute concentrations but much higher ultrafiltration rates. We have performed numerous comparative studies using various hemofilters and have found the total solute clearance in the predilution mode always greater than in the postdilution mode at identical blood flow rates and transmembrane pressures. This is true for urea, creatinine, and phosphorus clearances. To get the maximum amount of solute clearance over the shortest period of time, one should thus use the predilution mode with the blood flow at the highest obtainable rate and the transmembrane pressure set at the maximum level which is safe for the hemofilter. For any particular clearance, however, the quantity of infusion solution used in the predilution mode is almost double that used in the postdilution mode. If the cost of the infusion solution is a significant component in the total cost of the treatment (which it is not if on-line preparation and sterilization is used) then strong consideration to the postdilution mode must therefore be given.

HEMOFILTRATION EQUIPMENT

Figure 10-1 shows the Gambro HFM 10® hemofiltration unit (Gambro USA, Barrington, IL). It is currently the only federally approved hemofiltration apparatus available in the U.S. Basically this unit consists of two modules. The lower module controls and monitors the rates of fluid removal and infusion and the top module controls and monitors blood flow through the hemofilter. The top module is identical to that used with Gambro hemodialysis equipment. It has an adjustable blood pump which will pump at rates up to 500 cc/min and a heparin pump for continuous heparin infusion. An ultrasonic monitor is used for air embolism detection.

The lower unit contains the computerized hemofiltration module. It consists of two pumps: an ultrafiltration pump and an infusion pump. The ultrafiltration pump creates a negative pressure on the hemofilter.

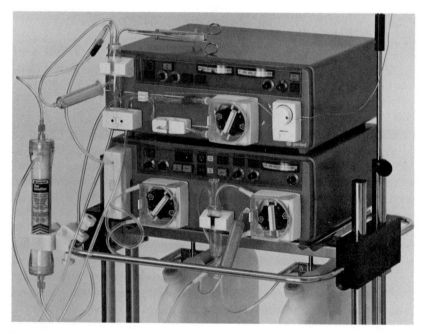

Figure 10-1. The Gambro HFM 10® hemofiltration unit (Gambro USA Barrington, IL).

The total transmembrane pressure is computed by the machine by adding the venous blood pressure to the ultrafiltration pressure and the speed of the ultrafiltration pump is automatically adjusted so as to maintain the transmembrane pressure at a preset value. The ultrafiltrate is monitored spectrophotometrically for blood leaks and then delivered into a carboy located beneath the hemofiltration module. The weight of this carboy is continually monitored by the computer. At the beginning of the treatment the fluid to be infused is placed in another carboy which is also hung below the monitor with its weight continuously monitored by the computer. If on-line sterilization is used, the fluid is pumped by the infusion pump through an ultrafilter into a heating block where its temperature is raised to between 35° and 40°C and finally is injected into the bloodstream, either immediately before or after the ultrafilter. The rate of infusion is determined by the computer on the basis of the ultrafiltration rate. In order that the amount of fluid gained between treatments can be removed during the treatment, the infusion rate must be lower than the ultrafiltration rate. At the beginning treatment, the nurse enters into the computer the total number of liters to be infused and the total amount of extra fluid to be removed. During the treatment the actual amount of weight loss is calculated by the computer from the difference in the ultrafiltration and infusion rates and is continuously shown on an indicator.

The length of the treatment is determined by the amount of fluid to be infused and is dependent on the infusion rate which in turn is dependent on the ultrafiltration rate. The ultrafiltration rate is continuously monitored and can be displayed on an indicator if desired as can the amount of time needed to infuse the remaining fluid. The rate of weight loss is monitored by the computer and if the equipment is working properly, should be linear with time. If the computer detects an excess amount of nonlinearity in the rate of weight loss, the machine will shut down and indicate the problem via a code on the indicator. The machine is very reliable and greatly simplifies the hemofiltration treatment.

ADVANTAGES AND DISADVANTAGES OF HEMOFILTRATION OVER HEMODIALYSIS

As with most new treatments, initially there were claims of many advantages of hemofiltration over hemodialysis.[3-11] Patients were noted to have a markedly reduced incidence of untoward symptoms during the treatments and blood pressure was found to be more stable during the treatments. Patients with uncontrollable hypertension when treated with hemodialysis were claimed to have their blood pressure easily controlled if placed on hemofiltration. Patients on hemofiltration, in addition, were said to have better phosphate control, a lower incidence of peripheral neuropathy, and decreased incidence of hyperlipidemia.

The major and most consistent advantage that hemofiltration appears to have over hemodialysis is the higher rate at which fluid can be removed without causing hypotension and untoward symptomatology. While the exact reasons are unclear at this time, studies have consistently demonstrated that high rates of ultrafiltration are better tolerated during the usual hemofiltration treatment compared to the usual hemodialysis treatment.

There are several possibilities as to the etiology of this improved fluid removal tolerance. First, small molecular weight clearances are generally much less with hemofiltration than with hemodialysis. With a blood flow of 200, urea clearance in hemofiltration is usually less than 100 ml/min whereas with hemodialysis urea clearances generally run in the range of 120–160 ml/min. This reduced urea clearance is thought by some to be the cause of the increased vascular stability seen with hemofiltration.

Second, the amount of acetate infused into the patient is less with hemofiltration than with most hemodialysis treatments. During hemofiltration the patient receives between 600 and 800 mEq of acetate while during many hemodialysis treatments greater than 1000 mEq of acetate is transferred across the dialyzer. As discussed in Chapter 5, acetate is a vasodilator, possibly a mild cardiac depressant, and at least in some patients contributes to the hypotension and symptomatology during hemodialysis.

Third, the amount of sodium lost with hemodialysis at any given fluid removal rate is usually greater than the amount of sodium lost with hemofiltration. Whereas an isonatric fluid is usually used for hemofiltration, the dialysate sodium concentration in most standard hemodialysis treatments is below the serum sodium concentration. As discussed in Chapter 5, this causes a shift of fluid from the extracellular compartment to the intracellular compartment and can aggravate the hypotension and symptomology during hemodialysis. With postdilution hemofiltration the Gibbs–Donnon effects caused by the high concentrations of the serum proteins result in the sodium concentration of the ultrafiltrate to be less than the plasma sodium concentration. Even if isonatric fluid, therefore, is used for both hemodialysis and hemofiltration the sodium loss during postdilution hemofiltration may be less than during hemodialysis.

Fourth, hemodialysis may remove a small molecular weight substance with vasoconstrictive activity. Since small molecular weight clearances are usually higher with hemodialysis than with hemofiltration, increased clearance of small vasoconstrictors may contribute to hypotension during hemodialysis. The catacholamines, epinephrine or norepinephrine (mol wt 200), would be prime candidates.

The final possibility is that hemofiltration removes vasodilatory toxin with a moderately high molecular weight which is not removed by hemodialysis. Whereas low molecular weight clearances with hemodialysis is usually better than with hemofiltration, the removal of middle molecules (1000 through 10,000 daltons) is much greater with hemofiltration than with hemodialysis. It is possible that a toxin in this molecular weight range accumulates in chronic renal failure and prevents the normal response to volume loss of an increase in vascular resistance from occurring during hemodialysis. Removal of this substance by hemofiltration would then allow vasoconstriction to occur. At this moment this is entirely theoretical and as yet no such substance has been identified in patients with renal insufficiency.

Shaldon and co-workers have performed some interesting comparative studies of hemodialysis and hemofiltration studies in attempt to shed light on the hemodynamic differences.[12] They determined cardiac outputs by lysamine green, both before and during tthe treatments. Peripheral resistance was calculated by dividing the blood pressure by the cardiac output. Similar to other studies they found that in response to fluid removal, cardiac output fell to a similar degree with both hemodialysis and hemofiltration. With hemofiltration, however, the peripheral resistance increased 25 perceent (a normal response to a reduction in cardiac output) while with hemodialysis, peripheral resistance actually fell a small amount.

In order to determine if this difference in peripheral resistance was due to the higher rates of small molecular weight removal during hemodialysis, they developed a method of high-efficiency hemofiltration. This method uses high blood flow rates in the range of 400 ml/min which were obtained from some patients' forearm fistulae and in other patients by placing a Thomas shunt in the lower extremity. With this high blood flow rate and a large surface area hemofilter, urea clearances were approximately 150 ml/min and not different from the urea clearance during hemodialysis. When this high-efficiency hemofiltration was compared to hemodialysis the results were identical to previous studies, with the peripheral resistance again increasing with hemofiltration but did not with hemodialysis. This suggests that differences in urea clearances are not the cause of the differences in vascular stability. It also suggests that increased hemodialysis clearances of other small molecular weight substances such as catacholamines are not the cause.

In order to determine if acetate is important in hemodynamic differences, they compared their high-efficiency hemofiltration using either an acetate or a bicarbonate infusion fluid to hemodialysis using either acetate or bicarbonate dialysate.[13] As can be seen in Figure 10-2, the response of the peripheral resistance to hemodialysis with bicarbonate dialysate was better than that with hemodialysis and acetate dialysate. In hemofiltration, peripheral resistance with bicarbonate infusion was also better than with acetate infusion. More importantly, however, there was still a large difference in peripheral resistance with hemofiltration using bicarbonate infusion fluid compared to hemodialysis using bicarbonate dialysate, suggesting that the basic differences in vascular responsiveness between hemofiltration and hemodialysis are not due to different acetate infusion rates.

To investigate the role of sodium in these differences the amount of sodium removed during the hemofiltration procedure was measured and compared to the calculated amount of sodium removed during the hemodialysis treatments.[14] Using both a dialysate sodium concentration and a hemofiltration infusion solution concentration of 140 mEq/ml, there was no significant difference in the amount of sodium

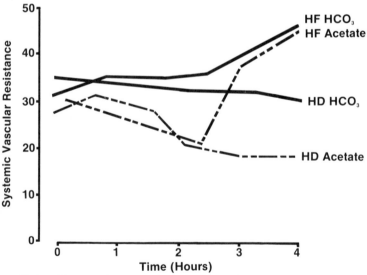

Figure 10-2. Changes in systemic vascular resistance during hemofiltration using bicarbonate or acetate infusion solution compared to hemodialysis using bicarbonate or acetate dialysate.

removed by the two procedures suggesting that the differences in blood pressure response and peripheral response to the two different treatment modes are not due to different sodium kinetics. A problem with this study is the possibility of large errors in the sodium balance calculations during hemodialysis. Small errors in dialysate sodium concentration may be amplified into large errors in sodium balance calculations. From a purely theoretical basis, the sodium loss should be greater during hemodialysis than hemofiltration. This casts some doubt on these data and more precise studies are needed in this area.

Shaldon and co-workers feel that the difference in vascular responsiveness may be related to the sympathetic nervous system. They measured plasma norepinephrine levels after hemodialysis and hemofiltration and found that there is a significant increase in norepinephrine in response to the decrease in cardiac output with hemofiltration, but with hemodialysis norepinephrine levels do not rise appropriately.[14] They suggest that the difference between hemofiltration and hemodialysis has to do with the adrenergic response to the two treatment modes. If this is true, the reason for the lack of increase in plasma norepinephrine during hemodialysis is not apparent at this time. It could be due either to a reduced production or an increased removal rate. Although the rates of removal of norepinephrine were not measured in the Shaldon studies, the rate of removal with hemodialysis should not be greater than that with hemofiltration.

Clearly the results of these investigators need to be confirmed by other investigators and further studies need to be performed to elucidate the etiology of these differences.

Hemofiltration for Uncontrollable Hypertension

Henderson suggests that there is a group of patients who have uncontrollable hypertension when treated with routine hemodialysis, but in whom the blood pressure can be controlled with hemofiltration treatments. Several noncontrolled studies in Europe have noted marked improvement in predialysis blood pressures upon switching the "uncontrollable" hypertensive hemodialysis patient to hemofiltration. The effect of the inevitable increased medical attention that these patients received upon switching from routine hemodialysis to the experimental hemofiltration treatments on the decrease in their bloood pressure is unknown, but may explain at least a portion of the differences.

Dr. Henderson performed a controlled study comparing hemofiltration to hemodialysis in hypertensive hemodialysis patients.[15] These patients received 3 months of hemodialysis treatments, 3 months of hemofiltration treatments, and another 3 months of hemodialysis. Results suggest that hypertensive dialysis patients fall into two groups. One group has better blood pressure control on hemofiltration and in the other group there is no apparent difference in blood pressure control between hemodialysis and hemofiltration. On close inspection of the data, however, it is not entirely clear that the two groups are distinct populations. It appears possible that the differences in blood pressure between the treatments is normally distributed and their "responsive" patients, arbitrarily defined as a lower mean pressure during the hemofiltration, were actually selected by chance. Further studies suggest, however, that there are other differences between the two groups of patients, adding validity to the separation, as the responses to epinephrine infusion were different between the two groups and there were some differences in the distribution of body fluids.

The better control of hypertension with hemofiltration, if true, may be related to the increased ease at which fluid is removed during hemofiltration allowing better control of extracellular fluid volume. Henderson, however, could not find a significant difference in the postdialysis weights or in the measured extracellular fluid volume between hemodialysis and hemofiltration treatments. Although further work needs to be done on the question of whether blood pressure is better controlled during hemofiltration than hemodialysis, it appears evident at this time that hemofiltration is not the sole answer for uncontrolled hypertension during hemodialysis. With the recent addition of more powerful antihypertensive agents the incidence of uncontrolled hypertension during dialysis is very low.

Several uncontrolled studies have suggested that serum lipids are lower with hemofiltration than with hemodialysis. Other studies, however, find no significant difference. Schneider found that markedly elevated serum triglycerides fell when patients were switched from hemodialysis to hemofiltration using a lactate or bicarbonate containing substitution fluid but rose again if an acetate containing fluid was used for fluid replacement, implying the possibility that acetate is involved in the hyperlipidemia.[16] The results of these studies are in conflict with hemodialysis studies which fail to demonstrate a difference in triglycerides between acetate dialysate and bicarbonate dialysate (see Chapter 5).

Initially a major disadvantage of hemofiltration was the cost and risk of producing and administering large amounts of intravenous fluids. Both the cost and the safety of the infusion fluid has been markedly improved by the on-line preparation of the fluid by ultrafiltration. The cost of the infusion solution prepared by this method is similar to the cost of dialysate for hemodialysis and in the range of 2 dollars each treatment. Over 3000 hemofiltration procedures have been performed by Drs. Henderson, Shaldon, and ourselves with this method without a single pyrogenic reaction. Dr. Shaldon has incorporated into his technique a continuous monitoring of the ultrafilter by recirculating Dextran blue in the fluid entering the ultrafilter and passing the outlet fluid through a photocell detector. The lack of detectable leaks by this method in over 1500 treatments may indicate that this precaution is not necessary. The intactness of the filter should, however, be checked on a regular basis by adding Dextran blue to the ultrafilter inflow and the visual observation of the ultrafiltrate during the set-up or clean-up procedure.

A theoretical disadvantage of postdilution hemofiltration is the possibility of harmful effects on the red blood cells by the very high protein concentrations reached during the procedure. Although there are no extensive, controlled studies of red cell kinetics, there does not appear to be any major red cell damage in that the anemia chronic renal failure does not deteriorate when switching from hemodialysis to postdilution hemofiltration.

Even though hemofiltration has been performed for over 15 years, it is still in the investigational stage. While in some patients it appears to have some definite advantages over hemodialysis as it is routinely performed now, it is not certain that modifications of hemodialysis might not produce similar results. Such modifications might include carefully controlled weight removal, changes in dialysate sodium concentration, and possible use of bicarbonate dialysate. Further studies into the pathophysiology of the differences between hemodialysis and hemofiltration may well lead to significant improvements in hemodialysis.

REFERENCES

1. Henderson LW, Besarab A, Michaels A, Bluemle Jr LW: Blood purification by ultrafiltration and fluid replacement (diafiltration). Trans Am Soc Artif Intern Organs 13:216–221, 1967
2. Henderson LW, Beans E: Successful production of sterile pyrogen-free electrolyte solution by ultrafiltration. Kidney Int 14:522–525, 1978
3. Henderson LW, Silverstein ME, Ford CA, Lysaght MJ: Clinical response to maintenance hemodiafiltration. Kidney Int (Suppl 2):558–563, 1975

4. Quellhorst E, Rieger J, Doht B, et al: Treatment of chronic uremia by an ultrafiltration kidney—First clinical experience. Proc Eur Dial Transplant Assoc 13:314–320, 1976
5. Quellhorst E, Schuenemann B, Doht B: Treatment of severe hypertension in chronic renal failure by haemofiltration. Proc Eur Dial Transplant Assoc 14:129–135, 1977
6. Schneider H, Streicher E, Hachmann H, Armiel H, von Mylius V: Clinical experience with haemofiltration. Proc Eur Dial Transplant Assoc 14:136–143 1977
7. Levy SB, Stone RA, Ford CA, Beans E, Henderson LW: The influence of hemodiafiltration on blood pressure regulation. Trans Am Soc Artif Intern Organs 23:691–693, 1977
8. Baldamus C, Bosch J, Funck-Brentano J, Shaldon S, Quellhorst E: Hemofiltration panel conference. Trans Am Soc Artif Intern Organs 25:502, 1979
9. Beckman H, Ossenkop C, Quellhorst E: Changes in peripheral nerve function with long-term hemofiltration. J Dial 1:585–594, 1977
10. Vantelon J, Laureat F, Perrone B, et al: Is it possible to treat uremia by hemofiltration: Initial clinical results obtained with polyacrylonytril membrane. Nov Presse Med 6:1117–1120, 1977
11. Von Herrath D, Schaefer K, Hofler M, et al: Clinical aspects of hemofiltration. J Dial 1:545–548, 1977
12. Shaldon S, Deschodt G, Beau MC, et al: Vascular resistance and stability during high flux haemofiltration compared to haemodialysis. Abst Am Soc Nephrol 12:129A, 1979
13. Shaldon S, Beau MC, Deschodt G, Ramperey P, Mion C: Vascular stability during hemofiltration. Trans Am Soc Artif Organs 26:391–393, 1980
14. Baldamus CA, Ernst W, Lysoyht M, Shaldon S, Koch: Is hemodynamic stability during hemofiltration a sodium balance related phenomenon. Proc Cin Dial Transplant Forum (in press)
15. Henderson L (submitted for publication)

Ted Groshong

11
Dialysis in Infants and Children

Experience with dialysis for children has been considerably less than that for adults. A number of technical factors, as well as a smaller patient population needing this treatment, has contributed to a relative lack of information regarding dialysis in the young.

Scattered use of both hemodialysis[1] and peritoneal dialysis[2] was reported in children before 1950. Serious technical problems with the former, related to equipment limitation and use of large extracorporeal blood volumes, severely limited artificial kidney utilization for treatment of acute and chronic renal disease until the mid-1960s, when large referral centers began developing chronic hemodialysis programs.[3,4]

Peritoneal dialysis received greater emphasis in the 1960s because of its requirement for less complex equipment, flexibility for accommodation to the small size and special metabolic requirements of children, and a general development of expertise.[5-7] By 1970 peritoneal dialysis was routinely used for treatment of acute renal failure in children as well as for the treatment of toxin ingestion when renal function was impaired.[8]

This chapter will review the use of peritoneal and extracorporeal hemodialysis for treatment of children with acute and chronic renal failure. Emphasis will be placed on specific issues concerning the use of these techniques in children, without reviewing the topics discussed in other chapters.

CAUSES OF RENAL FAILURE IN INFANTS AND CHILDREN

Acute Renal Failure

Acute cessation of renal function occurs in infants and children due to a widely varied group of diseases, each of which is relatively uncommon (Table 11-1). As a result, considerable diagnostic experience may be needed in determining the cause of acute renal failure in children, with the understanding that, on occasion, a specific etiology may never be determined.

The diseases which cause acute renal failure are frequently age dependent.[9] The hemolytic–uremic syndrome, for example, is by far the most common single cause of acute renal failure in infancy and childhood.[9,10] Its peak incidence is in children ages 1–3 years. It is encountered only infrequently in older children. Infants who develop a sudden reduction in renal function, especially those felt to be otherwise healthy, should therefore be considered likely victims of the hemolytic–uremic syndrome. Primary diagnostic considerations for acute renal failure in older children, however, tend to include acute poststreptococcal glomerulonephritis, Henoch-Schoenlein purpura, and acute tubular necrosis (vasomotor nephropathy), either due to volume depletion or toxic exposure. Full review of the differential

Table 11-1
Causes of Acute Renal Failure in Children*

Conditions	Percentage of Cases (162 total patients)
Hemolytic–uremic syndrome	40
Acute tubular disease	27
Glomerulonephritis	11
Cortical necrosis	6
Lithiasis	4
Nephrotic syndrome	3
Renal vein thrombosis	2
Nephroblastoma	2
Obstructive uropathy	1
Other	3

*Adapted from Lieberman E: Management of acute renal failure in infants and children. Nephron 11:193–208, 1973.

diagnosis, including the relative frequency of various renal diseases in children are beyond the scope of this chapter, and are available in pediatric nephrology texts.[9,11]

Chronic Renal Failure

The age dependency of diseases causing chronic renal failure is less obvious, and the variety of disorders is much greater than acute renal failure (Table 11-2). Chronic renal failure is a relatively uncommon problem in children, with an estimated annual incidence in the United States varying from 1.5–6/million total pop.[12-14] Congenital and structural abnormalities of the kidney generally tend to predominate as a cause of end-stage renal disease in early childhood, with acquired

Table 11-2
Causes of Chronic Renal Failure in Children

Congenital Disease
  Urinary tract malformations
  Renal hypoplasia dysplasia
  Hereditary diseases
    Congenital microcystic disease
    Cystinosis
    Juvenile nephronophthisis (Medullary cystic disease)
    Oxalosis
    Cystinuria
    Familial nephritis (Alport's disease)
    Renal tubular acidosis

Neoplastic Disease
  Wilm's tumor

Glomerular/Vascular Disease
  Hemolytic–uremic syndrome
  Henoch–Schoemlein purpura
  Renal vein thrombosis
  Membranoproliferative glomerulonephritis
  Focal glomerulosclerosis
  Renal cortical necrosis
  Minimal change nephrotic syndrome
  Membranous nephropathy
  Systemic lupus erythematosis
  Polyarteritis
  Familial nephritis
  Glomerulonephritis—other

Chronic Interstitial Nephritis

renal disease more likely in older children and adolescents. There is, however, great variation. Patients who have congenital diseases such as juvenile nephronophthisis and familial nephritis (Alport's disease) usually do not develop chronic renal insufficiency until adolescence. More than half of infants with autosomal-recessive polycystic kidney disease, conversely, will develop renal failure in infancy, with the remainder maintaining adequate renal function until late childhood. A high degree of diagnostic acumen and experience is therefore important when determining the etiology of chronic renal failure in infants and children.

The Neonate

Special diagnostic consideration must be made in the neonate with inadequate renal function. Historical facts which are commonly available to aid the physician in diagnosing renal disease in older children and infants are not available in the neonate. The differentiation between acute (self-limited) and chronic renal disease, often due to a congenital reduction or absence of renal tissue, may be difficult. Previous experience suggested that most newborn infants with renal failure appearing in the neonatal period likely suffered from a major congenital abnormality, frequently renal aplasia (Potter's syndrome). There were therefore, few reports of acute, self-limited renal failure in the neonatal period.[15] The major advances made in neonatology in the management of low birth weight infants during the 1970s, however, have resulted in an enormous increase in the frequency of acute renal failure.[16] The relative frequency of diseases causing renal failure in the neonate is noted in Table 11-3.
tab 11-2, 11-3

INDICATIONS FOR DIALYSIS

Standard therapeutic maneuvers used for conservative management of renal failure in adults may also be effective in the pediatric patient. Limited fluid and electrolyte administration should be used in most children with acute and some children with chronic renal failure. Dietary manipulation, ion-exchange resins, phosphate binders, calcium, bicarbonate, and diuretics may be helpful in patients with mild acute renal failure, or early chronic renal failure. Certain characteristics of infants and children, however, result in a requirement for earlier institution of dialysis than in adults. The immature individual has a

Table 11-3
Causes of Renal Failure in the Neonate*

Renal Failure in the Neonate	Number of Infants
Polycystic kidney disease	5
Renal dysgenesis	3
Hydronephrosis	1
Ureteral hypoplasia	1
Renal vein thrombosis	2
Acute tubular necrosis	20
Total	32

*Adapted from Jones AS, James E, Bland H, Groshong T: Renal failure in the newborn. Clin Pediat 18:286−291, 1979.

higher metabolic rate, with increased production of hydrogen ions and an accelerated rise in extracellular fluid concentrations of potassium ions. He also has an increased need for calories because of factors related to growth, development, and lifestyle. These factors cause the early use of dialysis to be more important in the child than in the adult.

Acute Renal Failure

While the duration of acute renal failure in infants and children may be somewhat shorter than in adults, depending upon the age of the patient, there is a greater likelihood that dialysis will be required for treatment, due to the factors noted above. Some children can be effectively treated with conservative medical management. Factors noted above, however, plus those associated with their prior state of health, character of their renal disease, and the presence or absence of coexisting illness determine the effectiveness and safety of conservative medical management. Maximizing caloric intake is helpful in reducing catabolic activity. Restriction of sodium, potassium, and fluids is mandatory unless the child in nonoliguric. Judicious treatment of hypertension and use of sodium−potassium exchange resins are occasionally successful, particularly in older children with renal failure due to acute poststreptococcal glomerulonephritis, Henoch-Schoelein purpura, or acute tubular necrosis.

Certain diseases are particularly likely to require dialysis. The hemolytic−uremic syndrome is invariably associated with major catabolic activity due to massive lyses of red blood cells and consequent release of potassium, phosphate, and other solutes into the body fluids. Early utilization of dialysis (when anuria or severe oliguria is initially present) has been advocated in these patients,[14,17] as this may improve their prognosis.[17,18] A similar situation exists in children following major cardiac surgery,[19] crush injuries, or ingestion of toxins which have general systemic effects.

Indications for dialysis in acute renal failure are relative, depending upon the rapidity of their development (Table 11-4).[20,21] Modifications can be made when there is a high likelihood that complications will be controlled with conservative management (Table 11-5). Patients whose serum potassium levels have risen slowly can be given Kayexelate by rectum or orally to lower the body's potassium load. Administration of insulin and glucose, calcium, and bicarbonate may be helpful in temporarily managing acute hyperkalemia. Should such a course be instituted, careful ECG monitoring should be used. Patients without excessive oliguria or fluid overload may respond to severe fluid restrictions, antihypertensive agents, and occasionally, diuretics. Finally, patients without major elevation of serum urea nitrogen, who are well into the course of their disease, may be closely monitored for complications of uremia.

Dialysis may be indicated under certain circumstances other than those noted Table 11-4. Patients developing acute renal failure due to hyperuricemia may not experience adequate control of serum uric acid levels with allopurinol. Massive hyperphosphatemia resulting from cytotoxic treatment for malignancy,[22] or ingestion of dialyzable toxins, may result in the need for prompt dialysis in the absence of other indications.

Chronic Renal Failure

Indications for dialysis in chronic renal failure are somewhat more complex. Dialysis generally should be initiated in patients with end-stage renal disease when it is determined that conservative medical management can no longer be expected to prevent the serious complications of uremia. For most children, vigorous predialysis therapy becomes ineffective when serum creatinine levels reach values greater than 10 mg/dl, or creatinine clearance drops to less than 5 ml/min/1.73 m^2 body surface area.[18]

Dialysis is frequently initiated in patients with less severe renal failure because of development of uremic symptoms. Patients who develop complications of severe uremia, such as uremic pericarditis, stomatitis, encephalopathy, neuropathy, or gastroenteropathy, should be started on a chronic dialysis program promptly. While most patients

Table 11-4
Indications for Dialysis in Acute Renal Failure

Elevated serum potassium (> 6.5–8 mEq/liter)

Severe acidosis (serum bicarbonate < 10 mEq/liter)

Fluid overload with hypertension, congestive heart failure, pulmonary edema

Profound hyponatremia (serum sodium < 120 mEq/liter with convulsions)

Increasing likelihood of uremic complications (serum urea concentrations 150–200 mg/dl)

Development of symptoms of uremia (encephalopathy, nausea, vomiting, stomatitis, etc.)

Table 11-5
Conservative Management of Acute Renal Failure

Indication	Treatment	Dosage
Hyperkalemia		
Brief reduction in level/effect	Calcium gluconate (10%)	1.0–2.0 ml/kg IV *slowly*
	Sodium bicarbonate	2 mEq/kg
	Insulin with glucose	0.2–0.5 U/kg 600–1500 mg/kg
Potassium removal	Sodium polystyrene sulfonate (Kayexlate)	1 gm/kg in 20–50% Sorbitol—oral or rectal
Hypertension	Hydralazine	1.7–3.5 mg/kg/day q 4–6 h IM or IV 1–7 mg/kg/day q 6 h PO
	Diazoxide	5 mg/kg/dose rapid IV push
	Methyldopa	10 mg/kg/day q 8–12 h PO
	Captopril	1–2 mg/kg/day q 6 h PO
	Minoxidil	0.1–0.5 mg/kg/day PO
Diuretics	Hydrochlorothiazide	0.5–1 mg/kg/day PO
	Furesomide	0.5–1 mg/kg/day PO q 12 h

Fluids should be administered at no more than 300 ml/m^2/day plus urinary output, and calories at 400 calories/m^2/day, primarily as glucose and fat.

with end-stage renal disease tend to excrete large quantities of potassium in their urine, severe reduction in renal function may result in hyperkalemia. Use of sodium-potassium exchange resins may be helpful as a temporizing measure; however, such treatment is generally not acceptable to patients for long-term therapy. Elevation of urea and of other products of protein metabolism often require reduction of protein intake to 0.5 g/kg/day. High-quality protein (a high concentration of essential amino acids) should be used when possible. Congestive heart failure resistant to medical management, as well as hypertension, acidosis, and refractory hyperphosphatemia are relative indications for beginning dialytic therapy.

Many pediatric nephrologists begin consideration of chronic dialysis when creatinine clearance drops below 10 ml/min/1.73 m^2 body surface area as a method of preventing the complications of uremia. This provides an opportunity to develop a smooth transition from conservative medical management to dialysis. Continuing experience with pediatric patients tends to support this impression.

One of the major factors of concern with children who have end-stage renal disease is growth failure, which rapidly occurs as renal function deteriorates. In theory, progressive dimunition of growth should be an indication for institution of dialysis. Growth in children receiving dialysis has been inconsistent, however, and frequently not equal to normal age-adjusted growth curves[23] (see below).

Recent experience with continuous ambulatory peritoneal dialysis has been cause for some encouragement, however, when amino acid supplementation of the dialysate is used.[24,25] Consistent improvement in growth with this form of treatment is controversial.[26] Further studies are needed before growth retardation can be utilized as an indication for institution of dialysis in chronic renal failure in children.

Finally most nephrologists have considered children with chronic renal failure to be candidates for dialysis only if they are also candidates for renal transplantation.[18,27] Poor growth and severe restrictions in the lifestyle of the children and their families has resulted in a perception that dialysis is inadequate in itself as a treatment for chronic renal failure in children. For many children, renal transplantation may be possible in the distant future, but only after a prolonged period of chronic dialysis. A significant percentage of children with chronic end-stage renal disease may be expected to be in this category, as transplantation in infants less than 2 years of age has generally been associated with a dismal prognosis.[28] Children with lower urinary tract disease not amenable to early surgery, and children with prior unsuccessful renal allografts and high titers of circulating antibodies, represent a population of pediatric patients whose lifestyle and lack of potential for growth created a dilemma regarding whether they were candidates for chronic dialysis. Long-standing experience in Europe,[23] however, as well as recent experience in the United States, especially with continuous ambulatory peritoneal dialysis (CAPD),[24,25] has renewed enthusiasm for chronic dialysis in small infants and children in whom considerable time must elapse prior to transplantation. As a result, while differing opinions exist, most programs are accepting patients into long-term dialysis programs in whom transplantation may be in the distant future.

Neonatal Renal Failure

The indications for initiation of dialysis in the neonate represents a special problem. Factors associated with enhanced metabolic activity in the young child are accentuated in the newborn infant. Acidosis, hyperkalemia, hyperphosphatemia, and hypocalcemia rapidly develop in an infant devoid of renal function.[16] The enhanced requirement for glucose administration and use of therapeutic agents necessary for treatment of coexistent diseases make the newborn infant particularly susceptible to fluid overload, with congestive heart failure, hypertension, and anasarca. While use of sodium–potassium exchange resins may delay the rise of serum potassium levels, the requirement for frequent administration, and the obligatory sodium absorption this causes, as well as the occurrence of rectal bleeding, makes this therapy less effective than in older infants and children. As a result, early institution of dialysis in the neonate with renal failure is frequently necessary.

A more complex technical and ethical issue arises in infants found to have severe, irreversible renal failure due to renal dysgenesis, aplasia, or acquired corticomedullary necrosis. Although some residual renal function may be present in patients with severe renal hypoplasia and dysgenesis, and occasionally infants with corticomedullary necrosis will have renal functional improvement,[29] for many of these infants, one is faced with the probability that growth to a size appropriate for transplantation and maintenance of a minimal quality of life will be very difficult. The moral dilemma regarding the value of maintaining life in these circumstances is not easily resolved. Recent experience with CAPD[25] offers some possibility of hope that will aid the physician in deciding this issue.

PERITONEAL DIALYSIS

The most extensive experience in the dialysis of pediatric patients by far has been with the use of peritoneal dialysis. Early studies in the childhood age group[5,6] indicate peritoneal dialysis is safe and effective in infants and children with acute renal failure. This technique is safe, easily instituted, and requires a minimum of equipment and paramedical expertise. It can be performed on an infant or child in any hospital in the country caring for children with acute disease. This treatment, in addition, is flexible. With modifications, peritoneal dialysis can be utilized as effectively in a premature infant as in an adolescent. It is therefore the dialytic treatment of choice for infants and children with acute renal failure.[30]

Widespread use of peritoneal dialysis for chronic renal failure in the pediatric age group is more recent. As a result, extensive experience is just now reaching prominent awareness. Enthusiastic nephrologists are reporting equivalent, perhaps even superior control of uremia in comparison with hemodialysis.[31]

Peritoneal Dialysis in Acute Renal Failure

Technique. Percutaneous placement of peritoneal catheters has been the traditional means of catheter insertion. Disposable, flexible peritoneal catheters are manufactured for adult and pediatric use. Prior to catheter placement, one must assure that the bladder is empty. As in adults, the site for catheter placement is the linea alba, ⅓ of the distance down from the umbilicus to the symphysis pubis. This will minimize bleeding. Sterile technique in catheter insertion is essential. The area is sterilized with povodone–iodine solution and alcohol, and draped. Lidocaine anesthesia is utilized.

Prior to insertion of the dialysis catheter itself, it is wise to fill the abdominal cavity with dialysis fluid to float the bowel and minimize the chance of perforation. Insertion of a 16- or 18-gauge needle is generally advocated for this purpose, but an intravenous type catheter of at least 18 gauge can be used. The catheter or needle is inserted so that the tip barely pierces the peritoneum. Thirty milliliters of dialysate per kilogram of body weight is then infused and the catheter removed.

A stab incision with a number 11 blade through the anesthetized area is necessary to permit easy placement of the peritoneal catheter. Care must be taken that the incision is no larger than necessary to permit its passage, or dialysis fluid will leak out. A blunt trocar is provided for placement in a dependent location, usually in the left pelvis. It is mandatory that the catheter be dependent in order to allow for suitable drainage.

Dialysis fluids are commercially available with a suitable concentration of sodium, chloride, bicarbonate, calcium, and magnesium. Usual dialysis exchange volumes vary from 30 to 50 ml/kg exchanged at 1-hour intervals. Larger volumes may cause respiratory embarrassment or even hydrothorax.[32]

Glucose concentration is available in either 1.5, 2.5 or 4.25 percent, the latter primarily used to aid in ultrafiltration. Potassium must be added to the fluid in appropriate concentrations, usually 2–4 mEq/liter. Addition of no potassium, or more frequent exchange intervals, can be utilized when potassium must be removed rapidly. Infants and children receiving potassium-free dialysis solution should be carefully monitored, however, for development of hypokalemia. Careful control of fluid intake and output can be monitored by using measuring devices placed in-line, as used in intravenous fluid administration, and carefully calibrated containers for outflow. Bed scales should ideally be used when major changes in fluid volumes are anticipated. At a minimum, frequent weights should be obtained, particularly on small infants, during the course of the dialysis.

Several pediatric nephrology centers have recently advocated use of in-dwelling Tenckhoff catheters for acute dialysis.[30,33] A major advantage of the use of a permanent catheter is that when acute renal failure is prolonged, constant dialysis can be performed during periods of oliguria. Placement under direct surgical observation additionally assures effective removal of dialysis fluid. Ultrafiltration and effective removal of dialysate is a particular problem in small infants, especially in the neonate. Even with the best technique, effective ultrafiltration may indeed not always be possible in newborns.[34] Routine use of very hyperosmotic fluids (2.5–4.25 percent glucose) is usually advisable in order to assure at least minimum filtration. Hyperglycemia may be a problem, particularly in the premature infant.

Effectiveness. Treatment of acute renal failure in childhood continues to be associated with a significant mortality rate. Judicious use of peritoneal dialysis has greatly improved long-term survival, however, so that as many as 80 percent or more of infants and children with acute renal failure from a variety of causes will survive,[35] even infants as small as 800 g.[36]

The efficiency with which peritoneal dialysis removes specific solutes from children has not been as extensively studied as in adults.[37] The peritoneal surface area of children and young infants is reported to be considerably larger, when compared by weight, than that in the adult.[38] Studies in puppies have demonstrated three times the urea clearance, by weight, when compared to adult dogs. Recent studies performed on infants and young children undergoing CAPD, however, did not confirm these results when ordinary infusion volumes were utilized.[39]

The methods of measurement of peritoneal clearance, however, are controversial. Because peritoneal clearance values are highly influenced by dialysate volume and by the time over which dialysis occurs, the "mass transfer coefficient," a measurement independent of these variables, is currently being utilized as the most effective method of evaluating solute clearances during peritoneal dialysis[40] (see Chapter 7). This is a theoretical measurement of the movement of a solute which would occur if dialysis solute concentration was maintained at zero during an entire exchange. It is directly proportional to the membrane area available for transfer, and inversely proportional to the sum of all resistances. Mass transfer coefficients for urea and creatinine in the child are roughly comparable to that expected in the adult. Ultrafiltration has not been as extensively studied in children as in adults either. It is generally assumed that a similar concentration of solute (glucose) added to dialysate in children will result in similar ultrafiltration characteristics as in adults. This is not always the case.[34] Studies on infants and small children have demonstrated that glucose transports across the peritoneal membrane in infants and young children at a faster rate than in adults. As a result, the osmotic gradient is rapidly lost and ultrafiltration is less effective. In very young infants, even very high concentrations of glucose (4.25 percent) are not consistently capable of inducing significant ultrafiltration.[34]

Current dialysis solutions contain either acetate or lactate as a source of bicarbonate. Otherwise healthy individuals should have no difficulty metabolizing these compounds to bicarbonate. There are reports, however, which question whether hypoxic newborn infants may be capable of metabolizing these compounds. Progressive lactic acidosis has been reported in hypoxic newborn infants subjected to peritoneal dialysis.[41] As a result, use of specially formulated dialysate using bicarbonate may be required in these infants, and can easily be made in most hospital pharmacies.

Peritoneal Dialysis in Chronic Renal Failure

Technique. In contrast to acute renal failure, the use of peritoneal dialysis in chronic renal failure is much more recent and much less extensive than hemodialysis. Early use of intermittent peritoneal dialysis was not notably successful.[42] Limitations on the length of time percutaneously placed peritoneal catheters could dwell resulted in infrequent dialysis treatments, too widely spaced to provide effective control of uremia, even with the use of extraordinarily strict diets. More satisfactory experience in a small number of pediatric nephrology centers was first published in the late 1970s and early 1980s.[43-45] Scattered reports of peritoneal dialysis as chronic treatment of ESRD in children has also been reported from predominately adult units.[46,47] While little long-term experience has yet been published, considerable enthusiasm has been generated by some of these techniques.

Utilization of chronic peritoneal dialysis has been highly dependent upon the development of a permanent indwelling peritoneal catheter.[32] Standard procedures for inserting these catheters have been modified for children.[48,49] Catheters of multiple sizes are now commercially available, but most chronic peritoneal dialysis is performed using adult-size Tenckhoff catheters.[49] Current practice[50] suggests the procedure be modified for children. Only one Dacron® cuff should be placed in the subcutaneous tunnel.[24,51] The function of the cuff is to develop a water-tight seal and with fibroblast infiltration into the mesh work, a permanent barrier which eliminates easy access of infectious agents into the peritoneum. The thin subcutaneous tissue of a child is generally not suitable for placement of two such cuffs.

Catheters are placed through an incision in the midline, under general anesthesia, in the operating room. Catheter tips are carefully directed into a dependent position. An exit site is created in the skin of the lateral abdomen, and the subcutaneous tunnel between the two incisions. In some children, in whom cosmetic factors may be significant, the exit site can be placed more laterally, in the flank.[44] A new technique has also been developed for catheter placement, using a special catheter guide under peritoneoscopic visualization.[52] To a limited degree, catheters may be used immediately following placement. It is generally recommended that exchanges of no more than 30 ml/kg of dialysis solution be utilized for the first week. Most centers use frequent exchanges (cycles of 1–2 hours) and do not allow the child out of bed with indwelling fluid until healing of the catheter incision has occurred.

Several methods for chronic peritoneal dialysis have been developed for use in children. Intermittent manual peritoneal dialysis, such as that conducted for acute renal failure, was initially used[42] and continues to be used at some centers.[53] This mechanism was improved upon with development of automated equipment for peritoneal exchanges, intermittent peritoneal dialysis known as (IPD).

Children are exposed to approximately 40 exchanges of dialysate, at 1-hour intervals, divided into several days (nights) each week. One advantage of this method is its use for home dialysis. Automated flow allows the child to be dialyzed during sleeping hours. Exchanges of 40–50 ml/kg at hourly intervals are usually used.

Continuous ambulatory peritoneal dialysis (CAPD) was developed in the mid-1970s.[54,55] This technique has the advantage of ambulatory dialysis. Individuals receiving this therapy have fluid exchanges performed 3–4 times during waking hours, with dialysis fluid indwelling for 3- to 4-hour periods. One exchange is allowed to dwell overnight. Children receiving this therapy are expected to attend regular school and participate in relatively normal activities.[25]

Continuous cycle peritoneal dialysis (CCPD) has recently been developed for use in adults, with very little experience reported in children.[56] CCPD is a combination of the above techniques (IPD and CAPD) that allows for 3–4 cycles during sleeping hours by an automated machine, and constant indwelling dialysate fluid during the daytime.

Enthusiasm for chronic peritoneal dialysis, particularly CAPD, among pediatric nephrologists has resulted from a perception that these children can sustain an improved lifestyle.

Children with constant indwelling fluid are usually able to attend school on a full-time basis without alteration in normal activities.[25,58] Little dietary manipulation is ordinarily necessary, as excessive intake of sodium and water can be managed by the family with intermittent use of hypertonic dialysis fluid. Visits to a nephrology center tend to be infrequent, not interfering with the child's lifestyle. Finally, the child and his or her family can assume the major responsibility for health maintenance. As of early 1982, approximately 100 children below age 18 were receiving CAPD maintenance therapy at 37 dialysis centers in the United States.[59]

The touchstone of successful dialysis therapy in children is the capacity of that therapy to provide growth. While some children treated with chronic peritoneal dialysis have demonstrated normal or supernormal growth,[24,44] growth is subnormal for most children.[26] Decreased appetite, presumably the result of the combined effects of uremia and abdominal fullness, inhibits normal dietary intake, despite few dietary restrictions. There is some evidence that, as in other forms of treatment for chronic renal disease in children, hyperparathyroidism may play a part in the growth process. If so, control of metabolic bone disease with vigorous attempts to reduce serum phosphate levels and promote calcium absorption with calcitriol may be successful in enhancing growth.[60]

As with adults, a major limiting factor in widespread use of chronic peritoneal dialysis is the constant risk of infection. Peritonitis, infection of the exit site, and infections of the subcutaneous catheter tunnel are a continuing problem. Of 12 patients receiving long-term CAPD at one center, 11 patients encountered at least one episode of peritonitis, 7 of exit site infections, and 6 of tunnel infections.[44]

HEMODIALYSIS

Scattered reports of hemodialysis for acute[61] and chronic[62,63] renal failure in children were published during the 1960s. With alteration in equipment and technique, hemodialysis can be effective and safe, in experienced hands, in infants as small as 1600–3000 g.[27,64] It is the fastest and probably the most efficient means of dialysis one can apply to the childhood age group. As a result, hemodialysis is the standard treatment for children with chronic renal failure.[65,66]

In large pediatric centers, with extensive experience in hemodialysis, this treatment has also become standard for acute renal failure.[14] Advantages, in comparison to peritoneal dialysis, include the ability to rapidly lower solutes and water from the extracellular fluid space, placement of a single surgically implanted shunt which allows dialysis for the entire course of a patient's disease, and the ability to carefully manage uremic symptoms.

Acute Hemodialysis

Technique. A variety of dialysis equipment is currently available for use in infants and children of almost any size. Essential for hemodialysis in children is a manageable extracorporeal volume.[27] No more than 10 percent of estimated blood volume should be utilized in the entire apparatus. Use of larger volumes predisposes to hypotension which seriously inhibits ability to ultrafilter water and potentially results in shock. Because of the relatively large priming volumes required and the marked compliance of the equipment, coil type dialyzers are generally not used in the pediatric age group. They have been replaced by small volume hollow fiber and parallel plate dialyzers. A listing of dialyzer priming volumes is noted on Table 11-6.

Blood tubing also constitutes a significant reservoir of extracor-

Table 11-6
Characteristics of Pediatric Dialyzers*

Manufacturer and Type	Dialyzer	Surface Area (m²)	Priming Volume (ml)†	Clearance of urea (ml/min) Blood Flow		Ultrafiltration‡ (ml/h/mm Hg TMP)
				100 ml/min	200 ml/min	
Hollow Fiber:						
Asahi–Medical (Tokyo, Japan)	AMO3	0.3	30	75	110	1.4
	AMO6	0.6	55	80	180	2.2
Cordis–Dow (Miami, FL)	CDAK 0.6	0.6	53	83	118	1.2
Erika (Rockleigh, NJ)	HPF 100	0.8	67	85	160	2.9
	HDF 200	1.0	78	90	170	3.2
Organon Teknika (Kansas City, MO)	Nephross Lento	0.7	65	—	142	2.8
	Nephross Andante	1.0	90	—	165	4.2
Terumo (Compton, CA)	TE07	0.7	60	80	140	2.8
	TE10	1.0	85	100	160	3.7
	TH10	1.0	100	80	140	2.5
Travenol (Deerfield, IL)	CF12–11	0.82	61	99	162	3.0

Parallel Plate:						
Cobe (Lakewood, CO)	PPD.8	0.8	45	70	115	2.0
Gambro (Barrington, IL)	Mini–Minor	0.28	20	51	61	0.4–0.6
	Minor	0.51	33	—	100	1.2–1.6

*Source—dialysis manufacturers.

†Priming volumes are determined under specific circumstances. Priming volumes will vary with TMP. Further information regarding alterations in priming volume can be obtained from the dialyzer manufacturer.

‡Ultrafiltration characteristics are determined in specific circumstances, and may vary considerably. Further information regarding ultrafiltration can be obtained from the dialyzer manufacturer.

poreal blood volume. The volume required for the tubing may indeed be greater than the priming volume for the dialyzer. Pediatric equipment is produced with widely varying volumes, depending upon the manufacturer. If one is not certain of the blood volume of dialysis tubing (including drip chamber), a sample tube should be filled with water and its contents carefully measured prior to instituting dialysis.

Children are extraordinarily susceptible to the development of the disequilibrium syndrome, a phenomena which occurs following overly efficient dialysis.[67,68] Rapid loss of measurable osmotic solutes results in a disequilibrium of osmols across the cell membrane. While this has little significance in most cells, swelling of brain cells may cause increased intracranial pressure. Within the brain, "idiogenic" osmols play the major role in this process. The result is progressive lethargy and/or seizures, either during or several hours after acute dialysis. Various methods have been developed to reduce the risk of the disequilibrium syndrome in children. Careful attention should be directed toward the efficiency of the dialyzer used (Table 11-6). Excessive urea clearance is generally recognized as the factor most closely associated with development of this syndrome. The anticipated clearance of urea should therefore be carefully determined by knowledge of blood flow and dialyzer efficiency.[14] The "clearance characteristic" has been developed as a measure of dialysis efficiency.[64] This number is an estimate of urea clearance per kilogram of body weight each hour (Curea/kg/h). A urea clearance characteristic of 3 ml/kg/h should be used for maximum safety. Children whose serum urea nitrogen values approach 200 mg/dl should, however, be dialyzed at the less efficient rate of 1.5 ml/kg/h or less.

Other maneuvers have been recommended for reducing the frequency of the disequilibrium syndrome. Some nephrologists[14] recommend routine use of mannitol, 1 gm/kg by intravenous infusion during the course of the dialysis. An increase in glucose concentration in the dialysis bath to 670 mg/dl and/or dialysis sodium of 140–144 mEq/liter has also been recommended.

Infants and small children undergoing hemodialysis are particularly prone to hypothermia. Even though the dialysis bath is usually maintained at body temperature, the relatively low flow through long dialysis lines may allow enough heat exchange to permit blood cooling, and cooling of the patient. As a result, overhead warmers are frequently required during dialysis for infants and small children.

Blood access is a major problem, and may be very difficult in infants below 10 kg. Traditional blood access has been provided by use of external Scribner type shunts.[69,70] While effective for acute hemodialysis, long-term use of these shunts is difficult because of clotting and infection. In older children (over 8–10 kg), shunts may be connected between the radial artery and cephalic vein in the arm or posterior tibial artery and long saphenous vein in the leg.[14] The arm is usually considered to be a superior site for shunt placement as this allows a child continued mobility. In smaller infants, however, blood flow through these shunts may not be adequate to prevent clotting. The brachial artery in the arm or superficial femoral artery in the leg may have to be used in these infants.

Acute dialysis may also be utilized through percutaneous placement of a Shaldon catheter, by Seldinger technique, into the femoral vein. In experienced hands, this technique is safe and effective even in small children. Dialysis may be conducted by using both femoral veins, or using a single catheter. A single catheter may also be used following placement in the subclavian vein.

Hemodialysis of new-born infants requires considerable experience. Adequate blood access can usually be obtained using umbilical vessels.

Meticulous sterile technique must be utilized in placement of all such catheters and shunts, and must be maintained for the entire shunt life. Heparinization is not ordinarily required, other than during the actual dialysis. When clotting occurs, however, removal of the clot with a Fogarty catheter may be followed by constant infusion of small amounts of heparin through a T-connector. Platelet inhibitors (dipyridamole and aspirin) may be utilized also.

Effectiveness of dialysis in acute renal failure. Hemodialysis is extraordinarily effective in maintaining most children who have suffered acute renal failure. The mortality rate of 40–50 percent in children with this condition is primarily related to the underlying disease process which caused acute renal failure. Ninety percent of children whose acute renal failure is primary (without significant extrarenal disease) should survive, with return of good renal function.[71] The mortality rate of infants and children with hemolytic–uremic syndrome may be even lower. Complications such as disequilibrium, volume overload or shock, and emboli are decreasing in frequency with increased experience with acute hemodialysis.

Chronic Hemodialysis

Technique. Chronic hemodialysis is technically similar to hemodialysis for acute renal failure. Because of the increased metabolic requirements of childhood, treatment must be somewhat more frequent in children than in adults. A minimum 5-hour dialysis, 3 times each week, is generally recommended.[14]

Vascular access may be somewhat difficult in infants and small children when chronic dialysis is required. Percutaneous catheter placement is usually not practical. Use of Brescia arterial-venous fistulas are an important alternative to the Scribner shunt in children weighing more than 20 kg. Fistulas are superior because there are no indwelling foreign bodies.[72] One can therefore minimize complications such as dislodging the catheters, infection, and trauma. A period of 6–8 weeks is usually required for full aging of the fistula for routine use. Large-bore (16 or 18 gauge) needles are needed for adequate blood flow. In some children, single-needle dialysis may be used so long as significant recycling does not take place within the tubing. While most children can be taught to overcome the fear of frequent fistula puncture for dialysis, in a small number of children, this is difficult. The Buselmeier shunt is an almost completely subcutaneously placed shunt and has been advocated for children 30 kg or greater.[73] Reduced blood flow through this shunt probably prevents its use in infants and smaller children. Use of this shunt removes the need for frequent skin puncture. Internal fistulas are now possible in many children, including toddlers, using expanded polytetrafluoroethylene[74] and bovine grafts.[75,76]

Studies in adults have shown that an improved lifestyle can be obtained and an increased survival expected, in people receiving home versus center dialysis.[77] Unfortunately, few children other than a small number of adolescents are candidates for home hemodialysis, though such efforts have been successful in England.[77,78]

Results of chronic hemodialysis therapy. Chronic hemodialysis has resulted in an impressive ability to sustain life. Overall survival of children, particularly those outside infancy, has been comparable or even superior to that expected from renal transplantation.[80] Actuarial survival of children undergoing hemodialysis is reported to approach 100 percent at 6 months and 95 percent at 5 years, in comparison to a somewhat lower survival of children undergoing transplantation.[81] Combined chronic dialysis-transplant programs are the usual pattern, however.[82]

Appropriate medical management is very important for the care of patients on chronic hemodialysis. Major problems with renal osteodystrophy are common[14] and vigorous efforts to reduce hyperphosphatemia to normal levels for age must be made. Phosphate binders (aluminum hydroxide) must be given to children on chronic hemodialysis regardless of the frequency or duration of treatment. Recent experience suggests 25-hydroxycholecalciferol[83] and particularly 1, 25-dihydroxycholecalcilerol[84] is helpful in healing osteodystrophy in many of these children. Vigorous attention must be paid to sodium and fluid balance, as hypertension and congestive heart failure can occur in patients vigorously dialyzed, but not sodium restricted. Hypertension is a common problem in such children and should be treated vigorously, and prevented when possible.

The diet of the child on chronic hemodialysis must be fairly strictly controlled. Dietary management includes a reduction of sodium, potassium, phosphate, and protein intake. Children should, however, receive a minimum of 2–2.5 gm/kg of high-quality protein in their diet each day.[14] Calories should be maximized using high carbohydrate and fat intake.

Long-term experience with children receiving chronic hemodialysis has shown disappointing growth. Studies have demonstrated a variety of metabolic abnormalities each of which is known to cause growth failure. These include acidosis, osteodystrophy, and endocrine disturbances.

The most important limitation to normal growth is, however, an inadequate caloric intake.[85,86] A combination of dietary restrictions and anorexia due to psychological and physiological factors is usually responsible for inadequate intake to support normal metabolic activities and growth. Calorie supplementation is possible in patients undergoing hemodialysis, but frequently is not successful. Vigorous efforts to control osteodystrophy have been helpful in some patients, but not clearly beneficial in others.[87] Growth retardation has also been affected by acidosis[88] and abnormalities in hormonal interaction.[89] Other factors, yet unknown, however, may contribute.[90] While these problems often limit growth in these children, dietary control has some potential for overcoming them, in part.

PSYCHOLOGICAL PROBLEMS

Children placed on chronic dialysis, while maintained with a low mortality, remain in a state of mild chronic uremia. The impact of various dietary and exercise limitations, and the dependence on dialysis equipment, may moreover result in major emotional problems.[91] These problems tend to be related to the age of the child.[92]

Children of all ages fear treatments which cause pain. Younger children and infants develop behavior patterns to painful procedures, however, that may be most threatening to the parents and dialysis staff, and result in considerable manipulative behavior or depression on the part of the child. In preschool children, honesty is as important as it is in older children. Young children should be constantly reassured and, when possible, allowed maximum contact with their mothers during frightening or painful procedures. The most pressing fear of the toddler, greater than fear of pain, is fear of separation from his mother. Allowing these children trivial participation in dialysis procedures may be most helpful in permitting the child to maintain a perception of self-control.

Children of school age tend to develop anxieties related to the threat of mutilation. This problem may develop into profound concerns regarding peer relationships in preadolescents. Constant reassurance is necessary. Efforts to maintain a relatively normal activity pattern (school, sports) consistent with physical capabilities are vital. Greater participation in procedures such as gathering materials, holding equipment during start-up, etc., may be very helpful.

Adolescent dialysis patients are a major concern. Their need for peer relationships and for increased self-control can be maximized by permitting them to take ever-increasing responsibility for their own care, and encouraging participation in making decisions.

Successful dialysis programs for children incorporate major involvement by nurse practitioners, social workers, and frequently, psychiatrists, as members of the health care team. Alteration in body image, personality maladjustments and behavioral problems, and development of psychosomatic disease are all common in children on chronic dialysis. Proponents of chronic peritoneal dialysis have stated that children receiving CAPD tend to have a lower frequency of such problems.[44] Constant attention to home dialysis procedures may result, however, in development of "family fatigue."[4,58] This problem is in no way exclusive for home-peritoneal dialysis, but rather any form of home dialysis.

Because of the well-recognized emotional problems seen in children, patients not considered to be imminent candidates for renal transplantation were not automatically considered chronic dialysis patients until recently. Improvements in dialysis capabilities and increased understanding of the emotional trauma undergone by children with chronic renal disease has resulted in a circumstance in which almost every child capable of functioning with a reasonable lifestyle is today considered to be a candidate for chronic dialysis.

Summary

Acute and chronic dialysis in children has become commonplace. The effectiveness of this treatment in maintaining life is outstanding. Children with acute renal failure may safely and effectively receive either hemodialysis or peritoneal dialysis depending primarily upon the experience of the patient's physician. Chronic hemodialysis, the standard therapy for life support in children with chronic renal failure for over 15 years, continues to be the standard therapy in most dialysis centers. Recent developments such as continuous ambulatory peritoneal dialysis presents a potential for supplanting this therapy in a large number of patients. The effectiveness of a dialysis program in children is based upon the experience of the dialysis team, their willingness to make provisions for the special needs of infants and children, and their ability to deal with the many emotional problems such children develop.

REFERENCES

1. Merrill JP, Smith S, Callahan EJ, Thorn GW: The use of an artificial kidney. II. Clinical experience. J Clin Invest 29:425, 1950
2. Swan H, Gordon HH: Peritoneal lavage in the treatment of anuric children. Pediatrics 4:586–595, 1949
3. Fine RM, DePalma JR, Lieberman E, et al: Extended hemodialysis in children with chronic renal failure. J Pediat 73:706–713, 1968
4. Fine RM, Korsch BM, Grushkin CM, Lieberman E: Hemodialysis in children. Am J Dis Child 119: 498–504, 1970
5. Segar WE, Gibson RK, Rhamy R: Peritoneal dialysis in infants and small children. Pediatrics 27:603–613, 1961
6. Etteldorf JN, Dobbins WT, Sweeney MJ, et al: Intermittent peritoneal dialysis in the management of acute renal failure in children. J Pediat 60:327–339, 1962
7. Lloyd-Still JD, Atwell JD: Renal failure in infants with special reference to the use of peritoneal dialysis. J Pediat Surg 1:466–475, 1966
8. Dobrin RS, Larson CB, Holliday MA: The critically ill child: acute renal failure. Pediatrics 48:286–293, 1971
9. Broyer M: Renal failure and arterial hypertension, in Royer P, Habbib R, Mathiew H, Broyer MWB (eds): Pediatric Nephrology. Philadelphia, Saunders, 1974, pp 343–357
10. Lieberman E: Management of acute renal failure in infants and children. Nephron 11:193–208, 1973
11. Lieberman E: Work-up of the child with azotemia, in: Clinical Pediatric Nephrology. Philadelphia, Lippincott, 1976, pp 45–64

12. Chan JCM: Hemodialysis in children: A 12 months experience. Virg Med J 107:141–142, 1980
13. Potter DE, Holliday MA, Piel CF, et al: Treatment of end-stage renal disease in children: A 15 year experience. Kidney Int 18:103–109, 1980
14. Mauer SM: Pediatric renal dialysis, in CM Edelmann Jr (ed): Pediatric Kidney Disease. Boston, Little, Brown, 1978, pp 487–502
15. Jain R: Acute renal failure in the neonate. Pediat Clin N Am 24:605–618, 1977
16. Jones AS, James E, Bland H, Groshong T: Renal failure in the newborn. Clin Pediat 18:286–291, 1979
17. Gianantonio CA, Vitacco M, Mendilaharzu F, et al: The hemolytic –uremic syndrome. Nephron 11:174–192, 1973
18. Fine RN: Treatment of end-stage renal disease in children. Pediat Ann 65–73, 1981
19. Chesney RW, Kaplan BS, Freedom RM, et al: Acute renal failure: An important complication of cardiac surgery in infants. J Pediat 87:381–388, 1975
20. Chan JCM: Acute renal failure in children: Diagnosis and treatment. Virg Med J 107:501–505, 1980
21. Kaplan BS, Datz J, Krawitz S, Lurie A: An analysis of the results of therapy in 67 cases of the hemolytic–uremic syndrome. J Pediat 78:420, 1971
22. Meyers L, Hakami N, Groshong TL: Acute renal failure due to massive hyperphosphatemia following treatment for malignancy (manuscript in preparation)
23. Broyer M, Kleinknecht C, Loirat C, et al: Growth in children treated in long term hemodialysis. J Pediat 84:642–649, 1974
24. Balfe JW, Irwin MA, Oreopoulos DG: An assessment of continuous ambulatory peritoneal dialysis (CAPD) in children, in Moncrief JW, Popovich RP (eds): CAPD Update. New York, Masson, 1981, pp 211–220
25. Alexander SR, Tseng CH, Maksym KA, et al: Clinical parameters in continuous ambulatory peritoneal dialysis for infants and children, in Moncrief JW, Popovich RP (eds): New York, Masson, 1981, pp 195–209
26. Salusky IB, Fine RN, Nelson P, et al: Nutritional status of pediatric patients undergoing CAPD. Kidney Int 21:177, 1982
27. Lynch RE, Mauer SM, Buselmeier TJ, Kjellstrand CM: Techniques, complications and results of chronic hemodialysis in children, in Straus J (ed): Pediatric Nephrology, Renal Failure. New York, Garland STM, 1978, p 195
28. Moel DI, Butt KNH: Renal transplantation in children less than 2 years of age. J Pediat 99:535–539, 1981
29. Groshong TD, Taylor AA, Nolph KD, et al: Renal function following cortical necrosis in childhood. J Pediat 79:267–275, 1971
30. Fine RN: Peritoneal dialysis update. J Pediat 100:7, 1982

31. Richardson MC, Harley RM: CAPD in children: treatment of choice. Dial Transplant 11:188, 1982
32. Lorentz WB: Acute hydrothorax during peritoneal dialysis. J Pediat 94:417–419, 1979
33. Tenckhoff H, Schecter H: A bacteriologically safe peritoneal access device. Trans Am Soc Artif Organs 16:181, 1968
34. Kohaut EC, Alexander SR: Ultrafiltration in the young patient on CAPD, in Moncrief JW, Popovich RP (eds): CAPD Update. New York, Masson, 1981, p 221
35. Griffin NK, McElena J, Barratt TM: Acute renal failure in early life. Arch Dis Child 51:459–462, 1976
36. Kanarek KS, Root E, Sidebottom RA, Williams, PR: Successful peritoneal dialysis in an infant weighing less than 800 grams. Clin Pediat 21:166–171, 1982
37. Grushkin AB, Elzouki AY, Baluarte HJ, et al: Periteonal dialysis kinetics—A pediatric perspective, in Straus J (ed): Pediatric Nephrology. New York, Plenum, 1981, pp 439–477
38. Esperance MJ, Collins DL: Peritoneal dialysis efficiency in relation to body weight. J Pediat Surg 1:162, 1966
39. Popovich RP, Pyle WK, Rosenthal DA, Alexander SR, Balfe JW, Moncrief JW: Kinetics of peritoneal dialysis in children, in Moncrief JW, Popovich RP (eds): CAPD Update. New York, Masson, 1980, p 227
40. Popovich RP, Moncrief JW: Kinetic modeling of peritoneal transport, in Trevino A (ed): Peritoneal Dialysis. New York, Karger, 1979
41. Nash NA, Russo JC: Neonatal lactic acidosis and renal failure: The role of peritoneal dialysis. J Pediat 95:101–105, 1977
42. Levin S, Winkelstein JA: Diet and infrequent peritoneal dialysis in chronic anuric uremia. New Eng J Med 277:619, 1967
43. Brouhard BH, Berger N, Cunningham RJ, Petrusick T, Allen W, Lynch RE, Travis LB: Home peritoneal dialysis in children. Trans Am Soc Artif Organs 25:90–93, 1979
44. Alexander SR: Pediatric CAPD: Three year's experience at one center. Second Annual National Conference on CAPD, Kansas City, Missouri, 1982
45. Potter DE: Comparison of peritoneal dialysis and hemodialysis in children. Dial Transplant 7:800–802, 1978
46. Oreopoulos EG, Clayton S, Dombros N, Zellerman G, Katirtzoglou A: Experience with continuous ambulatory peritoneal dialysis (CAPD). Trans Am Soc Artif Organs 15:95–97, 1978
47. Goka R, McHugh M, Frayer R, Ward JK, Kerr DNS: Continuous peritoneal dialysis: one year's experience in a UK dialysis unit. Brit Med J, p 474–477, August 16, 1980
48. Scott DF, Marsha VC: Insertion and complications of Tenckhoff catheters—Surgical aspect, Atkins RC, Thomson NM, Farrell PC (eds): Peritoneal Dialysis. New York, Churchill Livingstone, 1981, pp 61–72

49. Alexander SR, Tank ES: Surgical aspects of continuous ambulatory peritoneal dialysis in infants and children. J Urol 127:501, 1982
50. Tank ES: Catheter placement in children for CAPD. Second Annual National Conference on CAPD, Kansas City, Missouri, 1982
51. Balfe JW: The use of CAPD in the treatment of children with end-stage renal disease. Peri Dial Bull 1:35–38, 1982
52. Ash SR, Wolf GC, Bloch R: Placement of the tenckhoff peritoneal dialysis catheter under peritoneoscopic visualization. Dial Transplant 10:383–386, 1981
53. Lorentz WB, Hamilton RW, Disher B, Crater C: Home peritoneal dialysis during infancy. Clin Nephrol 15:194–197, 1981
54. Popovich RP, Moncrief JW, Nolph KD, Ghods AJ, Twardowski ZP, Pyle MK: Continuous ambulatory peritoneal dialysis. Ann Int Med 88:444–456, 1978
55. Oreopoulos DG, Robson M, Izatt S, et al: A simple and safe technique for continuous ambulatory peritoneal dialysis. Trans Am Soc Artif Organs 22:484–487, 1978
56. Lum GM: Peritoneal dialysis in children: A collaborative experience. Proceedings of the Clinical Dialysis and Transplant Forum, November 1981, p 18
57. Shmerling J, Kohaut E, Perry S: Cost and social benefits of CAPD in a pediatric population, in Moncrief JW, Popovich RP (eds): CAPD Update. New York, Masson, pp 1980, 189–193
58. Fine RN: Metabolism and growth in pediatric CAPD. Second National Annual Conference on CAPD, Kansas City, Missouri, 1982
59. Pyle K: National CAPD Registry, personal communication
60. Kohaut E: Growth in children with CAPD. Second Annual National Conference on CAPD, Kansas City, Missouri, 1982
61. Hickman RO, Scribner BH: Application of the pumpless hemodialysis system to infants and children. Trans Am Soc Artif Organs 8:309, 1962
62. Hutchings RH, Hickman RO, Scribner BH: Chronic Hemodialysis in a pre-adolescent. Pediatrics 37:68–73, 1966
63. Williams AB, Hargest TS, Wohltmann HJ: Chronic hemodialysis of a 2-year-old child. Pediatrics 43:116–122, 1969
64. Mauer SM, Lynch RE: Hemodialysis techniques for infants and children. Pediat Clin N Am 23:843–856, 1976
65. Potter D, Larson D, Leumann E, Perin D, Simmons J, Piel CF, Holliday MA: Treatment of chronic uremia in childhood. II. Hemodialysis. Pediatrics 46:678–689, 1970
66. Potter D: Management of the child on chronic dialysis, in Lieberman E (ed): Clinical Pediatric Nephrology. Philadelphia, Lippincott, 1976, pp 439–451
67. Hunter MB, Cole BR, Robson AM: Tactics for caring for children during hemodialysis. Dial Transplant 10:147–149, 1981
68. Johnson DL: The dialysis disequilibrium syndrome. Nephrol Nurse, p 27, January/February 1980

69. Franzone AJ, Tucker BL, Brennan LP, et al: Hemodialysis in children: Experience with arteriovenous shunts. Arch Surg 102:592, 1971
70. Buselmeier TJ, Santiago EA, Simmons RL, et al: Arteriovenous shunts for pediatric hemodialysis. Surgery 70:638, 1971
71. Hodson EM, Kjellstrand CM, Mauer SM: Acute renal failure in infants and children. Outcome of 53 patients requiring hemodialysis treatment. J Pediat 93:756–761, 1978
72. Arbus GS, Sniderman S, Trausler DA: Long-term experience with arterio venous fistulas in children on hemodialysis. Clin Nephrol 2:28, 1974
73. Buselmeier TJ, Kjellstrand CM, Simmons LC, Leonard AS, Najarian JS: A totally new subcutaneous prosthetic arteriovenous shunt. Trans Am Soc Artif Organs 19:25, 1973
74. Robinson HB, Wenzel JE, Williams GR: Internal vascular access for hemodialysis in children weighing less than 15 kg. Surgery 85:525–529, 1979
75. Arbus BS, Demaria JE, Galiwango J, Irwon MA, Churchill BM: The first 10 years of the dialysis-transplantation program at the hospital for sick children. Toronto I, Pre-Dialysis, CMAJ 120:655–664, 1980
76. Applebaum H, Shashikumar VL, Somers LA, Baluarte HJ, Gruskin AB, et al: Improved hemodialysis access in children. J Pediat Surg 15:764–769, 1980
77. Friedman EA: Introduction to dialysis, in Friedman EA (ed): Strategy in Renal Failure. New York, Wiley, 1978, p 4
78. Shaldon S, Ahmed R, Oog D, et al: The use of the A-V fistula in overnight home dialysis in children. Proc Eur Dial Transplant Assoc 8:65, 1971
79. Baillard RA, Ku G, Moorehead JF: Home dialysis in children and Adolescents. Proc Eur Dial Transplant Assoc 9:335, 1972
80. Avner ED, Harmon WE, Grupe WE, Ingelfinger JR, Eraklis AJ, Levey RH: Mortality of chronic hemodialysis in renal transplantation in pediatric end-stage renal disease. Pediatrics 67:412–416, 1981
81. Chantler CM, Carter JE, Bewick M, Counahan R, Cameron JS, Ogg CS, et al: Ten years of experience with regular hemodialysis and renal transplantation. Arch Dis Child 55:435–455, 1980
82. Fine RN, Grushkin CM: Hemodialysis and renal transplantation in children. Clin Nephrol 1:243–256, 1973
83. Luciani JC, Meunier PJ, Dumas R: Dialysis bone disease in childhood: Treatment with 25-hydroxcholecalciferol. Pediat Res 13:1105–1108, 1979
84. Chesney RW, Moorthy AB, Eisman JA, et al: Increased growth after long term oral 1, 25-vitamin D in childhood renal osteodystrophy. New Eng J Med 298:238, 1978
85. Simmons JM, Wilson CJ, Potter DE, Holliday MA: Relation of calorie deficiency to growth failure in children on hemodialysis and the growth response to calorie supplementation. New Eng J Med 285:653–656, 1971
86. Holliday MA: Calorie deficiency in children with uremia: Effect upon growth. Pediatrics 50:590–597, 1972
87. Broyer M, Kleinknecht C, Gagnadouy NF, et al: Growth in uremic

children, in: Pediatric Nephrology, Current Concepts in Diagnosis and Management, vol 4. New York, Garland, 1978, p 185
88. McSherry E: Acidosis and growth in non-uremic renal disease. Kidney Int 14:349–354, 1978
89. Lewy JE, VanWyk JJ: Somatomedin and growth retardation in children with chronic renal insufficiency. Kidney Int 14:361–364, 1978
90. El-Bisht M, Burke J, Gill D, et al: Body composition in children on regular hemodialysis. Clin Nephrol 15:53–60, 1981
91. Korsch BM, Fine RN, Grushkin CP, Negrete VF: Experiences with children and their families during extended hemodialysis and kidney transplantation. Pediat Clin N Am 18:625–638, 1971
92. Leumann EP, Merz-Ammann A: Psychological problems in children with chronic renal failure. Dial Transplant 10:813–814, 1981

John C. Van Stone

12
Acute Renal Failure

Acute renal failure is best defined as a rapid decline in renal function. It is invariably associated with increasing serum urea and creatinine concentrations. It is frequently, but not always, associated with oliguria, hyperkalemia, and sodium retention. There are numerous causes of acute renal failure. At the University of Missouri Medical Center, approximately 70 cases each year of acute renal failure are referred to the nephrology division. The incidence of the various causes are given in Table 12-1. Trauma and other causes of hypotension account for 24 percent. Prerenal refers to patients who are volume depleted and have immediate increase in renal function with fluid replacement. Since these patients do not truly have renal failure, sepsis is really the second leading cause of acute renal failure, accounting for about 12 percent of the patients seen in our medical center. Obstruction, glomerular disease, and drugs (predominantly the aminoglycoside antibiotics) each account for about 8 percent and the remaining patients have a variety of problems.

Many different kinds of renal insults such as hypotension and nephrotoxic drugs, result in a syndrome of prolonged, reduced renal function followed by the eventual return of normal or near normal function. This syndrome was originally referred to as acute tubular necrosis because of the necrosis of the tubular cells seen histologically at autopsy of fatal cases. With the advent of renal biopsy, however, it was found that tubular necrosis is only seen in about 15 percent of nonfatal cases and does not appear to be important in the pathogenesis of the decreased renal function. It has therefore been suggested that acute tubular necrosis is an inappropriate name and the syndrome has

Table 12-1
Causes of Acute Renal Failure at University of Missouri–Medical Center 1978–1981

Causes	Percentage
Trauma, hypotension	24
Prerenal	12
Sepsis	12
Obstruction	8
Glomerular disease	8
Drugs	7
Hypertension	5
Vasculitis	5
Rhabdomyalysis	4
Hepatorenal syndrome	3
Hyperuricemia	3
Postpartum	2
Unknown	7

been referred to as vasomotor nephropathy (implying that the major cause of decreased renal function is vascular in nature), lower nephron nephrosis (implying tubular dysfunction as a cause), or simply acute renal failure. Since there are many other causes of acute renal failure besides this syndrome and there is currently no agreement as to the actual cause of the decreased renal function, none of these terms are entirely satisfactory. In this text, we will refer to this entity by its original name, acute tubular necrosis.

PATHOGENESIS OF ACUTE TUBULAR NECROSIS

In spite of large amounts of research in the last 10 years, the mechanisms causing the decreased renal function in acute tubular necrosis are not well understood. There are several proposed theories, each with experimental evidence to support them and refute the others. It appears probable that the mechanism may differ on the basis of the underlying etiology. There is also some evidence suggesting that the mechanism initiating the decrease in renal function may differ from that which maintains the decrease.

The vascular hypothesis states that afferent arteriolar constriction and/or efferent arteriolar dilitation decreases the pressure in the glomerular capillary and reduces glomerular filtration.[1-4] It has been further suggested that these vascular changes are at least in part the result of the intrarenal release of renin with the formation of angiotension. In support of this theory is the fact that maneuvers which decrease renin stores, such as sodium loading, have a marked protective effect against the subsequent development of acute tubular necrosis. Against this theory is the fact that the administration of antibodies which destroy renin or angiotension antagonists have no effect on the development or resolution of acute renal failure. The evidence at this time suggest that this mechanism may be involved in the early development of acute tubular necrosis but it does not appear important in maintaining the prolonged period of decreased renal function.

Flores and Leaf examined biopsies of patients with acute tubular necrosis and found swelling of the glomerular endothelial cells.[5] They suggest that this is important in the pathogenesis of decreased renal function. They hypothesize that the cellular swelling is from an injury to the sodium–potassium pump which allows intracellular concentration to rise and results in the influx of water. The swollen endothelial cells then decrease the caliber of the capillary lumen which reduces blood flow and glomerular filtration. In support of this theory is the observation that hypertonic mannitol prevents the cellular swelling and attenuates the renal insufficiency. Against this theory is the fact that mannitol is only effective if given before or very early in the development of acute tubular necrosis.

A decrease in glomerular permeability has been found in some experimental models of acute tubular necrosis and has been proposed to be the cause of decreased renal function. The small reduction found, however, does not appear to be sufficient to explain the marked decrease in function. It is possible, however, that decreased glomerular permeability may play a supportive role.

There are several mechanisms by which the tubular damage which is frequently seen in this syndrome may cause a decrease in renal function. Sloughing of debris from the cells into the tubular lumen may cause an intrarenal obstruction to urine flow. In favor of this mechanism is the increased proximal intratubular pressure found by micropuncture study in some models of acute tubular necrosis.[6] This finding, however, is not consistent and in other models of acute tubular necrosis, intratubular pressures are normal or low.

The backleak theory hypothesizes that destruction of the tubular cells allows the glomerular filtrate to leak back into the peritubular capillaries.[7] In support of this theory is the observation that the clearance of neutral dextran exceeds inulin clearance in some clinical cases of acute tubular necrosis.[8] Normally their clearances are equal because both are freely filtered through the glomerulus and neither secreted nor absorbed by the tubules. The backleak theory hypothesizes that the rate of dextran reabsorption through the damaged tubule is slower because dextran is a larger molecule than inulin, therefore causing the increased dextran to inulin clearance ratio. In several models of experimental acute tubular necrosis, however, microinjection studies have not been able to demonstrate any significant reabsorption of radio-labeled inulin after direct injection into tubules.[9]

In conclusion, it appears likely that the pathogenesis of decreased renal function in acute tubular necrosis is multifactorial, with decreased filtration pressure, intratubular obstruction, and possibly decreased glomerular permeability and the backleak of glomerular filtrate all playing roles.

TREATMENT OF ACUTE RENAL FAILURE

The first step in the treatment of acute renal failure is the determination of the cause of the decrease in renal function. It is important to differentiate a primary renal problem from vascular volume depletion where the decrease in renal function is secondary to insufficient renal perfusion. The best method of evaluation of the volume status is the physical examination. Fluid depletion must be suspected in the patient with postural hypotension and tachycardia, whereas peripheral edema, pulmonary edema, and distended neck veins indicate that the patient is fluid overloaded. There are several biochemical tests which will help evaluate the acute renal failure patient with none of these physical signs. Table 12-2 lists biochemical data which are helpful in differentiating decreased renal function secondary to volume depletion from that caused by primary renal dysfunction.[10] A high plasma urea concentration to plasma creatinine concentration ratio, low urinary sodium concentration, high urine to plasma urea or creatinine ratios, and high urine osmolalities all suggest volume depletion. Calculation of the fractional excretion of sodium is helpful. Patients with prerenal azotemia usually excrete less than 1 percent of the filtered sodium whereas patients with primary renal dysfunction usually excrete more than 1 percent. Handa and Murrin have developed a "renal failure index" calculated as shown in Table

12-2. This index is based on the fractional sodium excretion but ignores the plasma sodium concentration.[11] Plasma sodium concentrations vary little and the values obtained are similar to fraction sodium excretion with prerenal patients usually having a value less than one whereas most patients with primary renal dysfunction have values greater than one. In the questionable patient, the careful administration of normal saline in 100- to 200-ml boluses with monitoring of the urine output may be helpful. Mannitol or a strong loop diuretic such as furosemide may also be administered. Patients with volume depletion will respond to either fluid administration or diuretics with a greater increase in urine volume than patients with primary renal dysfunction. The volume-depleted patient should be carefully repleted, but volume overload must be avoided in the patient with primary renal dysfunction.

The administration of mannitol or furosemide has been advocated for the treatment of acute renal failure.[11–14] Animal experiments and clinical studies indicate that diuretics can exert a protective effect from the development of acute renal failure if given before the inciting insult. There is, however, no evidence that the administration of diuretics will alter the course of established acute renal failure. Several prospective studies have been unable to demonstrate any decrease in morbidity or mortality from the administration of diuretics. Bichet and co-workers,

Table 12-2
Factors Differentiating Prerenal Causes of Oliguria from Primary Renal Dysfunction*

	Prerenal	Renal
1. Urine sodium concentration (mEq/liter)	<20	>40
2. Urine osmolality (mOsm)	>500	<350
3. Plasma urea: plasma creatinine ratio	>20:1	<15:1
4. Urine creatinine: plasma creatinine ratio	>40:1	<20:1
5. Fraction excretion of sodium (%)	<1.0	>1.0

$$\text{Fraction excretion of sodium} = \frac{U_{Na}}{P_{Na}} \times \frac{P_{cr}}{U_{cr}} \times 100$$

$$\text{Renal failure index} = \frac{U_{Na} \times P_{cr}}{U_{cr}}$$

*Adapted from Miller TR, Anderson RJ, Lionus SL, et al: Urinary diagnostic indices in acute renal failure a prospective study. Ann Intern Med 89:47–50, 1978.

however, suggest that furosemide can convert oliguric acute renal failure into nonoliguric acute renal failure.[4] Since nonoliguric acute renal failure is easier to manage and may have a better prognosis, this maneuver may be useful. Prospective, controlled studies are apparently in progress. If diuretics are used and increase urine output, it is important that the fluid and electrolytes be replaced so as to prevent further renal compromise from volume depletion. If there is no response to the administration of 25 g of mannitol or 200 mg of furosemide, it does not appear to be helpful to administer more.

Hyperkalemia

Hyperkalemia can be treated with the intravenous administration of sodium bicarbonate, glucose and insulin or the oral or rectal administration of cation exchange resins. Sodium bicarbonate and glucose decrease plasma potassium concentrations by shifting potassium into the intracellular compartment and are therefore only temporalizing measures. They cannot be expected to control serum potassium for prolonged periods of time. Cation exchange resins are very effective in reducing plasma potassium and are frequently useful in the patient with acute renal failure. However, since they increase total body sodium, they must be used with caution in the oliguric patient so as not to result in fluid overload. Dialysis is usually needed in the oliguric acute renal failure patient who is both hyperkalemic and fluid overloaded.

Dialysis

Even though the development of dialysis has had no large effect on the mortality of acute renal failure (see below), it is generally agreed that some patients with acute renal failure should be treated with dialysis. Indications for dialysis in acute renal failure are listed in Table 12-3. Dialysis should be strongly considered in the oliguric patient with a large degree of fluid overload, especially if there is pulmonary congestion.

It has been suggested that the early initiation of dialysis may decrease the morbidity and mortality of acute renal failure.[15,16] This is based on the facts that infection and hemorrhage are the leading causes of mortality in acute renal failure and that dialysis decreases the hemorrhagic abnormality and may improve the immunologic system in uremia (see Chapter 1). If the plasma urea or creatinine concentrations are increasing rapidly, dialysis should be started before the develop-

Table 12-3
Indications for Dialysis in Acute Renal Failure

1. Fluid overload
2. Refractory hyperkalemia
3. Overt uremia
4. BUN > 100 and/or plasma creatinine > 12

ment of uremic symptoms. In general it is probably wise to initiate dialysis if the blood urea nitrogen concentration is likely to exceed 100 to 120 mg/dl or the plasma creatinine 12–14 mg/dl within the next 24 hours. The development of uremic symptoms such as encephalopathy, pericarditis, gastritis, or colitis are indications for dialysis independent of plasma urea and creatinine concentrations.

Either hemodialysis or peritoneal dialysis may be used to treat acute renal failure. Although randomized, controlled studies have not been done, comparative studies do not show a consistent difference in morbidity or mortality between these two modes of therapy.[17] Peritoneal dialysis has the advantage of a more gradual decline in plasma urea concentrations avoiding the possibility of disequilibrium problems. There is also even, less rapid fluid removal rates with peritoneal dialysis which prevent fast intercompartmental fluid shifts in patients who are frequently already in an unstable cardiovascular state. The lack of the need for anticoagulation has definite advantages in some patients such as those with head trauma.

Hemodialysis, on the other hand, does not expose the patient to the possibility of peritonitis, With infection being the leading cause of mortality in acute renal failure this assumes a great importance. In patients with preexisting peritonitis, however, peritoneal dialysis offers the additional advantage of the local installation of antibiotics. There are rare patients who require hemodialysis because their rate of metabolism is so great that urea removal by peritoneal dialysis is insufficient to keep plasma concentrations at an acceptable levels. Hemodialysis is also much more effective for potassium removal in those patients with severe potassium problems. The vast majority of the patients with acute renal failure can be adequately treated by either hemodialysis or peritoneal and the degree of expertise that the medical facility has with each of these modes of therapy is an important determinant. In treating the acute renal failure patient with hemodialysis, low blood flow rates with a small to moderate surface area dialyzer should be used. In the normal-sized adult, 1.0 m^2 and

100–150 ml/min are usually sufficient. Dialysis should be performed at least every second day and may be required daily. The frequency and duration of the treatments should be adjusted so as to keep the predialysis serum urea concentration from rising above 80–100 mg/dl. Low dose or regional heparin therapy should be used in trauma, postoperative, or other patients predisposed to hemorrhage (Chapter 6). The dialysate sodium concentration should be equal to or greater than plasma sodium concentration and if possible bicarbonate dialysate should be used in the patient with cardiovascular instability.

If peritoneal dialysis is to be used to treat acute renal failure, continuous dialysis therapy should be considered. This is especially true if the patient's activities is already limited to his bed and a bedside chair. In the hospital setting, this is best accomplished with the use of an automated peritoneal dialysis machine which both decreases personnel time requirement and reduces the incidence of peritonitis. Careful monitoring of the patient's fluid and electrolyte status is necessary. If continuous dialysis is used, cycle length and dialysate glucose concentrations can be adjusted so as to control plasma urea concentrations and fluid balance.

Recently the technique of continuous hemofiltration for the treatment of acute renal failure has been described.[18] This technique uses a small, high-flux hemofilter. Blood access can be obtained by the use of an arteriovenous shunt or the percutaneous puncture of the femoral artery and femoral vein in these cases a blood pump is not required. Cannulas can alternatively be placed in the subclavian or femoral vein and either a double-loop catheter or peripheral vein used for blood return, but in this case, a blood pump is required. The treatments are performed in the intensive care unit without the continuous attendance of special dialysis personnel. Ultrafiltration rates of 10–20 ml/min are obtained and the fluid is replaced on an hourly basis. With this technique fluid balance is continuously maintained at an appropriate level and most patients need no other type of dialytic therapy. This technique is still in its infancy and needs further evaluation. (See Chapter 10 for a further discussion of hemofiltration.)

Nutrition

Nutrition plays a very important role in the patient with acute renal failure. Controlled studies indicate that hyperalimentation can decrease the mortality of acute renal failure. In a randomized study, Able and co-workers found a mortality of 25 percent in patients receiving glucose and amino acids compared to a 56 percent mortality in patients receiving glucose alone.[19] Others have found similar results.[20,21] Spreiter and co-workers have demonstrated that the administration of amino acids and glucose is capable of reducing the negative nitrogen and caloric balances in patients with acute renal failure.[22] They suggest that patients with acute renal failure should be given 1 g/kg of amino acids and greater than 12.5 g/kg of glucose each day.

If the patient with acute renal failure is unable to eat a sufficient diet, then hyperalimentation should strongly be considered. Because of the high risk of infection, a feeding tube should be used, if possible, instead of intravenous hyperalimentation. The varying and sometimes opposing effects of renal failure, hyperalimentation, and dialysis make it mandatory that serum electrolyte concentrations including phosphorus, magnesium, and calcium be carefully monitored.

Infection

Infection is the leading cause of death in acute renal failure, accounting for 60 to 75 percent of the total mortality.[23] Patients need to be carefully observed with appropriate cultures obtained when indicated. When antibiotics are needed, it is helpful to measure serum antibiotic concentrations in order to adjust the dosage. Intravenous, urinary, and other catheters should be avoided unless absolutely necessary and the use of the urinary catheter for the sole purpose of accurate determination of urine volume should be strongly discouraged. The patient should also be mobilized frequently so as to avoid pulmonary stasis.

PROGNOSIS

The mortality of acute renal failure is very high with most studies finding that less than 50 percent of patients survive.[23] Patients with acute tubular necrosis have the highest mortality whereas the prognosis of acute renal failure secondary to obstruction or glomerular disease is much better. The mortality of acute tubular necrosis is very dependent on the underlying disease. Surgical patients, especially abdominal and thoracic, have the highest mortality rates, whereas medical causes such as nephrotoxic agents have lower rates. The mortality rate is, surprisingly, relatively independent of age.

Infection is by far the leading cause of death in the patient with acute renal failure irrespective of the underlying cause. The combination of renal insufficiency with the stress and increased catabolism of the underlying disease process, whether it be postsurgery, postmyocardial infarction, or other, appears to produce a state of severe immunological supression. The pulmonary tree is the most frequent site of infection.

The second and a not uncommon cause of death is hemorrhage, usually in the gastrointestinal tract. Stress ulcers are frequent and the routine administration of cimetidine has been avocated by some. If cimetidine is administered, the dose must be reduced because of the renal insufficiency; 300–600 mg each day is adequate.

The onset of the availability of clinical dialysis to treat acute renal failure in the 1960s did not result in a large decrease in the mortality, nor has there been any decrease since.[23] This is somewhat surprising as there presently appears to be a significant number of patients who survive after several weeks of dialysis for severely compromised renal function. It appears unlikely that these patients would survive without dialysis treatment. If this is true, there are two possible explanations for the lack of a decrease in mortality. First, it may be that dialysis is causing the demise of patients who would have survived if not treated with dialysis. This could be due either to the procedure itself or by the dialysis treatment interfering with a proper administration of other important supportive measures. The latter appears more likely. Second, it may be that more patients with acute renal failure are critically ill now than before. It is probable that newer, more extensive recusitative measures and more risky and invasive surgical procedures have prolonged the life of patients who would not have previously lived long enough to develop renal failure. The mortality of patients with acute renal failure nevertheless remains high and dramatically points out the need for better methods of treating these patients.

REFERENCES

1. Smolens P, Stein JH: Pathophysiology of acute renal failure. Am J Med 70:479–482, 1981
2. Flamenbaum W: Pathophysiology of acute renal failure. Arch Intern Med 131:911–928, 1973
3. Hollenberg NK, Epstein M, Rosen SM: Acute oliguric renal failure in man. Evidence for preferential renal cortical ischemia. Medicine 47:455–475, 1968
4. Bichet DG, Burke TJ, Schrier RW: Prevention and pathogenesis of acute renal failure. Clin Exp Dial Apheresis 5:127–141, 1981
5. Flores JE, Dibona DR, Beck CH, Leaf A: The role of cell swelling in ischemic damage and the protective effect of hypertonic solute. J Clin Invest 51:118–126, 1972

6. Tanner GA, Steinhausen M: Tubular obstruction in ischemia-induced acute renal failure in the rat. Kidney Int 10:565–573, 1976
7. Bank N, Muly BF, Aynedjian HS: The role of "leakage" of tubular fluid in anuria due to mercury poisoning. J Clin Invest 46:695–704, 1967
8. Myers BD, Cance BJ, Yee RR, Hilberman M, Michaels AS: Pathophysiology of hemodynamically mediated acute renal failure in man. Kidney Int 18:495–504, 1980
9. Burke TJ, Cronin RE, Duchin KL, Peterson LN, Schrier RW: Ischemic and tubule obstruction during acute renal failure in dogs: Mannitol in protection. Am J Physiol 238:F305–F314, 1980
10. Miller TR, Anderson RJ, Linas SL, et al: Urinary diagnostic indices in acute renal failure, a prospective study. Ann Intern Med 89:47–50, 1978
11. Handa SP, Murrin PAF: Diagnostic indices in acute renal failure. Can Med Assoc J 96:78–82, 1967
12. Cantorovich F, Galli C, Benedetti L, et al: High dose furosemide in established acute renal failure. Brit Med J 4:449–450, 1973
13. Old CW, Lehrner LM 1: Prevention of radiocontrast induced acute renal failure with mannitol. Lancet 1:885, 1980
14. Barry KG, Cohen A, Knochel JP, et al: The prevention of acute renal failure during resection of an aneurism of the abdominal aorta. N Engl J Med 264:967–971, 1961
15. Conger JD: A controlled evaluation of prophylactic dialysis in post traumatic renal failure. J Trauma 15:1056–1063, 1975
16. Kleinknecht D, Jungers P, Chanard J, Barbanel C, Ganeval D: Uremic and nonuremic complications of acute renal failure, evaluation of early and frequent dialysis on prognosis. Kidney Int 1:190–196, 1972
17. Scott RB, Ogg CS, Cameron JS, Bewick M: Why persistently high mortality in acute renal failure? Lancet 2:75–78, 1972
18. Olbricht CH, Schurek JH, Muller C, Stolte H: Continuous spontaneous hemofiltration for acute renal failure in multi-organ-failure. Trans Am Soc Artif Intern Organs 28:33–37, 1982
19. Abel RM, Beck CH, Abbott WM, et al: Improved survival from acute renal failure after treatment with intravenous essential L-amino acids and glucose. N Engl J Med 288:696–699, 1973
20. Dudrick SJ, Steiger E, Long JM: Renal failure in surgical patients treatment with intravenous essential amino acids and hypertonic glucose. Surgery 68:180–186, 1970
21. Baek SM, Makabali GG, Bryan-Brown CW, Kusek J: The influence of parenteral nutrition on the course of acute renal failure. Surg Gynecol Obstet 141:405–408, 1975
22. Spreiter SC, Myers BD, Swenson RS: Protein-energy requirements in subjects with acute renal failure receiving intermittent hemodialysis. Am J Clin Nutr 33:1433–1437, 1980
23. Kjellstrand CM, Gornick C, Davin T: Recovery from acute renal failure. Clin Exper Dial Apheresis 5:143–161, 1981

John C. Van Stone

13

Treatment of Drug Intoxication with Dialysis and Hemoperfusion

Very soon after the demonstration that hemodialysis could effectively remove the endogenously generated toxins which accumulate in renal insufficiency, the possibility of treating exogenous drug intoxications with dialysis was explored.[1] The history of dialysis for drug intoxication has followed a course similar to that of many new treatments. There was at first great enthusiasm with some centers reporting success with its use for nearly all severe drug overdoses. The limitations and drawbacks of the technique soon became apparent, however, and the frequency that dialysis was performed for intoxication was greatly reduced. At this time it was even suggested that dialysis had no place in the treatment of any drug intoxication.[2] It is currently felt by many that dialysis and the more recently developed technique of hemoperfusion will reduce the morbidity and/or mortality of a limited number of drug intoxications.[3] There are, however, few well-controlled studies which the clinician can use to make the decision of whether to use one of these techniques in any particular case.

Neither hemodialysis nor hemoperfusion should be considered the primary mode of therapy for any drug intoxication. Proper medical management of the patient is usually far more important in determining the final outcome. The care of the comatose patient, which is frequently the case in drug intoxication, is a difficult medical task which requires the utmost in medical skills and the meticulous attention to detail. Since pulmonary complications account for the largest part of the morbidity and mortality, appropriate pulmonary care is exceedingly important. The position of the patient should be changed frequently to prevent fluid from pooling in the dependent portions of the lungs and the development of decubitus ulcers. Early intubation should be considered to provide ventilation support, prevent aspiration of stomach and oral secretions, and to allow for easy suctioning of pulmonary secretions.

Preventing further absorption of any portion of the drug remaining in the gastrointestinal tract is also important. If the ingestion was recent, the gastric contents should be removed. Because some drugs inhibit gastric emptying this may be helpful for long periods after ingestion. Samples of gastric contents should be sent to the toxicology lab for identification and quantification of the ingested drugs. In the conscious patient, emesis can be induced by the administration of syrup of ipecac. Gastric lavage with a large tube could be used in the comatose or semicomatose patient. Gastric lavage may induce vomiting and to prevent aspiration in the comatose patient, prior placement of an endotrachial tube is mandatory. Activated charcoal can be given after gastric lavage to prevent absorption of any remaining drug.

The cardiovascular system must be carefully monitored. Measurement of central venous and/or pulmonary wedge pressure is helpful in the hypotensive patient. Some drugs, like the barbituates, cause hypotension by vascular volume depletion from either a decrease in the actual vascular volume or an increase in the volume of the vascular bed. Other drugs decrease blood pressure by a decrease in vascular resistance. Volume depletion should be treated with colloid-containing fluids such as human serum albumin so as to replete the vascular volume without causing peripheral or pulmonary edema. Hypotension from decreased vascular resistance should be treated with vasoconstrictors.

While the extracorporeal removal of drugs is not indicated in all cases of intoxication it appears to be clearly of benefit in some instances. Serious consideration must be given to conservative management, however, and extracorporeal dialysis or hemoperfusion should not be performed on the premise that it can do no harm and there is an outside chance that it may help the patient. The potential benefits must outweigh the increased risk of a moderately complicated therapeutic procedure imposed on a critically ill patient. Schreiner has suggested 10 criteria for consideration of hemodialysis or hemoperfusion in drug overdose:[3]

1. Severe clinical intoxication with abnormal vital signs. Often this will include hypotension despite fluid replacement, apnea, or severe hypothermia.

2. Ingestion and probable absorption of a potentially lethal dose.
3. A blood level that is in the potentially fatal range.
4. A degree of intoxication or an underlying disease in the patient which reduces the normal route of excretion of the drug.
5. The presence of a significant quantity of a circulating substance which is metabolized to a more noxious compound.
6. Progressive clinical deterioration while the patient is under careful medical management.
7. Prolonged coma.
8. The presence of an underlying disease such as bronchitis or emphysema which increases the hazards of coma.
9. The development of a significant complication such as aspiration pneumonitis.
10. Poisoning by agents known to produce delayed toxicity such as paraquat, *Amanita phalloides,* and acetaminophen.

It is also important that the extracorporeal method will effectively remove significant quantities of the drug from the body. The clearance of the drug must be large enough to significantly increase the total rate of removal from the body. Sufficient quantities of the drug must be in the vascular space. If a drug is sequestered in the intracellular space, such as with digitalis, then hemodialysis and hemoperfusion will not remove significant amounts even though the blood clearance rates are high.

There are four common methods of actively increasing drug removal: forced diuresis, peritoneal dialysis, hemodialysis, and hemoperfusion. Urine flow may be enhanced by the use of mannitol, urea, or potent diuretics such as furosemide or ethacrynic acid. Urine flow rates of 500 ml to 1 liter each hour or greater are obtainable by these techniques. It is very important that, if a forced diuresis is initiated, the patient's fluid and electrolytes status be monitored very carefully to prevent severe imbalances. Forced diuresis is frequently inappropriately used. Although the excretion rate of some drugs can be significantly increased with the use of this technique, the rate of most intoxicants are not. If the pK of a basic toxin is between 6 and 8.5, then the excretion can be significantly increased by alkalizing the urine so that it is in its ionized form. This is true for some drugs such as phenobarbitol, however, if the pK is not in this range as in the case of most of the barbituates, then alkalinization is of no value. It is also of little value to increase the urine output greater than 400–500 ml/h. Although with aggressive diuresis urine flow greater than 1 liter can be obtained, the increase in toxin removal is minimal and the possibility of developing severe fluid or electrolyte problems is significantly increased.

While peritoneal dialysis is effective in increasing the clearance rate of many medications, it is seldom the procedure of choice. Either hemodialysis or hemoperfusion is usually many times more effective for most drug ingestions.

HEMOPERFUSION

Hemoperfusion is a therapeutic procedure with many similarities to hemodialysis. For this reason it is generally performed by the hemodialysis personnel. Similar to hemodialysis, hemoperfusion requires the availability of 200–300 ml/min of blood flow and the use of a blood pump. With hemoperfusion, however, the blood is passed through a column containing solid particles and the substances removed during the procedure are directly adsorbed onto these particles rather than diffusing through a membrane into dialysate fluid. In some cases, however, the particles are coated with a membrane that the toxins must diffuse through before absorption. There are two types of hemoperfusion cartridges commercially available in the United States: cellulose acetate-coated, activated charcoal sold by Gambro Inc. (Barrington, IL), and amberlite polystyrene resin sold by the Extracorporeal Corporation (King of Prussia, PA).

Charcoal has long been known for its capacity to adsorb large quantities of solutes from solutions. Charcoal adsorption is nonspecific and it is capable of adsorbing a large variety of substances. The direct perfusion of blood over charcoal is unfortunately associated with problems, such as platelet destruction and the microembolism of small particles of charcoal into the patient. These problems can be prevented by encapsulating the charcoal particles with a thin, semipermeable membrane.[4] Cellulose nitrate, albumin, acrylic hydrogel, and cellulose acetate have all been used to coat the charcoal. The charcoal in the currently available columns is coated with cellulose acetate which has been extensively hydrolyzed with sodium hydroxide so as to increase its diffusive capacity. Although the coating decreases the rate of solute removal, these columns are still capable of effectively adsorbing small and middle molecules and are very biocompatible.

Rosenbaum has extensively studied the use of amberlite XAD-2 and the more effective XAD-4 columns for hemoperfusion.[5] These are uncoated and uncharged polystyrene resins with a specific adsorption attraction for lipid soluable solutes. They are very biocompatible and the larger, more selective adsorption capacity of these resins prevents the large, progressive decrease in clearance which is frequently seen with charcoal columns. They also do not produce hypoglycemia or hypocalcemia which can occur with charcoal hemoperfusion. The adsorption capacity and clearance rate for most common drug intoxications is higher with the XAD-4 resin column than with the available charcoal columns. Some medications which are not absorbed by the XAD-4 columns, however, are absorbed by the charcoal columns.

Hemoperfusion has been used to treat not only drug intoxications, but also hepatic coma and as an adjuvant to dialysis in the treatment of uremia.[6] Although hemoperfusion may cause a temporary improvement in hepatic coma, there is no evidence it can change the ultimate prognosis or decrease the mortality and, while theoretically hemoperfusion may improve uremia by increased middle molecule removal, any potential benefit of its use as an adjuvant to hemodialysis remains to be demonstrated. At this time the use of hemoperfusion for purposes other than drug intoxication must be considered experimental.

TREATMENT OF SPECIFIC DRUG INTOXICATIONS

Sedatives

Barbituates continue to be responsible for a large number of acute drug intoxications and are not infrequently fatal, with the mortality rate of patients presenting in stage 4 coma being as high as 35 percent.[7] The early treatment of barbituate intoxication should include gastric lavage, oral charcoal administration, and respiratory and cardiovascular support. Identification of the offending toxin(s) from the gastric aspirate and serum is extremely important. Barbituate intoxications are frequently associated with hypotension secondary to a relative volume deficiency. This should be treated with the administration of colloid-containing fluids and monitoring of the fluid status with central venous or pulmonary artery pressure should be considered.

Forced alkaline diuresis has been advocated for acute barbituate overdose. The increase in renal clearance of the short- and intermediate-acting barbituates obtained by this method is minimal, but the urinary excretion of phenobarbitol can be increased several fold.[8] If this technique is used, careful monitoring of the patient is necessary so as not to increase the already present vascular instability. Even for phenobarbitol, hemodialysis and hemoperfusion are many times more effective.

Both hemodialysis and hemoperfusion are effective in removing short-, intermediate-, and long-acting barbituates.[3,5,8-10] Although there are no controlled studies, comparative studies suggest that the duration of coma can be significantly decreased, with patients frequently waking up after several hours of treatment. The clearance by XAD-4 resin hemoperfusion approaches that of blood flow (200–300 ml/min) and is considerably higher than charcoal hemoperfusion (100–150 ml/min) or hemodialysis (25–50 ml/min). Extracorporeal drug removal should strongly be considered in the patient with stage 3 or 4 coma, blood levels greater than 3.5 mg/dl for the short-acting barbituates or 8 mg/dl for the long-acting barbituates, or the ingestion of greater than 3 g of a short-acting or 5 g of a long-acting barbituate.

Chloral hydrate intoxication is clinically similar to that with barbituates. Fatalities are usually associated with the ingestion of greater than 10 g. Chloral hydrate is rapidly metabolized in the body to the alcohol, trichloroethanol, which is responsible for its therapeutic and toxic actions. Trichloroethanol, being very water soluble and of small molecular weight, is highly dialyzable. Hemodialysis clearances are 150–170 ml/min which is considerably greater than the charcoal hemoperfusion clearance of 100 ml/min.[3] Hemodialysis should be considered in patients with stage 3 or 4 coma.

Glutethimide (Doriden) intoxication was formerly very common, but is becoming less frequent. Glutethimide is highly lipid soluble and is concentrated in fatty tissues. Glutethimide overdose is frequently associated with marked fluctuations in the level of consciousness. The sudden onset of apnea must be carefully watched for and vascular instability is common. Clearances with hemodialysis are low at 20 ml/min and less than 10 percent of the ingested drug is removed in a 4-hour hemodialysis procedure. The clearance may be increased by using oil for the dialysate (lipid dialysis), but this is a very cumbersome procedure and is no longer indicated in view of the high clearances which can be obtained with resin hemoperfusion. Clearances with resin hemoperfusion are in the range of 200 to 300 ml/min and with charcoal hemoperfusion 125–150 ml/min.[3,5,14] There is frequently a rebound increase in the plasma concentration occurring after treatment has been terminated with a deepening of the coma, probably from the mobilization of the drug from fat stores. It is suggested that hemoperfusion be considered in the patient with stage 3 or 4 coma, ingestion of greater than 10 g of glutethimide or a blood concentration greater than 3 mg/dl.

Tranquilizers

Diazepam (Valium) is a very common drug seen in overdoses. It has a low fatality rate, usually only producing stage 1 or 2 coma, from which the patient can easily be aroused. It seldom results in respiratory depression or vascular instability. Supportive care is generally the treatment of choice and hemodialysis or hemoperfusion is seldom indicated. If extracorporeal drug removal is desired, charcoal hemoperfusion appears to have higher clearances than resin hemoperfusion or hemodialysis.[3]

Chlordiazepoxide (Librium) intoxication is similar to diazepam intoxication in that, while it is commonly encountered, it seldom results in fatality. Supportive therapy is again usually adequate but, if extracorporeal removal is necessary, charcoal hemoperfusion would appear to be the method of choice.[3]

Meprobamate (Miltown) overdose can result in coma, respiratory depression, vascular collapse, and death. Hypotension is usually the result of decreased vascular resistance rather than fluid depletion and should be treated with vasopressors.[11] Fatalities are usually associated with the ingestion of greater than 8 g and/or blood concentrations above 12 mg/dl. Meprobamate is metabolized by the liver fairly rapidly with a plasma disappearance rate of 8 percent each hour. For this reason hemodialysis and/or hemoperfusion is seldom indicated unless there is reason to believe that the normal metabolic pathways are compromised. The clearance for hemodialysis is in the range of 50–75 ml/h and for charcoal hemoperfusion 175–200 ml/min.[3-12]

Phenothiazines: chlorpromazine (Thorazine), promazine (Sparine), and trifluoperazine (Stelazine). Fatalities from phenothiazines overdose are extremely unusual. Toxicity is usually limited to acute neurologic symptoms, frequently extrapyramidal in nature and responds to benztropine (Cogentin). The phenothiazines are highly tissue bound and the amounts removed by hemodialysis or hemoperfusion are very limited.

Methaqualone (Quaalude) intoxication is associated with severe central nervous system depression, but hyperactive deep tendon reflexes. It is a commonly abused drug and intoxication from methaqualone obtained from illegal sources is not uncommon. Metabolism of the drug, at least at therapeutic blood levels, is rapid with a drug half-life of 2.6 hours. Clearances with hemodialysis (20–30 ml/min) are much less than with hemoperfusion, where clearances of 200–300 ml/min are obtainable. The clearance with charcoal hemoperfusion decreases rapidly with time and resin hemoperfusion appears to be preferable.[3,13,14] There are no comparative studies to determine if hemoperfusion or hemodialysis can reduce the mortality or morbidity, but with the rapid endogenous clearance rate it is likely that conservative management is adequate in most cases.

Methyprylon (Noludar) overdose is associated with coma, respiratory depression, and severe hypotension. Dramatic improvements have been reported with hemodialysis.[15] Clearances with hemodialysis are 80 ml/min and with charcoal hemoperfusion are 150–200 ml/min.[14,15] It has been recommended that hemodialysis or hemoperfusion be considered when the ingested dose is greater than 6 g or the serum concentration over 5 mg/dl.

Ethchlorvynl (Placidyl) is very slowly metabolized by the body (half-life 72 hours) and similarly to glutethimide is sequestered away from the plasma compartment. Intoxication is associated with deep coma, hypothermia, respiratory depression, and hypotension. It is not infrequently fatal. Clearance by resin hemoperfusion (175–225 ml/min) is better than that by charcoal hemoperfusion (115–140 ml/min) or hemodialysis (50–100 ml/min).[3,10,16-18] Patients ingesting more than 10 g of ethchlorvynl or with blood levels greater than 7 mg/dl should be considered for hemoperfusion or hemodialysis.

Tricyclic drugs: imipramine (Tofranil), amitriptyline (Elavil), doxepin (Sinequan). Intoxication with the antidepressant tricyclic amines results in coma, hyperactive tendon reflexes, muscle twitching, seizures, hyperpyrexia, vascular instability with either hypertension or hypotension, metabolic acidosis, hypokalemia, and severe cardiac arrythmias. The correlation between plasma concentrations and the severity of coma is poor. These drugs are rapidly tissue bound and it is unlikely that hemodialysis or hemoperfusion will significantly decrease the morbidity or mortality. This has generally been the experience when they have been tried.[3] Lidocaine is helpful in treating the cardiac arrythmias and diazepam, paraldehyde, or phenobarbitol may be used for seizure activity.

Monoamine oxidase inhibitors: paragyline (Eutonyl), nialamide (Niamid), isocarboxazid (Marplen), phenelzine (Nardil), tranylcypromine (Parnate). Acute intoxication with monoamine oxidase inhibitors is associated with agitation, hallucination, hyperreflexia, hyperpyrexia, cardiovascular instability with hypertension or hypotension, convulsions, and coma. It may cause death. There are no good data available on the use of hemodialysis or hemoperfusion, but several clinical reports suggest that hemodialysis or peritoneal dialysis may be associated with clinical improvement.[3,19] Hypertension, when it occurs should be treated with an alpha blocking agent and phenothiazines may be used to treat the hyperactivity.

Amphetamine intoxication is associated with hyperpyrexia, convulsions, hypotension, coma, and death. Hyperpyrexia may cause rhabdomyolysis with acute renal failure. The drug is quickly tissue bound with very small amounts remaining in the vascular compartment and hemodialysis or hemoperfusion are probably of little use for its removal. The phenothiazines will counteract much of the toxicity.

Analgesics

Salicylate (Aspirin) is the leading cause of poisoning in children and is not infrequent in adults. The diagnosis in adults is frequently not considered and delay in diagnosis will significantly increase the mortality. Salicylate intoxication is associated with tachycardia, initial respiratory alkalosis from hyperventilation followed by metabolic acidosis with a large anion gap, hyperpyrexia, fluid depletion, hypokalemia, hemorrhage, coma, and death. Salicylate excretion can be increased 10-fold by alkalinazation of the urine. Mild diuresis is helpful, but extremely high urine rates (greater than 1 liter/h) are no more effective than the more moderate flow rates of 200 ml/min. Hemodialysis effectively removes large amounts of drug and probably decreases the morbidity and mortality.[3,20] Peritoneal dialysis is only 25 percent as effective as hemodialysis, but is more effective than forced diuresis. Both charcoal hemoperfusion and resin hemoperfusion remove salicylate but less effectively than hemodialysis. Hemodialysis should be considered when greater than 0.5 g/kg of salicylate has been ingested or blood concentrations are above 80 mg/dl. With smaller ingestions and blood concentrations between 20 and 80 mg/dl mild forced diuresis should be considered.

Acetaminophen (Tylenol) ingestion in large amounts is associated with mortalities as high as 20 percent.[3] Early clinical signs are mild and consist mainly of vomiting. Two or three days after ingestion, however, signs of hepatic dysfunction occur with hyperbilirubinemia, increased transaminase, and increased prothrombin time. Acetaminophen causes hepatic necrosis with collapse of the central lobular reticulum and patient's dying of hepatic coma 1–2 weeks after ingestion. Those that recover may develop permanent hepatic fibrosis. The toxicity of acetaminophen is related to hepatic glutathione depletion and experimental evidence in animals suggest that preventing this depletion by the administration of glutathione or its precursors can decrease toxicity. Cystamine, methionine, and N-acetyl cysteine has been used clinically with encouraging results.[3,21]

Acetaminophen is rapidly metabolized in the body with a half-life of 4 hours. Plasma concentrations greater than 30 mg/dl usually result in sustained liver damage and concentrations below 12 mg/dl do not. Acetaminophen can be removed by hemodialysis (clearance 120 ml/min), but charcoal hemoperfusion is more effective at 200–300 ml/min.[3,20] A controlled study was unable to demonstrate any benefit of charcoal hemoperfusion, but many of the patients were treated late.[22] In view of the severe toxicity it might be of value to use charcoal hemoperfusion, if it can be instituted within the first few hours of ingestion.

Propoxyphene (Darvon) intoxication is associated with the rapid onset of coma, respiratory depression, pulmonary edema, convulsions, and death. The narcotic antagonist nalorphine will reverse most of the effects. Propoxyphene is sequestered in many tissues and plasma concentrations are very low. Hemodialysis and hemoperfusion remove minimal amounts of the drug and are of little or no value.[3]

Narcotics: morphine, heroin, methadone, meperidine (Demerol). Narcotics rapidly leave the vascular system and are concentrated in the liver, kidney, skeletal muscle, and brain. Plasma concentrations are low and metabolism is rapid with half-lives of 1–2 hours. Dialysis and hemoperfusion are probably of no value and intoxication should be treated with specific antagonists like nalorphine or naloxone.[3]

Alcohols

Methanol ingestion is associated with central nervous system depression similar to that produced by ethanol, severe metabolic acidosis from the formation of formic acid, and blindness caused by retinal toxicity from the metabolite formaldehyde. Ingestion of a few ounces may produce permanent retinal damage. There are two components to the treatment of methanol ingestion. The first is to inhibit the formation of the toxic metabolites. Methanol and ethanol are both metabolized by the same hepatic dehydrogenase. Ethanol causes a competitive inhibition of this enzyme and prevents the formation of the more toxic methanol metabolites. Ethanol should be administered in doses of 5–10 g/h so as to maintain blood concentrations of 100 mg/dl. The second part of the treatment is the removal of methanol and its metabolites. Peritoneal dialysis, hemodialysis, and charcoal hemoperfusion all remove methanol with hemodialysis being more effective and resulting in rapid clinical improvement.[3,23] A concentration of 1.5 ml/liter of ethanol in the dialysate will maintain appropriate blood ethanol levels during the procedure. Dialysis will also correct the metabolic acidosis, although intravenous sodium bicarbonate may also be given. Dialysis should be considered if more than 1 ounce is ingested, blood methanol levels are above 100 mg/dl or severe acidosis is present. Dialysis shold be continued until blood methanol concentrations are below 50 mg/dl.

Ethylene glycol ingestion is similar to methanol ingestion in that the toxicity is primarily due to a metabolite, in this case oxalic acid. Toxicity is manifested by metabolic acidosis, mental confusion, ataxia, convulsions, occular palsy, pulmonary edema, and nephrotoxicity. The nephrotoxicity is the result of the deposition of oxalate which causes an interstitial nephritis. The metabolism of ethylene glycol by alcohol dehydrogenase can be competitively inhibited by ethanol and blood concentrations of 100 mg/dl of ethanol should be maintained. Hemodialysis will remove both ethylene glycol and oxalate and should be considered for ingestions greater than 1 ounce or blood concentrations greater than 100 mg/dl.[3,24] Ethanol may be added to the dialysate see methanol ingestion). Forced diuresis may be helpful in preventing renal damage.

Isopropyl alcohol toxicity is associated with coma, respiratory depression, areflexia, hypothermia, and hypotension. Isopropyl alcohol is metabolized to acetone which may be responsible for some of the toxicity. Hemodialysis effectively removes the alcohol, will remove some of the acetone, and should be considered for alcohol blood levels greater than 100 mg/dl.[3]

Arsenic

There is some evidence that hemodialysis may be effective in treating acute arsenic and arsine poisoning. Arsine (AsH_3) is a gas generated when arsenic is present in a strong reducing environment. Arsenic is present in many industrial situations and arsine is not infrequently produced during industrial accidents. Both arsenic and arsine poisoning acutely cause vomiting, headache, abdominal and skeletal cramps, and acute renal failure. Arsine is also associated with marked hemolysis and hemoglobinuria. Hemodialysis will remove arsenic with clearances of 80–100 ml/min, but is probably not indicated if the patient has normal renal function.[3,25] Although the objective evidence suggests that arsine complexes with hemoglobin and is not removed by dialysis, hemodialysis has been claimed to decrease the mortality of arsine poisoning.[3,26] Exchange transfusion has also been suggested for arsine poisoning. Dimercaprol (BAL) will bind arsenic, promote its excretion, and should be used in both acute and chronic arsenic poisoning.

Herbicides

Paraquat and *diquat* are dipyridium compounds frequently found in herbicides. Ingestion acutely produces shock, acute renal failure, and local ulcerations in the mouth, pharynx, and esophagus. The drug appears to be slowly concentrated in the lungs where it produces pulmonary failure from progressive pulmonary fibrosis a few days after ingestion. Death from pulmonary insufficiency is common. Paraquat may be absorbed from the gastrointestinal tract several days after ingestion and gastric lavage, sorbants, and aggressive catharsis are indicated. Renal paraquat clearances are in the order of 10 ml/min. Hemodialysis (70–100 ml/min), charcoal hemoperfusion (100–150 ml/min), and the cation exchange resin, zerolit 225 (200 ml/min), are effective in removing paraquat. Diquat has been shown to be less dialyzable than paraquat, but removal by hemoperfusion should be similar to paraquat. Since there is evidence that both these agents are concentrated from the blood into the lungs for several days after ingestion, active removal from the blood should strongly be considered and is felt by many to decrease the otherwise very high mortality.[3] Oxygen administration increases the pulmonary toxicity in animal studies and should be administered only if absolutely necessary.

Insecticides

The organophosphate compounds *parathion, malathion, diazinone, nitrostigmine,* and *demeton* are cholinesterase inhibitors which are frequently found in insecticides. They produce poisoning by absorption through the skin or oral ingestion. Toxicity is associated with vomiting, diarrhea, urinary and fecal incontinence, blurred vision, sweating, lacrimation, excessive salivation, muscle twitching, and flaccid paralysis. Red cell or plasma analysis reveal low cholinesterase activity. Atropine is a specific antidote and its aggressive administration is indicated. Respiratory support may be needed. The oxime compounds can reactivate the cholinesterase and 1–2 g of pralidoxine should be slowly administered intravenously. This will usually reverse the muscle weakness and can be repeated as needed. Most, but not all, of the organophosphate compounds are removed by hemodialysis (clearance 25–50 ml/min) but charcoal hemoperfusion is more efficient (clearance 75 to 100 ml/min).[3] Charcoal hemoperfusion has been associated with clinical improvement.

Mushroom Poisoning

Two types of poison mushrooms grow in North America. *Amanita muscaria* produces an acute toxic syndrome which begins shortly after ingestion (2 minutes to 2 hours). The symptoms are due to muscarine and consist of marked lacrimation, salivation, sweating, myosis, dyspnea, abdominal pain, severe diarrhea, vascular collapse, coma, and death. Atropine is a specific antidote and the prognosis is good even in severe cases if the diagnosis is recognized and atropine administered. Dialysis and hemoperfusion are not indicated.

The second type of mushroom poisoning is much more common and is caused by the mushroom *Am. phalloides*. This mushroom has two toxins, phalloidine and amanitine. Symptoms are delayed and occur 6–15 hours after ingestion. They consist of severe abdominal pain, nausea, vomiting, and diarrhea. Severe dehydration occurs accompanied by extreme thirst. There is marked hepatic toxicity with liver dysfunction developing 2 to 3 days after ingestion. Acute yellow atrophy of the liver may develop with death occurring 5–8 days after ingestion. The mortality rate of untreated cases is between 50 and 100 percent. Treatment should consist of gastric lavage, oral charcoal administration, correction of fluid and electrolyte depletion, and cardiovascular support. The administration of thioctic acid and high doses of penicillin which inhibits the binding of amanitine should be considered.[27] Hemodialysis, resin and charcoal hemoperfusion will remove both toxins from the blood with hemoperfusion being more efficient.[3,28] Although comparative studies are lacking, both modalities have been used in *A. phalloides* intoxication and have been thought to reduce the incidence and severity of hepatotoxicity.

Quinine intoxication is associated with tinnitus, visual disturbances, headache, nausea, vomiting, and diarrhea. In more severe cases coma and blindness from optic atrophy may occur. The fatal dose is approximately 8 g with death from respiratory and cardiovascular depression. Neither hemodialysis nor peritoneal dialysis are very effective.[29] The effect of hemoperfusion is not known. In patients with normal renal function large amounts of quinine can be eliminated by forced diuresis.[29]

Disopyramide (Norpace) induces early and severe cardiogenic shock. Resin hemoperfusion is more effective than hemodialysis and has resulted in dramatic clinical results.[30]

Theophylline intoxication can lead to vomiting, unusual thirst, agitation, convulsions, shock, and death. It is very effectively removed by charcoal hemoperfusion, which should be instituted as soon after intoxication as possible.[31]

REFERENCES

1. Schreiner GE, Maher JF: The dialysis of poisons. Bull New Jersey Acad Med 6:310, 1960
2. Merrill RL: Treatment of drug intoxications by hemoperfusion. N Engl J Med 284:911–912, 1971
3. Winchester JF, Gelford MC, Knepshield JH, Schreiner GE: Dialysis and hemoperfusion of poisons and drugs. Trans Am Soc Artif Intern Organs 23:762–842, 1977
4. Walker JM, Denti E, Van Wagenen R, Andrade JD: Evaluation and selection of activated carbon for hemoperfusion. Kidney Int (Suppl 7) 10:S320–S327, 1976
5. Rosenbaum JC, Kramer MS, Raja R: Resin hemoperfusion for acute drug intoxication. Arch Intern Med 136:263–266, 1976
6. Chang TMS: Hemoperfusion alone and in series with ultrafiltration or dialysis for uremia, poisoning and liver failure. Kidney Int (Suppl 7) 10:S305–S311, 1976
7. Arieff AI, Friedman EA: Coma following non-narcotic drug overdosage. Management of 208 patients. Am J Med Sci 266:405–426, 1973
8. Setter JG, Maher JF, Schreiner GF: Barbituate intoxication. Evaluation of therapy including dialysis in a larger series selectively referred because of severity. Arch Intern Med 117:224–236, 1966
9. Adandi AD, Oehme FW: An activated charcoal hemoperfusion system for the treatment of barbitol or ethylene glycol poisoning in dogs. Clin Toxicol 18:1105–1115, 1981
10. Crome P, Hampel G, Widdop B, Goulding R: Experience with cellulose acetate-coated activated charcoal haemoperfusion in the treatment of severe hypnotic drug intoxication. Postgrad Med J 56:763–766, 1980
11. Ferguson MJ, Germanos S, Grace WJ: Meprobamate overdosage, a report on the management of five cases. Arch Intern Med 106:237–239, 1960
12. Lobo PI, Spyker D, Surratt P, Westervelt FB: Use of hemodialysis in meprobamate overdosage. Clin Nephrol 7:73–78, 1977
13. Baggish D, Gray S, Jallow P, Bia MJ: Treatment of methaqualone overdose with resin hemoperfusion. Yale J Biol Med 54:147–150, 1981
14. Chang TMS, Coffery J, Lister C, Stalk A, Taroy E: The efficiency of the ACAC microcapsule artificial kidney for the removal of glutethimide, methyprylon and methaqualone in patients with acute intoxication. Trans Am Soc Artif Intern Organs 19:87–91, 1973
15. Yudis M, Swartz C, Onesti G, et al: Hemodialysis for methyprylon (Noludar) poisoning. Ann Intern Med 68:1301–1304, 1968

16. Zmuda MJ: Resin hemoperfusion in dogs intoxicated with ethylchlorvynl (Placidyl). Kidney Int 17:303–311, 1980
17. Lynn RI, Honig CL, Jatlow PI, Kliger AS: Resin hemoperfusion for treatment of ethylchlorvynl overdose. Ann Intern Med 91:549–553, 1979
18. Benowitz N, Abolin C, Toyer T, et al: Resin hemoperfusion in ethychlorvynl overdose. Clin Pharmacol Ther 27:236–242, 1980
19. Matter BJ, Donat PE, Bull ML, Ginn HE: Tranylcypromine sulfate poisoning, successful treatment by hemodialysis. Arch Intern Med 116:18–20, 1965
20. Winchester JF, Gelfand MC, Helliwell M, et al: Extracorporeal treatment of salicylate or acetaminophen poisoning—Is there a role? Arch Intern Med 23:370–374, 1981
21. Sellers EM, Freedman F: Treatment of acetaminophen poisoning. Can Med Assoc J 125:827–829, 1981
22. Gazzard BG, Willson RA, Weston MJ, Thompson RPH, Williams R: Charcoal haemoperfusion for paracetamol overdose. Br J Clin Pharmacol 1:271–277, 1974
23. Lins RL, Zachee P, Christiaens M, et al: Prognosis and treatment of methanol intoxication. Dev Toxicol Environ Sci 8:415–421, 1980
24. Peterson CD, Collins AJ, Himes JM, Bullock ML, Keane WF: Ethylene glycol poisoning: Pharmacokinetics during therapy with ethanol and hemodialysis. N Eng J Med 304, 21–23, 1981
25. Vaziri ND, Upham T, Barton CH: Hemodialysis clearances of arsenic. Clin Toxicol 17:451–456, 1980
26. Uldall PR, Khan HA, Ennis JE, McCallum RI, Grimson TA: Renal damage from industrial arsine poisoning. Br J Ind Med 27:372–377, 1970
27. Mitchel DH: Amanita mushroom poisoning. Ann Rev Med 31:51–57, 1980
28. Heath A, Delin R, Eden E, et al: Hemoperfusion with amberlite resin in the treatment of self-poisoning. Acta Med Scand 207:455–460, 1980
29. Sabts JK, Pierce RM, West RH, Gan FW: Hemodialysis, peritoneal dialysis, plasmaphoresis, and forced diuresis for the treatment of quinine overdose. Clin Nephrol 16:264–268, 1981
30. Gosselin B, Mathieu D, Chopin C, et al: Acute intoxication with disopyramide. Clinical and experimental study by hemoperfusion with amberlite XAD4 resin. Clin Toxicol 17:439–449, 1980
31. Chang TM, Espinosa-Melendez E, Francoeur TE, Eade NR: Albumin-collodion activated charcoal hemoperfusion in the treatment of severe theophylline intoxication in a 3-year-old patient. Pediatrics 65:811–814, 1980

Anne Campbell

14

Education of the Renal Patient: Assistance for Change

End-stage renal disease (ESRD) affects every aspect of a patient's life. Normal daily activities, work and leisure activities, family roles and relationships, and self-concept are disrupted in varying amounts and intensities. Probably no other chronic disease requires such a complicated treatment regimen based upon constantly changing metabolic balances.

A vital need of all patients with renal failure is to receive individualized instruction concerning the effects of renal disease and changes that must be made to accommodate the regimens necessary for survival. Education must be made available to patients, families, and significant others if they are to adjust their lives successfully to a permanent, serious health problem. Planning and delivering education to renal patients is a complex and time-consuming task. It requires effort to properly assess the needs of the patient and family and to individualize a program for them. Understanding the nature of the educational task and the proper creation and coordination of the educational aspect of patient care are thus necessities for ensuring that such a program is organized and feasible for team members to deliver effectively.

Although it may at times seem demanding just to teach complicated regimens and their rationales in an effective manner, the challenge of educating renal patients increases when one adds the diversity of patients, the effects of uremic toxins on learning ability, and the frequent need to describe and compare three very different treatments.

This chapter discusses several aspects of planning and implementing education for the adult ESRD patient. Education for adult patients has been chosen for discussion because the majority of renal patients are adults whose median age is greater than 50 years. Considerations and activities for the development and implementation of educational programs for renal patients will be emphasized rather than precise content and objectives. Specific content and objectives must be individualized for each facility's patient population and needs.

BACKGROUND OF PATIENT EDUCATION

Patient education is not a new concept within medical care settings. Education has been offered through the years by many health care personnel in contact with patients and has been viewed primarily as information given to patients about certain aspects of their conditions and the resulting implications. This information was generally provided by the physician and/or nurse in the usual course of contact with the patient. The quality of education varied tremendously according to the practitioner's belief in the importance of education, the time available, and the skill level one possessed for assessing educational needs and delivering appropriate information. Patient education, at best, was often done sporadically and without a planned, consistent approach.[1,2]

While physicians are still very important sources of information for patients, several changes have occurred in recent decades which have paved the way for the current emphasis on delivering systematic, professionally planned programs for patient education rather than depending upon episodic and fragmented delivery of information by many health care personnel.

The first change has been the transformation of the field of health care through continual scientific and technological advances. The capacity now exists for sophisticated diagnosis, management, and life-prolonging treatments for diseases which once meant certain death. Second, as health care has become more complex, new doors have been opened for people with a wide variety of specialized skills to participate in and augment the delivery of care to the patient. Third, as medical advances have provided ways of prolonging the lives of vast numbers of patients with chronic illnesses, it has become apparent that there is a great need to educate people in the skills needed to manage and cope with diseases that profoundly alter their lives in multiple ways. A final influence for change in the delivery of patient education has been the activation of health care consumers who have become increasingly assertive about their rights to be well informed and participate in their health care.

Today's patient education is designed to provide a systematic, well-planned learning experience for the patient in which formalized objectives and content are individualized for each patient's needs. Basic to all definitions of health education in general, and patient education in particular, is the goal of assisting the individual with attitudinal and behavioral changes that will enhance his ability to reach and maintain an optimal state of health and well-being.[1,3,4]

While health education is often aimed at prevention of disease, avoidance of risk factors, and promotion of wellness in the general population, patient education differs in that it is provided as a response to a particular diagnosis or disease state. Patient education is employed for many types of diseases and situations. Whether a patient needs education for a normal condition such as pregnancy, an acute condition such as gallbladder surgery, or a chronic condition such as renal failure, the initial goal of each type of patient education is to impart new knowledge and skills that assist the patient in coping with an immediate medical problem with which he has little or no experience. The ultimate goal of all patient education, however, lies in the broader context of helping people not only to understand their diagnosis and immediate problem, but to plan ways of integrating new health-enhancing ways of thinking and behaving into their lifestyles.

ACUTE AND CHRONIC DISEASE EDUCATION

A patient with a short-term, or acute, health problem has vastly different needs for learning than a patient with a long-term, or chronic, health problem. The specific goals and content of patient education programs must be designed to reflect such differences. Until recently, patient education for acute problems has been more prevalent in many hospitals than education for chronic conditions. Nurses on surgical floors, for example, frequently teach skills such as relaxation and breathing techniques that will be helpful postsurgery, while physicians, nurses, and anesthesiologists may provide information about the purpose and risks of surgery. This type of education is structured to assist the patient in maintaining control and briefly adapting his behavior to promote a rapid recovery. The goals are short-term and specific to recovery and resumption of normal activities.

Bonnie Sturdevant, an instructor in both a school of nursing and education department of a teaching hospital, discusses a common misconception many professionals have of assuming that acute care information-giving is the same as a planned educational program.[5]

> For one thing, many nurses think that giving information is teaching. It is not. Information giving is usually done by one person to another, with little or no feedback required. Its primary purpose is to gain support or cooperation for a short period of time. In many situations, it is provided during high anxiety periods when patients hear only a portion of what is said. Information nearly always bears repeating.*

In contrast to the short-term goal of gaining cooperation for an acute procedure, the overall goal of chronic illness education is to teach the management of a medical condition and the changes in lifestyle resulting from a disease that never leads to total recovery and resumption of normal activities. Educating the patient regarding management skills and lifestyle changes requires a more highly sophisticated and coordinated approach than information-giving.

Sturdevant emphasizes the essential ingredients that characterize learning as a tool for change.

> Learning's objective is to change behavior. This includes achieving a degree of understanding about one's illness; identifying strengths and weaknesses; identifying the need to know; and utilizing the knowledge, skills, supports, and supporting persons in one's life style. Changing behavior is a slow process.*

Chronic renal disease entails many losses of physical and social functioning which were once taken for granted. Loss of certain functions and resulting changes in a patient's life can be overwhelming, particularly if one lacks an understanding of the cause of the present distress. In addition to current losses and changes, concern about future losses of one's health and possible implications may at times produce inordinate amounts of fear and denial, factors that may paralyze a person's ability to cope with the disease.

The patient with a chronic disease needs both medical and educational assistance. While receiving basic facts about the disease and its treatment, each patient needs to be assisted in regaining a sense of control over his or her own life in understanding the changes that need to be made. An understanding of what to expect and what is expected of the patient provides a framework for important decision making about his or her treatment and life.

---

*Reprinted with permission from Sturdevant B: Why don't adult patients learn? Supervisor Nurse 5:44, 1977.

While a review of the literature indicates that some facilities provide high-quality educational programs for patients with chronic health problems such as diabetes, arthritis, chronic lung disease, malignancies, and renal failure, this is still not universally the case. According to Kasch, a major complaint of persons seeking health care for chronic diseases is the difficulty they have in obtaining and understanding information about their conditions and what to expect. She also indicates that many studies have found a high percentage of patients dissatisfied with the information they do receive.[6] Patients may experience difficulties, for example, with such factors as (1) contradictory advice from medical personnel, (2) use of unfamiliar terminology in a discussion of their diagnosis, (3) lack of time for adequate discussion and answering of questions, (4) lack of a general framework into which is placed medical information such as test results, (5) uncertainty concerning their future course, and (6) uncertainty about what behavior is expected of them.

When needs for education are not recognized or met, problems may arise or become exacerbated. Patients may become fearful, anxious, and show adjustment difficulties such as denial or anger. These problems in turn may play roles in nonadherence to regimens and poor adaptation to the meaning of illness and changes that may need to be made.[6,7] Patients with progressive renal disease have educational needs that are important to address even before end-stage renal failure occurs if good adherence and adaptation are to be facilitated. For example, patients with normal blood chemistries who are hypertensive and losing a great deal of protein in the urine must be assisted in recognizing the seriousness of the diagnosis and the possibility of future problems including renal failure and its treatment. They need help in understanding the medical condition and their current responsibilities with diet and medication. Without careful education, patients are very likely to deny problems or react with anger or nonadherence to prescribed changes.

While education is an essential tool in helping patients comprehend the necessity of following prescribed regimens in order to avoid serious complications of their disease, it is essential to realize three important points. First, chronic illnesses such as renal failure are very intrusive upon patients' lives and require them to make more numerous and complex behavioral changes than acute illnesses. For example, there are enormous differences between taking antibiotic medications for 10 days and taking multiple medications every day for the rest of one's life. Second, teaching patients about their disease does not always guarantee that they will be able to understand the treatment and adjust to its demands. Third, many times patients' values and philosophy of life, health beliefs, motivational level, environment, and support systems play larger roles than educational intervention in determining the decisions and adjustments made. While patient education strives to enhance the patient's knowledge and ability to adapt to chronic illness, it must be viewed in a framework of many factors influencing the patient at a critical time.

Despite the fact that education alone cannot assure perfect outcomes, chronically ill patients who receive planned educational experiences and take an active participatory role in their care are able to cope with their illness and comply with their regimens more adequately than patients not offered comparable experiences.[6] An educational program for renal patients should emphasize coping skills and strategies for adapting to required changes in addition to the provision of information. The usefulness of this endeavor can be maximized by a thorough understanding of the background the patient brings with him to the illness experience, features of the disease and treatments, and strengths and weaknesses of educational intervention.

A quality educational program for renal patients should include adequate time for the educator(s) to assess each patient, plan the educational intervention, deliver and document the education, and evaluate the results. Figure 14-1 illustrates a flowchart of each step in the educational process.

If the steps in Figure 14-1 were condensed, it could be stated that patient educators use a similar basic approach to educational intervention that a physician would use in planning clinical therapy. Both diagnose needs, decide on acceptable outcomes, select methods appropriate to the patient and his condition, administer the treatment or education, and observe the results.[8] While the professional task differs between physicians and educators in many ways, it is possible to select similarities and observe that both specialties thoroughly investigate the need for their services and select the best methods of meeting client needs.

The time and effort spent with every step of patient education, not merely the teaching step, is well repaid in terms of both patient satisfaction and overall program results. Due to the required investment of time and effort, many renal facilities have one or more staff members hired to coordinate patient education. Depending on the size and needs of each facility and renal population, the educator may be responsible for the total patient education program, including the actual teaching, or may serve as coordinator and provide material and inservice education to assist renal nurses, social workers, and other

Plan educational program to meet needs and goals of specific population
↓
Assess each patient's knowledge, skills, lifestyle, medical condition, and support system
↓
Determine educational needs
↓
Set educational goals
↓
Establish an individualized teaching plan through use of a formalized, structured program modified by patient's needs, attitudes, capabilities, motivational level, cultural background, and readiness to learn
↓
Implement the teaching plan
↓
Evaluate patient's response to educational program
↓
Revise plan as necessary
↓
Document patient's educational progress and communicate with other team members regarding educational status
↓
Provide ongoing follow-up and support of patient

Figure 14-1. Sequential steps of patient education.

health professionals in the implementation of each step of the educational program.

The remainder of the chapter will focus attention on five of the steps outlined in Figure 14-1: patient assessment, program goals, planning the program, teaching implementation, and evaluation. The assumption is made that although the nephrologist is still educating his or her patients as part of professional care, the typical renal program is of sufficient size and scope to warrant staff members who design and supervise further in-depth education of the patients.

The first step is patient assessment. Patient educators are constantly called upon to make learning assessments. Proper assessment is vital for effective education. It basically involves careful observation and the asking of specific questions. When an educator assesses a renal patient, there are several key areas of inquiry. It must be determined what the patient wants to know; whether the patient is physically and emotionally ready to learn; and how the patient can best be assisted through education to understand the disease and live with it.

Table 14-1 presents major areas of assessment for planning and implementing renal education. Sources for some of the information regarding the patient may be the patient's medical record, conferences with other renal team members who have had contact with the patient, or conferences with the patient's family or significant others. Other information can only be obtained through direct interviewing of the patient while closely observing his reactions and recording his statements about his experiences and knowledge of renal disease.

These areas of assessment have a bearing on a renal patient's ability to learn and on the design of the individualized educational program. Assessment is a continuous endeavor throughout the patient's treatment course that demands involvement of all renal team members. It takes time to assess a patient's learning potential and identify possible barriers to education, and the educator must be prepared to reassess and revise teaching plans more than once as the patient and his or her needs become better known.

If assessment is important for the success of all patient education, it is doubly important for renal education. There are at least four factors that make renal patients one of the most difficult of all chronically ill groups of patients to educate. (1) The effects of uremia and electrolyte imbalance can have a profound impact on the patient's energy level, mental alertness, and ability to concentrate and recall information. Dialysis is generally initiated before uremia is severe, yet even mild chemical imbalance in some patients can make them less than ideal learning candidates. Uremia can complicate accurate assessment of learning ability and must be accommodated in the teaching plan. (2) Renal patients have the most visible and complex treatment regimen to follow. No other patient group must adhere to the multiple and time-consuming regimens that are required of both hemodialysis and peritoneal dialysis patients. The regimens can be quite intrusive upon patients' lives and patients vary tremendously in their ability to learn to manage and adjust to the disease. (3) Many renal patients also have concurrent chronic health problems such as diabetes which may have caused their renal failure and which demand separate treatment regimens of their own. Multiple factors will influence these patients' ability to learn and take on additional responsibilities for failing health. (4) A final factor that makes renal education difficult is the potential need to teach three very different and complex treatments to those

Table 14-1
Assessment for Patient Education—Patient's Background

Medical History	Education
Age	Level of formal education
Renal diagnosis	Reading ability
Presence of other medical conditions	Enjoyment of school and learning experiences
Level of renal function	
Results of lab tests and diagnostic procedures	Additional educational experiences since formal schooling
Presence of uremia	Feelings of adequacy or inadequacy as a learner
Presence of fatigue (uremia, tests, postdialysis)	Extent of vocabulary
Past and present medical regimens	major language spoken
Vision	ability to articulate on medical and nonmedical subjects
Hearing	
Renal Disease	Extent of curiosity about illness and motivation to learn
Length of time patient has known about presence of renal disease	Level of intelligence or mental capacity
Previous sources of information regarding disease and treatments	recall ability
	learning handicaps
Level of sophistication of medical knowledge in general, renal in particular	understanding of concepts
	Social Background
	Employment status
Description of renal problems and their implications	Socioeconomic background
	Cultural background
Presence of misconceptions regarding renal disease and treatments	Type and extent of family or other support system
Emotions	Routine daily activities
Response to illness	Internal or external locus of control
Beliefs regarding diagnosis and present situation	Adherence to medical and health regimens in the past
Coping patterns for other problems	
Coping patterns for illness	
Emotional support system available	

patients who are candidates for more than one treatment. The existence of hemodialysis, peritoneal dialysis, and transplantation, plus the regimens which must be followed for each, create a volume of material for the patient to master.

Due to the amount of material, team members must continually assess the patient and the educational plan to prevent the patient from becoming totally overwhelmed. The educational efforts of nurses, dietitians, and social workers should be integrated so that education is delivered sequentially and with appropriate timing. The patient will otherwise despair of learning the medical, technical, dietary, social, and financial details concerning his renal disease.

Careful assessment can assist the educator in planning, timing, and delivering education to the patient. The following are several suggestions to assure more successful assessment of the patient and his problems and capabilities:

1. Read the medical chart and social history if available to get an idea of the patient and his health and other problems before initiating contact.
2. Confer with other team members who may have already worked with patient.
3. Allow enough time to get to know the patient before rushing into teaching content areas.
4. Avoid snap judgements and labeling of patients.
5. Remember that a person who is under stress and possibly uremic may have difficulty showing his or her normal personality and coping mechanisms.
6. Be open to change in the assessment of the patient and the patient's abilities. For example, poor compliance in the past does not always correlate with future compliance. Be flexible and give the patient a chance.
7. Listen intently to the patient, family members, and significant others.
8. Observe the patient's body language, gestures, and facial expressions.
9. Check for misconceptions when assessing level of medical and renal disease knowledge. Quickly correct misconceptions before proceeding.
10. Do not overestimate a patient's medical knowledge or sophistication about renal disease and dialysis on the basis of formal education or occupation. Often a college graduate or nurse who is a renal patient needs to cover the same basics as those with less education. Conversely, do not underestimate the learning ability of an adult who received very little formal education and/or cannot read. Formal education level and ability to learn are very different entities.
11. Prepare a form or checklist for help with assessment, consequent educational planning, and later transfer of a new patient to treatment.

SELECTED PSYCHOSOCIAL ISSUES OF PATIENTS WITH ESRD

Much has been researched and written about the renal patient's psychosocial problems in adjustment to chronic disease and treatment.[9,10,11] Although psychosocial issues are not the emphasis of this chapter, a brief review of this area is necessary to understand the effects of such problems on the patient's ability to learn and comply. "The impact of any chronic illness occurs when the patient begins to recognize that his symptoms have long-range meaning for his subsequent life."[9] When a patient is first told that he or she has renal disease and there is a possibility of renal failure and dialysis, it is important for the staff to know some psychosocial information about the person. Social and emotional factors play an extremely important role in the patient's overall acceptance of the diagnosis and in his or her ability to learn and make appropriate behavioral changes. The new renal patient experiences deteriorating health, an increasingly complex medical regimen, and may also experience the effects of uremia—all accompanied with fear and uncertainty about these experiences and the future. The patient may have difficulty in functioning in his or her job, in household and parental tasks, in sexual performance, and/or in enjoyment of social life. If the loss of function is profound, the patient may become depressed and suffer greatly from the changes in performance and consequent self-esteem. The patient's family also suffers. The months preceding and immediately following the initiation of dialysis can be full of problems for family members as they watch the changes without the patient.

A social worker is invaluable for social and emotional assessment of both the patient and the family. Factors such as cultural background, age, socioeconomic status, employment status, experience with other health problems, and extent of support system all affect the patient's response to renal disease. Three additional factors are helpful to know when planning the educationl approach: (1) locus of control, (2) beliefs regarding illness, and (3) emotional reactions to illness, particularly denial.

Locus of Control

What is the predominant locus of control for the patient? Does the patient accept responsibility and is he or she self-reliant, or does the patient depend heavily on others? How independent has the patient been with daily activities? It is important to know how much control the patient has exercised in managing his or her adult life in nonmedical areas. Most adults have a certain amount of control over their lives; they have power to regulate events in order to feel comfortable in a given situation. When adults lose control or feel they have fewer options, even on a temporary basis, they struggle in many ways to regain choices and a sense of control.

The adult renal patient generally perceives the news of his or her diagnosis and regimen in terms of loss of control. For the patient who is seen for several months or even years on an outpatient basis prior to dialysis, this loss of control may be gradual—first a need for medications, then a need for some dietary restrictions and more frequent clinic visits, and finally a decrease in stamina and the need to discuss treatment options. Although this gradual loss of control can be difficult for many patients, the problem is often exacerbated for those who enter the hospital needing immediate treatment for renal failure without any previous warning or education. If the renal patient is not helped to understand the purpose of the regimen and how it relates to his or her disease and overall well-being, multiple instructions from others are apt to be viewed as unnecessary impositions with resultant further loss of control.[12]

Health Beliefs

What are the patient's beliefs regarding his or her health problem? A patient's health beliefs have a major influence on the amount of benefit he or she can gain from education regarding illness and change. The Health Belief Model developed by Hochbaum and Rosenstock and elaborated by Becker, uses motivational theory to explain an emotional arousal that occurs in response to illness.[13,14,15] This model focuses on perceptions of susceptibility, severity, benefits, and barriers. It assumes that an individual's beliefs about health are as important as cognitive knowledge about health. Dracup and Meleis discuss the individual's emotional response to illness:[16]

An individual, once aroused, is likely to engage in health-seeking behavior depending on two variables: the amount of threat perceived by the individual and the attractiveness or value of the action in question. The degree of perceived threat, in turn, is determined by the feeling of vulnerability to the specific disease state in question and to illness in general, the perceived extent of bodily harm, the extent of possible disruption of social roles, the presence of symptoms, and past experience with symptoms.*

---

*Reprinted with permission from Dracup KA, Meleis O: Compliance: An interactionist approach. Nursing Research 31:32, 1982.

An educational presentation to a renal patient concerning hyperkalemia might incorporate the Health Belief Model by helping the patient to comprehend his or her susceptibility to the serious consequences of high potassium. Education should include discussion of the difficulty (barriers) of reducing potassium intake, but should also recommend actions that would reduce the perceived barriers. If the patient is assisted to perceive the benefit (increased survival) as outweighing the barriers (limiting of dietary potassium), he or she has a greater chance of adopting a restricted potassium diet. In any such presentation, a realistic assessment of risk is a far better initiator of behavior change than a high fear arousal technique.

Emotional Reactions to Illness

The educator should identify the patient's response to renal failure; the patient may experience denial, anger, fear, depression, acceptance, optimism, or confusion. The patient's reaction to diagnosis of renal failure depends on many factors including age, philosophy of life, ethnic background, previous coping patterns with other problems, and his or her support system. The patient educator should have a firm understanding of anticipated reactions to a diagnosis such as renal failure and be prepared to adjust educational plans accordingly. Initial intake interviews should assess not only the learning abilities and needs of the patient, but also the primary method of adjustment the patient is using to deal with the news of renal disease. Most people have elaborate mechanisms that serve to protect them from the impact of unpleasant news. These are termed defense mechanisms because they help individuals to reduce anxiety and regain control in periods of extreme stress.

Some commonly documented defenses are denial of a problem, displacement or projection of a problem onto something else, regression of personality back to an earlier developmental stage, intellectualization of the problem, and withdrawal, or isolation of affect. Many renal patients use various defense mechanisms during the course of their illness. It is imperative to understand the functional purpose of defense mechanisms as they have a profound influence on the patient's ultimate ability to deal with the reality of the disease, symptoms, and the disillusionment that he or she may never again feel completely well or regain all previously enjoyed freedoms. Eccard discusses the importance of understanding and working around defenses.[9]

The defenses mentioned are adaptive for the patient, depending on the degree of their use and the effect they have on the patient's adaptation to his illness. Regardless of the value the nurse places on the defense the patient is using, she must not tamper with the mechanism until she has a clear understanding of the patient's ability to cope with the anxiety produced by the situation in a more healthy manner. Clearly, the mechanism the patient utilizes wards off anxiety that would otherwise affect his functioning and allows him a sense of equilibrium and the ability to function . . . Working around these defenses rather than confronting them is probably the best approach.*

Of all the defense mechanisms, denial is of special significance to the educator of new renal patients. Cohen and Lazarus interviewed patients the night before they underwent surgery for minor conditions like hernia repair or gallbladder removal.[17] They found two main coping strategies: vigilance and avoidance.

The avoiders weren't interested in thinking about, or listening to, anything that related to their illness or the surgery. They'd say things like, "I have the best doctor in the world. He knows what he's doing." They had no idea of the nature of their problem, and no inclination to find out.

The vigilant types, however, were extremely alert to everything. Their way of coping was to get as much information as they could. They tried to control the situation and were alert to any dangers. They said things like, "Is there an article I can read about this? I'd like to find out more." Or, "I asked the doctor the other day what kind of incision he's going to make and what kind of anesthesia they'll use."*

Despite the widespread idea that the work of worrying and gathering information produces successful resolutions to problems, Cohen and Lazarus found that in situations where vigilance could not lead to patient action (such as minor surgery), a patient was better off denying what was happening and allowing the hospital staff to administer care. They found that denial was a hindrance, however, for chronically ill patients who repeatedly needed to take various actions to ensure survival.

What is the significance of such a finding for those involved with the education of renal patients? Clearly, not all end-stage renal patients place control of their lives within the realm of their own responsibility. Some even deny they could be susceptible to renal failure or to consequences of neglecting aspects of their chronic medical regimen.

When initial assessment indicates a patient is unable to benefit

---

*Reprinted with permission from Eccard M: Psychosocial aspects of end stage renal disease, in Lancaster LE (ed): The Patient with End Stage Renal Disease. New York, Wiley 1979, p 67.

*Reprinted with permission from Lazarus RS (interviewed by Daniel Coleman): Positive denial: The case for not facing reality. Psychology Today, Nov, 1979, p 51.

from education due to extreme avoidance or denial of the problem, three approaches can be utilized by the educator.

First, the educator can probe to understand the cause of the denial. If the avoidance of the subject is based on misconceptions or negative information received from the media or from knowing kidney patients who have had difficulty with treatments, the provision of accurate and current information or a discussion of the patients' fears can help increase readiness to learn.

Second, a possible approach is to work with a patient's family or significant others to assess and respond to their needs for education. Although families are often highly anxious, they do not have to contend with the fear of death or the effects of uremia upon their ability to learn. Many family members derive benefits from education and are able to calmly and slowly assist in informing the patient of his situation. Use of these individuals is very instrumental because they can serve as teachers and reinforcers on a continual basis. Often when the family responds with more control, calmness, and optimism, the patient will become more open to learning.

Third, the timing and content of education are of great importance. The patient in denial can deal only with the initial problem. Denial can, in fact, help to keep morale up when the patient is very vulnerable. Discussion of the future and treatment choices should be postponed until the patient has time to come to terms with the diagnosis. Information should be as simple and nonthreatening as possible. A uremic predialysis patient in denial, for example, can be taught that his or her symptoms are signs of uremia. The patient should understand that his or her difficulties are connected with a very real medical problem, yet the teaching approach can also relieve anxiety over the possibility of other diseases or that symptoms may be permanent. If the educator can show benefits of education by explaining even a small amount about renal disease and offering positive suggestions on dealing with the problem area, this can begin to show the patient that avoidance of information in chronic illness hinders rather than helps adjustment.

At times, education can break through denial and be therapeutic in promoting a more active response to illness. In some cases, however, education must not be initiated until the patient is ready to learn, even if it means waiting for severe symptoms or initiation of treatments. The educator can teach more effectively in such cases when the patient is given more time to realize the seriousness of the condition and see the need to deal with it. All patients deserve an individualized approach and should be given every opportunity to show readiness to learn and to manage their health at the optimal level possible for them.

The specific goals for renal patient education, the planning and implementation of education, and the ultimate success or failure of the venture largely depend on taking the time to determine the needs of the patient and family.

The author was once asked to initiate education with a 45-year-old man and his wife. Knowing that renal function was deteriorating rapidly and the attending nephrologist wanted the patient educated as quickly as possible, the temptation existed not to take the time for preliminary assessment and to begin teaching content immediately. The initial session, however, revealed a couple dealing with severe stress and multiple problems, only one of which was renal failure. A hurried, unplanned approach would have been doomed from the start. The case study in Table 14-2 illustrates areas of vital importance for assessment before and during delivery of education to a renal patient and his or her family.

Educational plans were markedly altered in terms of content, timing, emphasis, and sequence of subjects to fit the problems and needs of this patient and wife. The case was closely coordinated with other renal team members and learning needs were continually reassessed. A slide program, a booklet, or an unadapted, information-giving approach to renal disease for this couple could have been disastrous. Instead, six individualized sessions were held to assist this couple in gaining control and preparing for peritoneal dialysis. While education certainly did not solve all the myriad problems this patient had, it enabled him to know what to expect and plan for the initiation of dialysis. Continuous ambulatory peritoneal dialysis (CAPD) training went smoothly and the patient learned to manage his care independently. To accomplish such an outcome required much more than just adequate assessment. If renal education is to be successful, program goals must be formulated and teaching plans implemented to achieve the stated goals.

GOALS OF A PREDIALYSIS RENAL EDUCATION PROGRAM

The patient and family facing dialysis often have multiple difficulties that may affect their ability to cope and make appropriate decisions concerning their situation. As stated, a well-planned educational program can contribute substantially toward reducing certain problems and easing the transition to treatment. Figure 14-2 illustrates one way of viewing the process of employing selected educational mechanisms

Table 14-2
Case Study Illustrating Assessment

Patient's Background	Assessment
Medical history	The patient has a history of two myocardial infarctions in the past 9 months and was turned down for coronary bypass surgery. He is not a transplant candidate and probably not a hemodialysis candidate at the present time. The patient has rapidly progressive glomerulonephritis and is also nephrotic, edematous, hypertensive, and mildly uremic. The patient is obese and has a speech impediment.
Knowledge of renal disease	The patient knows very little about the body in general, and his knowledge of renal disease is confined to, "They clean blood." His knowledge of dialysis came from driving a van for a state mental hospital that brought a schizophrenic dialysis patient for treatments. He never saw dialysis but envisions a machine like a CAT scan that drains all the blood from the body. His passenger did poorly and died—he does not know the cause of death. He states, "Just shoot me before I have to have dialysis."
Education	Patient has a 7th-grade education.
Social background	The patient has been married 25 years and has 5 children. There are multiple problems with adolescent and newly married children. He has been disabled since his first heart attack and has been told he can never work again. The patient sees sex roles very traditionally. He is filing for bankruptcy because of no income, no insurance, and thousands of dollars of unpaid hospital and other bills. His wife is unable to work due to a back injury. He is living in a van in a daughter's yard and is looking for a trailer to rent. He has been eating soup and lunch meat due to habit, financial problems, and living arrangements. He is a chain smoker. His wife cries easily and nags him to "stop smoking and eating salt or you'll die." There is bickering over compliance problems and perceptions of patient's illness. The patient acknowledges sexual problems and asks if these are related to kidney disease. He fears his wife will leave. He notes previous infidelities.
Emotions	Both he and his wife are emotionally out of control, very anxious, frightened, and using a variety of defense mechanisms.

Educational Mechanisms →	Educational Program Goals →	Anticipated Outcomes
Provision of education concerning renal disease, its treatments, and regimens	Increased:	Increased:
Provision of education concerning structure and function of renal health care system	Knowledge of renal disease and treatments	Selection of self-care treatments whenever possible (CAPD, home hemodialysis, self-care within a center)
Provision of discussion concerning patient's affective responses to diagnosis and need for behavioral changes	Recognition of diagnosis and implications for changing role and behavior	Predialysis management phase
Provision of support and encouragement of positive changes and decision-making on part of patient and family during time of transition	Realistic and positive attitudes concerning treatments and future	Self-esteem through increased control and participation
	Personal control and responsibility for health	Adherence to treatment regimens
	Mutual participation of patient and staff in health care decisions	Avoidance of preventable medical problems
	Decreased:	Cost effectiveness
	Unnecessary fear and anxiety	Longevity
		Quality of life
		Decreased:
		Use of defense mechanisms

Figure 14-2. Patient education goals and outcomes for predialysis and new dialysis patients.

to achieve goals which will hopefully enhance the realization of specific desired outcomes within the patient population.

Referring to Figure 14-2, certain educational mechanisms are used to meet program goals. When educational program goals are met effectively, the probability of reaching positive outcomes is increased. Upon examining the anticipated outcomes of patient education in Figure 14-2, it can be seen that such outcomes would be beneficial to both patients and the renal care system.

Educational Mechanisms

Renal patients have a right to know what to expect from their disease and what is expected of them prior to dialysis and after the initiation of treatments. They should be informed about the disease process, their specific diagnosis, the symptoms of renal failure, the need for dialysis or transplantation, the types of treatment available, and the interrelated aspects of the medical regimen.

The provision of education should also include other elements. Many patients are not only confronted with a complicated and frightening health problem to learn about, but are often also thrust into a large, complex health care system for which they may have little or no preparation. They may need education concerning the ways in which teaching and tertiary care hospitals differ markedly from community hospitals, the reasons there may be changes in teams and physicians when they may be accustomed to one primary physician, the length of time often necessary for testing and preparation for dialysis, and the multiple disciplines and skills of staff and members of the renal team. The demystification of the renal care system is essential in aiding the patient to become a partner in his or her care and in decreasing negative reactions toward care.

The inclusion of affective subjects is essential not only for the social worker but for all team members involved with the renal patient. Affective subjects concern the patient's feelings, attitudes, and values. The patient must be given opportunities to state his or her feelings about his or her health situation and what he or she is learning as education progresses. Of particular relevance are feelings concerning the patient's ability to change behavior and accommodate new realities.

A final educational mechanism is support by the educator and other team members. The educator serves in a support position primarily in the areas of positive behavioral changes and decision making. The elements of support and encouragement of patient responsibility are as essential to the realization of goals as the provision of cognitive information.

Educational Program Goals

A primary goal of patient education is the reduction of unnecessary fear and anxiety with the replacement of more positive and realistic attitudes regarding renal disease and treatments. A certain amount of fear and anxiety is natural in new situations, particularly when confronting a serious health problem. Some anxiety can even be functional as a motivating factor in helping the patient to learn. An excessive amount of fear and anxiety, however, especially if based on misconceptions, can be crippling. Education alone cannot be expected to eliminate all fear and anxiety as some is rooted in factors that knowledge acquisition does not affect. Despite this, much of the misconception and distorted information new patients have about dialysis patients and treatments can often be corrected and replaced with more positive viewpoints. Another goal is the recognition of the disease and its implications. Unless the patient comes to terms with the health problem and its meaning, there will never be a successful adaptation to living with renal failure. Although this task often takes time due to existence of defense mechanisms, one of the major purposes of providing education for renal patients is to make sure that the patient (1) recognizes that he or she has a kidney disease; (2) incorporates a role of serious health problems into his or her role repertoire; (3) receives information on his or her problems and possible solutions; (4) is helped to believe that treatment and behavior change can be of benefit; and (5) receives support for his or her decisions and adherence.

The goal of assisting patients to incorporate a new role is discussed by Dracup and Meleis:

> Counseling strategies generally have been directed toward giving patients information. But the poor correlation that exists between increased knowledge and compliant behavior is well established. If counseling strategies were directed instead toward helping the person incorporate the sick role or the at-risk role into their repertoire of roles, that is, purposeful socialization and dealing with the feelings that such an incorporation engendered, this strategy might be extremely effective. Compliance is enhanced by the patient's increased knowledge and competency in the enactment of the at-risk, sick or well roles.*

---

*Reprinted with permission from Dracup KA, Meleis O: Compliance: An interactionist approach. Nursing Research 31:34, 1982.

The educational mechanisms designed to be supportive and increase a patient's understanding of his or her disease, feelings, and place within the health care system are also designed to realize goals of more participation and control by the patient. From initial contact, emphasis should be placed on helping the patient to have a maximal amount of control and participation. Although acknowledging the fact that some patients are not very capable of active participation and that education cannot transform many of the life circumstances that may contribute to feelings of chaos or loss of control, it is nevertheless important to verbalize and encourage these goals at whatever level of participation and control possible.

The task of educating patients to assume responsibility and control is not an easy one. Many renal patients are suffering from multiple chronic diseases and disabilities. Some are elderly persons who are losing control in many aspects of their lives and often have been socialized to "let the doctor or nurse take care of them" long before today's emphasis on consumerism and the patient's right to know and participate. An additional difficulty in promoting control is that most hospitals and health care settings are structured in ways that promote dependency in the service of more efficient professional care.

Despite these problems, it is again important to emphasize the vital necessity for all personnel to be constantly alert for ways of enhancing patient control. Whenever possible present the patient with information on what is happening and what will possibly happen in the future, along with specific recommendations about actions and decisions he or she can participate in. A discussion on anemia, for example, can relieve anxiety about symptoms the patient may have experienced such as fatigue upon exertion, yet the discussion will be far more helpful by incuding advice about the benefits of exercise and activity upon red cell production and giving specific suggestions of possible activities for the patient. Information can also be provided on pacing of activities and on the availability of certain medications for treatment of anemia. Such discussion encourages the patient to take responsibility and gives him control by knowing that something can be done about his problem.

Anticipated Outcomes

It is anticipated that a successful patient education program will increase the likelihood of positive patient outcomes. Well-informed patients who feel they have personal control and the right to participate in health care activities and decisions generally can be expected to fare better than patients without these assets.

One positive outcome of renal patient education would be the increased selection of self-care dialysis options. Judy Tyler studied the significance of educational programs to selection of self-care dialysis and discovered that centers which encouraged patient participation in selection of treatment options had a significantly higher percentage of self-care patients than the national average.[18]

In addition to greater selection of self-care treatments, a good patient education program may prolong the predialysis management phase. Some patients can be successfully educated to follow strict dietary and medication regimens and to recognize dangerous symptoms. They are taught to control blood pressure plus potassium, phosphorus, and BUN levels. Although outcomes partially depend on type and progression of their underlying disease, some patients have participated in delaying the onset of dialysis through motivation and careful education.

Further anticipated outcomes of patient education would be greater adherence to treatment regimens by patients with concomitant avoidance of preventable medical problems. Clotted vascular access, bone disease, congestive heart failure, and hyperkalemia are examples of medical problems often related to lack of patient adherence. Achieving higher adherence is a major reason many patient education programs are initiated. Yet the realization of this outcome must not depend solely on educational intervention since adherence is difficult to achieve and is related to many variables, the most important of which may be the quality of interaction and support the patient has with family and staff members. Education also should seek to assist patients in developing ways of increasing their self-esteem, gaining control over their lives, and participating in their medical care. All of these in turn influence adherence rates. Successful outcomes are not always realized due to several forces. For example, continual losses of function and medical complications such as those a diabetic renal patient might encounter can decrease self-esteem and control. Successful outcomes are sometimes not realized due to staff members who may be threatened by well-informed patients. The entire staff must believe in the importance of such goals and outcomes and be willing to share participation and control with their patients.

Cost effectiveness, increased longevity, and quality of life are the final three outcomes discussed in Figure 14-2. The subject of cost effectiveness often appears in discussions of patient education. The author is not aware of specific research published on the subject of cost effectiveness of renal education, although it seems very probable that cost effectiveness is realized through greater selection of self-care dialysis, longer predialysis management, adherence to regimens, and avoidance of preventable medical problems. Documented patient education also has the potential to reduce malpractice suits. Since education is not the sole factor influencing outcome, measurement of cost effectiveness due to educational intervention per se is difficult. The human benefits of patient education are also difficult to measure directly, but it is anticipated that the ultimate benefits of education are enhanced quality of life and longevity for renal patients.

This section has discussed some possible goals of a renal education program. Much of the discussion was specific to predialysis patients, yet the same or similar goals apply to chronic hemodialysis and self-care training programs. More specific goals, of course, may be developed for each stage and type of treatment. Predialysis goals of decreased anxiety, learning general concepts of renal disease, and choosing the best treatment are quite different from self-care training goals of the development of basic motor skills used for performing hemodialysis or peritoneal dialysis and the development of sound judgment and problem-solving techniques. Finally, the goals of chronic center hemodialysis education are also somewhat different. Emphasis is placed upon learning to live with the reality of restrictions and changes brought by dialysis, achieving the maximum rehabilitation possible, and avoiding complications. Coordination and continuation of educational efforts between these stages and types of treatments are essential.

PLANNING THE EDUCATIONAL PROGRAM

After assessment has begun and goals are set, an educator needs to spend time planning a program that will best suit the needs of individual patients and the renal population as a whole. When planning an educational program for renal patients for the first time, several factors need to be considered by a variety of professionals within nephrology. What needs does the program have for patient education? Is there support and interest? Will an education coordinator be used? Will adequate time, resources, and facilities be allocated? Once the decision is made to include an educational component within patient care, planning the approach depends on the type of education needed, the population served, and the overall goals to be accomplished.

It is essential to remember that people learn in several ways. They learn cognitively from lectures, they learn affectively from discussions, and they learn performance skills through demonstrations and practice. Well-planned programs often make use of all three styles of learning and adapt the mixture to fit the needs of the patient group and the learning situation.

When the need for education and the educational goals have been established for the target patient population(s), the next step in planning is to determine what the patients need to know. In other words, one must develop the content of the program. Some suggestions are (1) interview various staff members and current dialysis patients and families for what they think patients need to know; for example, question those involved or formerly involved in self-care training programs, or chronic hemodialysis patients for their thoughts on learning needs of patients; (2) conduct a literature search concerning the renal population; and (3) observe other educational programs for renal patients or those for patients with other chronic health problems such as diabetes, arthritis, and so forth. Using results of the needs survey, an educational plan can be created. If desired, a pilot program often helps determine content appropriateness and acceptability to patients. Continued further refinement is necessary utilizing feedback from both patients and staff members.

Content for any educational program basically arises from learning needs. A learning need has been defined as "a lack of knowledge, skill or attitude that prevents a patient from learning how to live with his illness, or that interferes with his potential for assuming greater responsibility in his care."[19] Existence of such needs means that understanding and change must come from new learning. Learning needs can be detected directly from comments by patients such as "I've been feeling pretty badly. I can't go on this way. Is there anything that can be done?" They can also be detected indirectly through physical parameters that are constantly elevated such as blood pressure, potassium or phosphorus, or other variables such as hospitalization for a potentially avoidable problem.[19] Direct learning needs are generally initiated by patients' perceived problems while indirect needs arise from staff observations. These may or may not coincide. Both types of needs are useful to consider in the formulation of educational objectives and content.

The Modular Format

One method of arranging the content for the education program is the modular format. Modules are designed for topical areas such as vascular access, laboratory tests, principles of dialysis, medications, and so forth. Each module should have an overall goal stating the teaching emphasis plus objectives stating what the patient should be able to do at the completion of the module. An example of an overall goal of a vascular access module might be: To assist the patient in understanding the types of access and their care. Examples of objectives for patients to meet might be (1) states the purpose of vascular access for hemodialysis; (2) describes situations in which a synthetic graft might be necessary; (3) lists precautions to observe in caring for fistula arm; (4) demonstrates ability to properly check thrill; and (5) indicates problems concerning vascular access requiring contact of a physician. In addition to stating the goal and objectives, modules frequently include suggested content to be taught to the patient and any written or audiovisual resources that can be used to supplement the verbal instruction given to the patient.[4,20] A sample of a module for teaching medications is shown in Table 14-3.

Developing Educational Objectives

The health education literature frequently discusses the importance of writing and using objectives as an aid to organization and measurement of educational programs.[4,20,21] Despite the coverage in the literature, many educators resist writing objectives. The process is not difficult in practice. Objectives are derived from learning needs and state what is to be taught and what the patient is expected to learn. Whenever possible they should be stated in behavioral terms which can be directly measured.

Referring to the medication module in Table 14-3, objectives are generally stated in measurable terms such as describes, lists, and states. An objective that states "Patient understands medications" is subjective and cannot be measured. The use of objectives helps keep learning on track and documents for the renal team what is being taught and learned. Objectives also lay the groundwork for future evaluations of knowledge acquisition.

Many educators do not understand how to use objectives for the types of teaching they routinely do. In this context, one misconception is that every subject presented to a patient needs a behavioral objective. When one is giving an overview of a subject there is generally no need to make detailed objectives. Certain skills and knowledge are crucial for the renal patient to have, however, and their presence or absence must be documented. It must be documented, for example, whether a hemodialysis patient is able or unable to meet the

Table 14-3
Medication Module

Goal: To provide the patient with instruction on his medications and to enhance the likelihood of the medication regimen being incorporated into his or her lifestyle

Objectives	Content	Teaching Aids
Lists names of all medications taken	Teach recognition of medications by sight, names, and purposes	Medication cards for each drug giving name, purpose and any side-effects of the medications. Slide tape on categories of meds for renal patients
Describes the purpose of each medication and how it relates to renal disease and/or dialysis		
States that certain medications or dosages may change if physical parameters or type of treatments change	Rationale for decisions on what medications are necessary (teach when feasible)	Patient's medical chart to correlate lab and medications
States and follows special instructions for timing of certain medications such as phosphate binders and antihypertensive medications	Rationale for timing and consequences explained	Noted on patient's daily medication schedule
Discusses rationale for medications that need to be taken at certain times Explains consequences of inaccuracy with these medications		Use of clinical measures to demonstrate consequences if meds such as phosphate binders taken incorrectly

Describes any side-effects relevant to his medications	Inform which medications may have side-effects; distinguish dangerous vs annoying effects	Medication cards, phone numbers to contact physicians if problems
Recognizes each medication by sight, especially while in hospital	Situation-check as nurse brings medications	Teach with actual medications
States rationale for avoidance of nonprescription drugs	Explains dangers of self-medication. Encourage to check with physician	
Follows a medication schedule at home for proper dosage	Assist patient in making a schedule and keeping it current	Medication schedule
Integrates taking of medications into lifestyle	Suggestions for purchasing, storing, timing, and remembering to take medications at home and away	Slide tape presentation illustrating these concepts

objectives concerning vascular access by properly checking the flow in his or her access and by listing precautions to observe and problems requiring physician notification. Other examples would be recognizing signs of peritonitis, listing medications, and listing high potassium foods. Such objectives need documentation of whether or not they have been met.

Another common misconception is that separate lists of behavioral objectives must be written out separately for every patient in order to create an individualized learning package for each teaching encounter. In searching the literature, one discovers extremely opposing viewpoints in this regard. Some authors describe educational programs without mention of assessing needs or considering objectives.[12,18,22,23,24] At the opposite extreme are authors such as Donald Bille who insist that not only must objectives be created for each patient, but that the educator and patient must write them out together in contract form and then proceed to measure each with written pre- and posttests to show accomplishment.[21]

A compromise may be found along the continuum between these two extremes. A general teaching plan can be designed that shows the major content areas and skills that most renal patients need to know. This can be reviewed with a new patient along with a discussion of major goals of the educational program and his or her individualized learning needs. A copy of the plan may be given to the patient if desired.

This approach allows the new patient to begin formulating questions, to see what is expected, and begin to negotiate his or her capacity for learning and changing behavior to meet the needs of the health problem. It also recognizes the current level of knowledge and notes accomplishment. For example, if the patient is already able to state his or her medications properly and shows good comprehension of their purposes and doses, this behavior is documented in the medication module. Content and objectives are standardized for all patients through the modular format. The educator and individual patient then adapt each module in terms of methods and complexity to the special needs of the patient, taking into account the many social, medical, educational, and emotional factors that make each patient unique. The final result is a standardized educational format which can be customized for each patient and one that allows both assessment by the educator and maximal input from the learner.

One final misconception concerning objectives is their formality. While they look very formal in writing, they do not need to be presented to a patient in a formal manner. "Tell me some things you should do to take care of your fistula arm," or "How can you tell if it is clotted?" are conversationally simple and informal ways of measuring the formal objectives: "Patient states precautions for caring for fistula arm," or "Patient demonstrates ability to properly check thrill."

Other considerations determine the final approach used when planning educational programs. Thought must be given to time, personnel and resources available, written and audiovisual materials that will effectively supplement learning, the stage of renal failure present or the type of treatment patient is on, the size of the group needing education, and differences in outpatient versus hospital-based education. Before looking at some common barriers to the success of educational programs, this part of the planning section will conclude with a summary of the essential elements of an educational program.

Each patient education program ideally should include:

an interview or assessment form to be used to determine educational needs;
a teaching plan to document the patient's educational needs;
a teaching manual to divide all content in single concept modules;
and documentation of what the patient was taught and his or her response to it.[21]

BARRIERS TO EFFECTIVE PATIENT EDUCATION

While inadequate planning and assessment can decrease the potential effectiveness of an educational program, there are also other barriers that interfere with adult renal patients' ability to learn and change. Barriers may exist within the teacher(s), within the learner(s), and within the organizational structure in which the education is conducted. Table 14-4 lists some common problems that often reduce effectiveness of patient education.

It is possible to reduce barriers within teachers and teaching techniques, but effort is required. Not many persons are natural-born teachers. Teaching is a developed skill. It takes time, dedication, and patience to learn the correct content to teach, methods of assessment and teaching, and evaluation of successful patient education. Teacher barriers can be decreased by inservice education emphasizing educational skills and the importance of planned and documented teaching. Patient feedback plus openness to new skills and approaches are also ways of reducing barriers to effectiveness within teachers. To be successful as a teacher of renal patients, perhaps the two most

Table 14-4
Barriers to Patient Education

Teacher	Learner	Organization
Lack of adequate assessment of learner	Physical barriers:	Frequent interruptions during educational sessions
Teaching bits and pieces—no overall plan	Uremia	Lack of separate and quiet place for teaching
Use of wrong objectives or no objectives	Extremely aged	
Contradictions between teaching content of team members	Poor physical condition	Daily routine of hospital
	Other barriers:	Hospital increases passivity, dependency
Insufficient knowledge for teaching	Low mental capacity	Lack of continuity between inpatient and outpatient status
Staff beliefs—desire to withhold control and knowledge from patients	Lack of support system	Lack of coordination of dialysis, dietary, and other education
	Poor self image as learner	
No involvement of family or significant other (support group)	Excess fear and anxiety	Poor team communication
	Excess use of defense mechanisms, especially denial	Lack of administrative or physician support
Overwhelm with too much teaching at once	does not view self as susceptible to renal problems	Role conflict between patients and providers
Use of overly technical vocabulary	unconvinced of use of education	
	Lack of personal interest or responsibility for health	
	Inflexibility to change in habits and lifestyle	

important skills one can develop are thorough assessment of the learner—including careful listening—and creative presentation of renal disease and treatments to a wide variety of clients.

Barriers within learners are linked to many of the factors discussed in the section on assessment of the patient. While the total elimination of learner barriers is of course not possible, the educator should attempt to present the teaching at whatever level of physical and mental capacity the patient possesses. Defense mechanisms and personality characteristics need to be understood, and physical limitations such as hearing and vision impairment require adaptation of teaching methods. Not all renal patients are able to benefit equally from an education program, but barriers can often be reduced and learning enhanced if educators give attention to the following:

1. Establish rapport. Show a genuine interest in the patient and in his or her perceived needs and problems.
2. Determine the wants and needs of each patient and establish the relevance of education and the need for behavioral change to meet his or her particular needs.
3. Minimize high anxiety levels and fears of failure. Maximize feelings of self-worth whenever possible.
4. Develop special teaching approaches for special groups such as low intelligence, blindness, deafness, illiteracy, and ethnic minorities. For example, consider pediatric-level material for some adults, liberal use of pictures, tactile items for the blind, an interpreter to sign for deaf patients, the use of ethnic staff members when rapport is needed by minorities, and so forth.
5. Involve other people with a patient's education. Use relatives or significant others. If the patient has no support group, consider including him or her when education is given to another person or to a group.
6. Inform the patient of others who are doing well with the same problem. Involve the patient in group discussions with other renal disease patients, if possible, to build hope and to provide positive role models.
7. Give each patient the opportunity to verbalize negative feelings.
8. Build self-esteem by reinforcing and praising any positive response, changed behavior, or intention to change on part of the patient.
9. Encourage learning as a two-way street. Provide time and encouragement for discussions concerning health problems, lifestyle, and educational needs as the patient faces a new experience.

10. Reassure the patient that he or she can learn and that grade level achieved or prior negative learning experiences are not correlated with intelligence and ability to learn. Build learning confidence by reminding the patient of the many things he or she may have already learned.
11. When helping the patient to set goals, be aware that the patient must believe the effort needed to change is worthwhile and should set realistic goals for learning and behavioral change. Goals should be "owned" by the patient so that his actions show that he understands and wants to change.

Organizational barriers are often the most frustrating to contend with on a daily basis. Hospital and dialysis center procedures and schedules rarely provide quiet, private, uninterrupted opportunities for patient education. The scheduling difficulties inherent in multiple tests, procedures, and clinical appointments can fatigue patients and make educational sessions difficult to schedule.

Barriers of scheduling may be reduced by (1) formally scheduling educational sessions because they are as important as tests and procedures, and (2) scheduling education away from the patient's room in a separate education room if available, or whenever possible, scheduling education away from the hospital or outpatient clinical areas. Since organizational structures that promote passivity and dependency are the antithesis of desired adult behavior, it is important to separate education from treatment areas if at all possible.

Finally, barriers such as the lack of communication and coordination of educational activities by staff members and lack of overall support for the importance of patient education can reduce effectiveness of the effort. These barriers can be reduced by (1) frequent sessions to plan educational strategy during which team members comment on patients' needs and progress and coordinate types and amount of education given, and (2) communication of the status of patient education with physicians and team members to gain support.

A final organizational barrier may be role conflict. Role conflict can develop as the priorities and organization of health care change rapidly. It can develop in both the staff and in patients. In the past, for example, physicians and nurses were seen as sole providers of patient education. Currently new types of professionals have claimed some educational territory and may be viewed as a threat unless careful support is gathered and expectations concerning duties, territories, and exact roles of all health professionals are carefully discussed and made known.

Role conflict not only affects the staff. Patients, too, can be involved in conflicting roles. Patients formerly were expected to be submissive and compliant. Now they are often expected to take an active role in learning about and participating in their health care. An activated patient may be threatening to staff members who may view increased knowledge in patients as an invasion of territory and loss of total professional control of the patient. The patient also may feel threatened by the conflict of old versus new role expectations if education encourages him to put aside a comfortable passive role for one of responsibility.[25] These conflicts are easing as more people see the benefits rather than the disadvantages of the cooperation of a variety of professionals, of planned educational programs, and of involved patients. With increased time, discussion, and experience with these new changing roles, it is anticipated that they will no longer be viewed as conflicts.

IMPLEMENTATION OF THE RENAL EDUCATION PROGRAM

Theories of Adult Learning

The delivery of instruction to renal patients may vary somewhat according to needs and characteristics of the patient population, values and styles of teaching of the educator(s), the setting and timing of the education, and the methods and materials selected. While the educational program needs to be flexible to adjust to such variables, it must be grounded firmly in theories of how learning occurs and ways in which learning can be enhanced. This section on implementation will discuss adult learning theory (andragogy), methods of using and adapting this theory for a chronically ill population, and suggestions for increasing the effectiveness of education for patients and families. Theories and methods of teaching pediatric and adolescent renal patients are very different from those used with adults, and discussion of nonadult education has been excluded only because of space constraints and the wish to make the content apply to the large majority of renal patients.

Background of Adult Learning Theory

Since the turn of this century, there have been two predominant views, or schools, of learning that have developed in the field of psychology. The first view stresses behaviorism and is exemplified by

Pavlov's experiments demonstrating operant conditioning as a means of behavioral modification.

The second view stresses the idea of a cognitive field, or gestalt. It differs from the behaviorist view of learning in that individuals are seen as far more complex in their learning than simply responding to stimuli in predictable ways. Kurt Lewin and Jerome Bruner were the originators of cognitive field theories.[26] They believed that each person had a cognitive field of knowledge to which new insight and knowledge could be added by rearranging and building upon previous experiences and ideas. They also believed that in order to understand a person's behavior in any given time or situation, one had to know as much as possible about that person. The word gestalt referred to all influences in an individual's life. Since the development of cognitive field theory, many psychologists and educators have studied developmental stages of learning, differences in the education of children and adults, and methods of enhancing education.

Building upon these previous psychological and educational theories, Knowles postulated four principles of adult learning:

As individuals mature:

1. Their self-esteem moves from dependence toward self-direction.
2. They experience a variety of life situations that may serve as a learning resource.
3. Their readiness to learn is closely related to developmental tasks of their social roles.
4. Their time perspective changes to an immediate application of knowledge, and orientation to learning becomes problem-centered.[27]

While the author does not deny the research and applications to health care made by behaviorists, particularly in the use of behavior modification for certain conditions, it is thought that learning theory based upon adaptations of cognitive field theory offers broader explanations for complex health behaviors.

Knowle's principles of adult learning can be restated and expanded so that a theoretical base can be more readily understood and applied by individuals responsible for educating adults about chronic renal disease.

Learning Principles for Adult Patients

1. Learning should be problem centered. Interest and learning are heightened if the education is situation-oriented rather than subject-oriented.

2. Learning should be experience-centered. Previous adult learning and life experiences should be utilized during education.
3. Education should be usable to solve current problems. Adults must quickly see the relevance of what is proposed or it may be ignored. Learning is more apt to be done for the meeting of a need than for the pleasure of learning per se.
4. Adults may have somewhat negative feelings about other adults having authority over them concerning their health since most view themselves as independent and self-directing in other areas of life.
5. Many adults have strong opinions about their beliefs, values and behavior. Fixed attitudes and behavior are more difficult to influence in an adult than in a child.
6. Sharing and interaction among adult learners increases motivation and the rate of learning.
7. Participation in decisions about their learning is vital for effective learning.[3,28]

Breckon sums up the central theme of these principles in the following way:

> The key to adult education, then, is helping adults see the relevance of what they need to know, so that in their own self-directing way, they will choose to learn about regaining or maintaining their health. Stated differently, the central purpose of health education is to bring valid knowledge to bear on the decisions that clients must make. In so doing, it is aimed at achieving the needs and goals that the individual specifies, and if possible, to also satisfy the needs and goals of the hospital and society.*

Central concepts from the principles of adult learning will be discussed in more detail as they specifically relate to the teaching of renal patients.

Self-Directed Learning

Knowles based his theories on the fact that as the child matures into an adult he learns more readily in an open, informal manner from life's experiences. He has an increasing amount of control over decisions concerning what he wants to learn and ways in which he desires to learn. Health education literature often speaks in terms of assessing and responding to what the learner "wants" to know about health rather than what he "needs" to know. The assumption is made

---

*Reprinted with permission from Breckon DJ: Hospital Health Education. Rockville, Maryland, Aspen Systems Corp., 1982 p 178.

that clients should have autonomy concerning content of their learning rather than relying on health care providers to determine learning needs and content.

Most health education, in contrast to patient education, activities deal with healthy adults. The concept of "wanting" information is thus relevant when applied to adults who initiate attending a class on prevention of risk factors in heart disease or a class modifying a behavior they would like to change such as smoking or overeating. Levin discusses features of self-care health education that illustrate this concept:

> Self-care education . . . derives its goals from the learner's perceived needs and preferences, regardless of whether or not they conform to professional perceptions of the learner's needs. It is the learner who determines the desired outcomes in accordance with his or her decision on which risks to avoid (or not to avoid); similarly, content is learner determined; learner preferences for education methods are honored; and evaluation is in terms of criteria proposed by the learner.*

With the diagnosis of a serious, potentially fatal disease such as renal failure, the scenario changes from a healthy adult voluntarily "wanting" or seeking information to an unhealthy adult now "needing" information to help him or her solve problems and survive. The potential or new dialysis patient receives education because of the presence of a disease, not because of intrinsic choice or eagerness to learn about renal disease and treatments. The patient may want no information about renal subjects or he or she initially may want to know things such as: "Will my kidneys recover? How can I feel better? Why do I have to learn about dialysis—can't I just have a transplant?" and so forth.

Despite the fact that some viewpoints, including Knowles', emphasize that all teaching should be in response to learner-induced "wants," patient education must also teach certain content the patient "needs" to know. Adding to the dilemma concerning wants and needs is the fact that the lay public generally does not possess much information about renal disease and thus the patient may have little or no idea of what he or she needs to know. Because the experience of renal disease is new to each person, the educator must seek to blend what the patient needs to know as determined by staff, literature, and

---

*Reprinted with permission from Levin LS: Patient education and self-care: how do they differ? American Journal of Nursing Co., Nursing Outlook 26(3): 171, 1978.

former patients with what this individual patient and new patients in general, want to know.

The fact that clients for renal education are not healthy adults choosing to seek information affects their motivation to learn and their perception that they may not be in total control of their learning experience. It is therefore essential for the educator and renal patient to negotiate a blend of the program content for effective delivery of both "wanted" and "needed" information as the education proceeds. Control of the process must be shared or as Levin observed, ". . . professional regulation of the process and outcomes keeps the control in professional hands and does not transfer skills to the patient".[8]

Implications for hospitalized patients. Knowles' self-directed learning principles must be adapted to hospitalized patients. It can be difficult to encourage control and independent decision-making behavior in a hospital situation. The hospital environment is often the antithesis of the educational goal of increasing independent behavior. The patient is likely to be more passive, dependent, and uncertain than he or she would be in a normal adult setting and role. This may necessitate giving the patient more support, patience, and reassurance than one would usually give an adult because hospitalization can bring out the child within the adult. While respecting some degree of childlike emotional reactions, the educator should make every attempt to reduce dependency and to encourage self-control. For this reason, introducing concepts during hospitalization and later following with indepth education on an outpatient basis can be very beneficial.

Implications for behavior change. Self-direction of the learner also denotes taking responsibility for one's learning and behavior. While personal responsibility is welcomed by some patients, to others it is very threatening. Adults are often quite set in their ways. They derive control and security from habitual ways of thinking and behaving. A new renal patient may want to be in control of the situation yet see risk, burden, and the threat of further loss of control in the midst of unwelcomed change and stress. Learning new knowledge and skills is not always appealing, especially in times of crisis.

Reaching positive outcomes in renal disease treatment often requires behavioral change. For example, the patient may have to add behavior such as checking a fistula or blood pressure, or delete behavior such as freely eating and drinking with no attention to food composition or amount of fluid.

Even if the patient wants to change, he or she may need help knowing how to change. There must be emphasis placed upon ways of changing as well as statements concerning the need to change. Telling the new patient that intake of phosphorus must be reduced is very ineffective if the patient has a limited grasp of food content, meal planning for low phosphate foods, and use of phosphate binders.

Change of behavior needs concrete information and the material needs repetition and support. This is often painstakingly slow work for the entire renal team. Educating both the new renal patient and the dialysis patient often involves far more than delivering facts. It means interaction and feedback, mutual respect, humor, sympathy, empathy, listening, teaching, demonstrating, giving emotional support, and providing suggestions of new ideas and methods of change to meet goals.

Life Experiences

Most adults have a wealth of accumulated experiences and wisdom to draw upon in assisting them in understanding renal disease and treatments. Cognitive field theory originated in the belief that one could learn by reorganizing and building upon already existent knowledge. New educational experiences must make contact with the patient's previous lifestyle, experiences, and knowledge.

The only way to establish contact is through adequate assessment of the patient. The more that is known about the patient, the more his education can be customized to familiar events, experiences and ideas in his life. Relationships and analogies always strengthen learning and recall. This accomplishes two major goals: (1) it demystifies the new subject be contacting more established ideas, and (2) it also recognizes the patient as an independent adult having many competencies and interests apart from his or her health problem.

Readiness to Learn and Problem-Oriented Learning

The renal patient is ready to learn when faced with a concern that needs answering. This may or may not occur at the time of diagnosis. It often takes time to adjust to the news of the diagnosis, to begin to see onself in a new role as patient and perhaps to feel the symptomatic effects of one's disease. Timing is important. An educator probably should avoid teaching in depth about dialysis and transplant if such treatments are more than a year away, unless asked specific questions. The education must be done when the patient accepts the problem as reality and is open to information. For maximal effectiveness education should center on a patient's immediate problems and must be viewed as useful to the patient.

Listening is the best way to assess readiness to learn and problems that need to be answered. Examples of patients' statements illustrating these ideas would be: (1) "There's no use wasting your breath on what's wrong with my kidneys. I've heard those dialysis treatments cost thousands of dollars and I'll just have to die because I'm disabled and don't have much money." (2) "My local doctor told me when the BUN gets to 100 you're dead. When I came here to the hospital a doctor told me I'm 90. What's a BUN? If I'm so close to dead, why don't I feel worse? What will it feel like?"

Special Teaching Suggestions and Considerations

The following section is designed to give the educator practical ideas for implementing some of the theoretical concepts previously discussed. Suggestions are offered under the topics of emotions, structural elements of teaching, family education, and dialysis options.

Emotional Suggestions and Considerations

- Acknowledge with the patient that many people have difficulties dealing with illness, the amount of material to learn, and the necessity to make changes and decisions.
- Use humor as often as possible.
- Instill confidence as a learner. Praise any learning and changes taking place. Pride and self-esteem are wonderful motivators for more learning. Tragically, many people feel inadequate at learning and state that no one ever before complimented them on their learning ability.
- Educate the patient about other types of renal patients and problems he or she may see when treatment begins. Prepare the patient to expect occasional times of reduced stamina, problems, and discouragement as part of any treatment from time to time, and that good and bad days are characteristic.
- Be as honest with the patient as possible. All nephrology personnel at times have a dilemma of emphasizing hopefulness versus the reality of the situation. Be realistic about the possibility of problems so the patient won't feel betrayed in the future if problems occur, yet attempt to maintain an overall sense of hopefulness and the possibility of better control in the future. This is not always easy, especially with those who have systemic diseases and multiple organ damage.
- Introduce new patients and their families to people who are doing well with dialysis. Choose these "models" carefully.

Structural Suggestions and Considerations

- Review the medical record and question other staff members, if possible, before meeting a new patient to facilitate assessment and education.
- Coordinate teaching plans with other team members and with the patient's medical procedures. No one should have to undergo dialysis, a renal biopsy, and visits by two or three team members for various educational topics in one day, yet it happens if proper planning is not done.
- Inform the patient of the purpose of patient education. Share the teaching plan if appropriate.
- Concentrate first on needs assessment, reduction of anxiety, and answering the patient's most important questions. Assess the person's present knowledge on renal subjects and correct his or her misconceptions.
- Be alert to the possible effects of uremia on a patient's retention and alertness. If uremia symptoms are mild, proceed with short sessions; if the symptoms are severe, work with the patient's family or wait until dialysis reduces uremia.
- Teach new patients individually or in small groups. Some patients feel threatened by group experiences until they have some time to adjust. Groups can be very beneficial when patients are ready to share, however, such as during self-care training.
- When time is limited, the content of sessions can be condensed. The presentation of some education about the functions of real kidneys is necessary, however, or dialysis descriptions will make very little sense to the patient.
- Recap important points within each session or module. Leave reading material if appropriate. Written material is not necessarily helpful to all patients. Assess patient preference and select material carefully.
- Review key points of previous session(s) before proceeding. Ask questions and repeat the instruction if necessary.
- Consider using a notebook that the patient can add to as he or she collects educational material from various team members.
- Use understandable vocabulary that is consistent with the patient's medical sophistication and amount of experience with renal disease. New patients need an explanation of basic concepts and overviews of renal disease and treatments.
- Use jargon sparingly and only if the terms are essential to the patient's current treatment (fistula, ultrasound, and so forth).

Concepts such as principles of both hemodialysis and peritoneal dialysis can be described with everyday words and analogies at differing levels of complexity yet without terms such as semipermeable, diffusion, and so forth.
- Develop analogies based on experiences familiar to the patient—machinery, animals, cars, cooking, and so forth—that will lessen the foreign nature of the content.
- Use visual items, pictures, slides, and real equipment to encourage more active interest. Media should be used as a supplement to human contact and interaction with the patient, never as a sole method of teaching.
- Use sensory information while teaching. This is particularly important when patients face procedures such as biopsies, difficult tests, surgeries, and/or initiation of dialysis. Interview others who have undergone such procedures and relay to new patients the sensations they may feel.
- Prepare a copy of predialysis educational content and evaluation for primary nurses in the hemodialysis unit or self-care training unit to assist in continuity.
- When learning ability is very limited, select only the most essential material from learning modules. Concentrate on emphasizing the patient's responsibilities while away from the dialysis unit, such as checking the fistula or graft, taking medication accurately, avoiding specific foods, and the importance of not skipping dialysis treatments.

Suggestions and Considerations for Education of Families and Significant Others

Encourage family involvement in the educational process because the entire family is affected by renal failure. Families or significant others have learning needs of their own when a patient is diagnosed with renal disease. These needs, while similar, are not identical to the patient's needs. Families can be very helpful in the patient's adjustment, rehabilitation, and adherence to regimens if they understand the disease process and its effects, the treatments, and what to expect. In addition to educational sessions for the patient, families often need separate help from the staff in understanding their own feelings, needs, and reactions to illness. They may have many questions, doubts, and concerns that need attention if they are to cope successfully and be supportive of the patient.

While social workers play the predominant role in helping the family adjust, those who provide education regarding the current situation and future expectations also play a vital role. Education can be helpful: (1) in the predialysis phase to assist the family in understanding the difficulties of living with a uremic individual and learning to tolerate certain symptoms and/or work around them; (2) in the initial dialysis treatment stage to help the family with concerns such as how to treat the patient, timetables for increasing activity, and so forth; and (3) during the chronic therapy stage of either type of dialysis to provide groups and sessions to help in sharing of experiences and maximizing coping.

Education of families and significant others should be of a continuing nature as they need to know the changing status of the patient, their role responsibilities, and ways in which they can more effectively handle chronic illness in the family. In summary, the following are reasons to include the family in education:

- A calm, knowledgeable family helps the patient to cope.
- Family support is crucial to patient success.
- The patient feels less alone; misunderstanding is reduced.
- Two or more individuals listening can remember more than one since hearing is not a strongly developed sense.
- The family can often be used to assist in teaching the patient.
- Role conflict is reduced through understanding and negotiation of responsiblities.

Suggestions and Considerations when Presenting Overviews of Dialysis Treatments

Since CAPD (and in some cases continuous cycling peritoneal dialysis [CCPD]) is rapidly expanding in many parts of the nation as a dialysis option, these suggestions are given for use in settings where both hemodialysis and peritoneal dialysis are available as patient choices. It is understood that a patient's medical condition or availability of treatment options may preclude the possibility of a choice being made based solely upon patient preferences.

- Avoid presenting hemodialysis and peritoneal dialysis at once. It is far too confusing to the patient. Avoid any comparisons until finished with each as a separate entity.
- Inform the patient that the order of presentation does not reflect staff bias. Present treatments, including advantages and disadvantages, with as much neutrality as possible.
- Desensitize the patient who may be apprehensive about dialysis. While each aspect of dialysis is explained, the patient can examine a book of color photographs showing the steps and

equipment used for treatment. The patient then can view dialysis and speak with other patients and staff members. Careful preparation makes the observation and initiation of dialysis far more positive and helpful.
- Emphasize that no treatment for renal failure is perfect. Offer some historical perspectives on progress in all treatments and emphasize the hope for further research and changes within treatment modalities.
- Compare the dialysis decision to making other consumer decisions. Emphasize lifestyle implications and that treatments involve a whole "package" of benefits, risks, and responsibilities.
- Carefully evaluate written and video materials on dialysis treatments. They can have very biased viewpoints that unfairly influence patients who cannot evaluate total implications.

EVALUATION OF RENAL EDUCATION PROGRAMS

The establishment of a renal education program in response to learning needs implies the expectation that learning will occur and hopefully will be measurable. The process of creating learning objectives in behavioral terms sets the stage for the eventual measuring, or evaluation, of learning that takes place.

According to Green, evaluation is defined as "the comparison of an object of interest against a standard of acceptability."[29] The word evaluation implies a judgement of worth. With patient education there is a desire to know what teaching has been done, what level of competency the learner has achieved, areas of educational strengths and weaknesses in both the patients and the program, and ultimately if the educational program is a worthwhile effort.

Evaluation can be beneficial in adapting the program to meet the needs of renal patients and their families, to increase effectiveness, and to promote staff efficiency. Evaluation can furthermore prevent liability cases, determine if learning is occurring, promote quality and continuity of patient care through documentation of teaching and outcomes, and can judge the long-range effects of education in terms of patient satisfaction and behavior.

Despite these benefits, some educators find reasons not to evaluate their programs. Some are concerned that evaluation will involve use of complex statistics, computer, and paperwork that may be too unmanageable. Some are concerned that inadequate time and funding exists for this part of their work. There is also a frequent concern that the evaluation will be negative and force changes in the way the educational program is provided. These concerns can be overcome by realizing that adequate evaluation can be done without great amounts of expense or staff effort and that there is room for improvement in any endeavor.

There are two basic types of evaluation, formative and summative. Formative evaluation is used throughout the phases of program development to evaluate if learning objectives are being met, if the program goals are on the right track, and if the program needs revision in its content or teaching methods. Often educators can use this form of evaluation by a "pilot test" of various educational methods and materials and comparing effectiveness of each.

Formative evaluation implies a continual monitoring of the educational process. Of particular concern is whether or not learning objectives are being met. To determine if the patient and family are learning, written testing, direct observation of behavior, or oral questioning are possible methods of evaluation.

Written testing is a widely used method of measuring knowledge acquisition. Written tests require skill to construct, however, and they require concentration, reading, and visual ability on the part of the patient. Their use and interpretation should be carefully evaluated by the staff because of potential difficulties in a renal population such as uremia and decreased vision secondary to other medical conditions.

Observation and documentation of behavior by anecdotal notes, or by noting a level of skill achievement or completion of an educational module, is a feasible evaluation method. Learning and competency levels can also be evaluated effectively by the following oral questioning methods: (1) quizzing during teaching or at end of a session; (2) situation problem solving ("It is 10 o'clock at night and you notice your fistula is not buzzing. What are you going to do?"); (3) questions about previous sessions to determine if patient needs review or a different approach; and (4) return demonstration ("Can you show me how to check your dialysate drainage bag for signs of peritonitis?").

Summative evaluation is not concerned with the nuts and bolts of running the program and measuring the patient learning. It centers on the overall impact of the program. Is it worthwhile in terms of time, efficiency, and effectiveness? Record keeping of the staff hours spent on education; age, sex, and types of patients; and the number of people served can help to evaluate the effort being expended. Efficiency can be evaluated by an annual meeting to discuss whether any staffing, funding, or procedural changes would aid the reaching of program goals.

When evaluating the impact of education, many people think in terms of long-range effectiveness. In other words, programs can be efficient and individuals can be expending effort, but effectiveness is often difficult to prove. Because of the presence of many variables affecting patients, measures of educational effectiveness are not valid proof of effectiveness when used alone.

Rather than attempt to "prove" effectiveness, educators can collect evaluation data that suggest the impact of education. It is possible to develop, a simple evaluation instrument to get feedback on the patient's satisfaction with and estimation of usefulness of various aspects of the program.

Long-range effectiveness can be evaluated by random sampling of the dialysis population every few years and checking for such things as compliance to the dialysis regimen, hospitalizations for complications that might have been prevented, and ability to take appropriate action if problems arise. This type of evaluation takes time to complete. If results are not encouraging, it is important to keep in mind that education alone is not the sole determining influence on a patient's clinical course and ability to deal with dialysis.[3]

In conclusion, evaluation can be incorporated successfully into a renal education program. As educators create and use various evaluation methods to fit their programs, they will be rewarded by increased professional skills, the knowledge with which to provide better patient education programs, and a more effective influence on patient behavior and satisfaction.

REFERENCES

1. Fylling C: A comprehensive system for patient education—Guidelines for development, in Bille DA (ed): Practical Approachs to Patient Teaching. Boston, Little, Brown, 1981, pp 15–25
2. Leman NJ, Reynolds AJ: Patient education as a part of patient care. Carle Selected Papers, nos 1, 2, 27, 1974, pp 15–24
3. Breckon DJ: Hospital Health Education. Rockville, Maryland, Aspen Systems Corporation, 1982
4. DeJoseph JF: Writing and evaluating educational protocols, in Squyres, WD (ed): Patient Education: An Inquiry into the State of the Art. New York, Springer, 1980, pp 45–109
5. Sturdevant B: Why don't adult patients learn? Supervisor Nurse, 5:44–46, 1977
6. Kasch CK: Some Thoughts on Patient Education, DAY (Dialysis and You), Spring/Summer 1980, p. 9
7. Green L: What is quality in patient education and how do we assess it? in

Squyres WD (ed): Patient Education: An Inquiry into the State of the Art. New York, Springer, 1980, pp 137–156
8. Levin LS: Patient education and self-care: how do they differ? Nursing Outlook 26(3): 170–175, 1978.
9. Eccard M: Psychosocial aspects of end stage renal disease, in Lancaster LE (ed): The Patient with End Stage Renal Disease. New York, Wiley, 1979, pp 61–81
10. Gelfman M, Wilson EJ: Emotional reactions in a renal unit, in Garfield CA, (ed): Stress and Survival: The Emotional Realities of Life-Threatening Illness. St. Louis, Mosby, 1979, pp 219–225
11. Levy NB: Coping with maintenance hemodialysis—Psychological considerations in the care of patients, in Massry SG, Sellers AL (eds): Clinical Aspects of Uremia and Dialysis. Illinois, Charles C Thomas, 1976, pp 53–67
12. Morris JE: Patient education: Nursing intervention for control-seeking behaviors. Nephrology Nurse 3(5):20–23, 1981
13. Hochbaum GM: Why people seek diagnostic x-rays. Public Health Rep 71:377–380, 1956
14. Rosenstock IM: What research in motivation suggests for public health. American Journal of Health and Human Behavior 4:166–173, 1960
15. Becker MH et al: Motivations as predictions of health behavior. Health Services Research 87:852–862, 1972
16. Dracup KA, Meleis O: Compliance: An interactionist approach. Nursing Research 31:31–36, 1982
17. Lazarus RS (interviewed by Daniel Coleman): Positive denial: The case for not facing reality. Psychology Today, Nov, pp 44–60, 1979
18. Tyler J: Patient education programs: Their significance to home dialysis and self care. Contemp Dial 1:41–44, 1980
19. Kucha D: The health education of patients: Assessing their needs. Supervisor Nurse, Apr, pp 26–35, 1974
20. Hekelman FP, Ostendarp CA: Designing educational activities for health care learners, in Lancaster LE (ed): The Patient with End Stage Renal Disease, New York, Wiley, 1979, pp 258–268
21. Bille, Donald A: An overview of patient teaching in: Practical Approaches to Patient Teaching. Boston, Little, Brown, 1981, pp 1–14
22. Coover D, Lewis S: Pre-treatment patient education for dialysis. Nephrol Nurse 3 (3):12–18, 1981
23. Crandell L: Plato system training: A new aid to patients and support staff. Contemp Dial 2 (9):53–54, 1981
24. Ferguson G: A guide to patient teaching. Nephrol Nurse 1 (4):24–26, 1979
25. Bernheimer E: Working through the territorial imperative in a hospital setting, in Squyres WD (ed): Patient Education: An Inquiry into the State of the Art. New York, Springer, 1980, pp 181–192

26. Bruner J: Toward a Theory of Instruction. Cambridge, Mass., Belknap Press, 1966
27. Knowles M: The Modern Practice of Adult Education, New York, Association Press, 1970, cited by Hekelman FP, Ostendorp CA: Designing educational activities for health care learners, in Lancaster LE (ed): The Patient with End Stage Renal Disease, New York, Wiley, 1979, p 260
28. Battista L: Design process for continuing education. Nephrol Nurse 1 (4):13–18, 1979
29. Green L, Squyres W, D'Altroy L, et al: What do recent evaluations of patient education tell us? in Squyres WD (ed): Patient Education: An Inquiry into the State of the Art. New York, Springer, 1980, pp 11–36

E. Ann Murray

15
Dietary Management

In the past 15 years there has been an increased appreciation of the importance of the diet in renal failure, both for dialysis and predialysis patients. The increase in both duration and quality of life produced by modern technology has increased the importance of appropriate dietary therapy for the patient with chronic renal failure. The diet is important in preventing malnutrition, uremic bone disease, hyperkalemia, congestive heart failure, and even death. A small percentage of patients die every year from dietary abuse.

THE RENAL FAILURE DIET

There are seven major considerations in the renal failure diet: protein, calories, potassium, sodium, calcium, phosphorus, and vitamins. When formulating a diet for the renal failure patient these aspects must all be considered and adjusted on the basis of the individual patient's needs. These needs will change periodically and need to be assessed continuously.

Protein

Little was known about protein restrictions in renal failure prior to the early 1960s. In 1963 Giordano showed that the blood urea concentration in patients with advanced renal insufficiency could be decreased by restricting protein intake, giving 2 g of essential amino acids daily and providing an adequate amount of calories, vitamins, and minerals.[1] Giovannetti and Maggiore, provided a two-stage diet to their patients in 1964.[2] The first stage provided only the minimum requirements of essential amino acids and was given until the BUN decreased. The patients were then maintained on a 20-g protein diet. There have been many modifications of these diets which confirm the observation that decreasing protein intake can lower the BUN and suggest that providing essential amino acids can maintain the renal failure patient in positive or neutral nitrogen balance and improve the sense of well-being. Some investigators suggest that by lowering the protein intake and providing the minimum amount of essential amino acids, the body can form the nonessential amino acids from the excess urea. This hypothesis has yet to be proved.

The body requires protein for the growth and maintenance of tissue. Each protein is composed of amino acids. Humans require nine essential amino acids: valine, leucine, isolencine, threonine, methionine, phenylalanine, tryptophan, lysine, and histidine. Sufficient quantities of these amino acids must be provided in the diet daily. The remainder of the 22 amino acids can be synthesized in the body from carbon and nitrogen precursors obtained in the diet.

When a protein is being synthesized, sufficient quantities of the required amino acids must all be available at the same time. An adequate amount of calories and certain vitamins must also be available or protein formation will be inhibited. When protein synthesis is inhibited, increased amounts of amino acids are degraded to urea.

Proteins can be classified on the basis of their biologic value. High-biologic-value proteins provide the most complete pattern of essential amino acids. Egg whites have the highest biologic value, then milk, followed by beef, poultry, pork, and fish. Fruits, vegetables, and grains have low-biologic-value proteins since they lack in one or more of the essential amino acids.

Calories

An adequate caloric intake should be emphasized to the renal patient in order to maintain their ideal body weight and to provide a protein sparing effect. If the patient ingests an inadequate amount of calories then protein will be used for some of the balance of the energy required. This not only limits protein use for growth and maintenance of body tissues but the metabolism of protein also increases the blood urea level. This compares with the by-products of water and carbon dioxide produced by the metabolism of carbohydrates and fats when they are used for energy. Concentrated sources of calories are jams, jellies, honeys, hard candies, sugar, and butter.

There is an increase in serum triglyceride concentrations in many dialysis patients. This may be partially influenced by high carbohydrate intake, obesity, and alcohol consumption.[3] Reaven and associates have demonstrated in renal failure patients that a 15 percent reduction in carbohydrate intake can decrease postprandial insulin response, very low-density lipoprotein (VLDL) secretion, and plasma triglyceride concentration.[3] Concentrated sources of carbohydrates, such as jams, jellies, candy, and sugar, should be avoided if there is a problem with high triglycerides. The patient should also be encouraged to increase their polyunsaturated fat intake by the use of more oils from plant origin and trimming excess fat from meats.

Potassium

Potassium is the chief cation found in the intracellular fluid. Major functions of potassium are transmission of nerve impulses and muscle contraction. Potassium is also a major contributor in maintaining a normal fluid pH and osmolarity. Symptoms of hypokalemia are muscle weakness, intestinal ilieus, and paralysis. Symptoms of hyperkalemia are muscle weakness and cardiac arrhythmias. High serum potassium can result in cardiac arrest.

Potassium restriction is usually not necessary until the patient becomes oliguric and chronic dialysis is required. After chronic dialysis is started patients who maintain a fairly high urine output may still have a more liberal intake of potassium because of their capability of excreting some of the potassium in their urine.

The majority of potassium in the diet should be obtained from high-biological-value protein foods. Other foods that are high in potassium are nuts, legumes, and some fruits and vegetables. Potassium is also found in salt substitutes and some low-sodium products (see Table 15-1).

Sodium

Sodium is the chief cation found in the extracellular fluid. Its main function is in the control of body fluid osmolarity and, therefore, body fluid volume. Sodium is also involved in nerve transmission and muscle contraction by temporarily replacing potassium in the intracellular fluid. Excess amounts of sodium cause hypertension, edema, and pulmonary congestion. Sodium deficiency results in hypotension.

Dietary restrictions of patients with renal failure depend on the patient's renal disease; some patients are sodium losers and some are sodium retainers. Factors that will determine the sodium prescription

Table 15-1
High Potassium Foods*

Food	Serving	mgK/Serving
Almonds	1 oz	220
Apricots (dried)	10 halves	340
Apricot nectar	6 oz	280
Artichokes	1 bud	360
Avocado	½	680
Banana	1 medium	440
Cantaloupe	1 cup	400
Cashews	1 oz	130
Dandelion greens	1 cup	240
Dates	10	520
Figs	1 large	130
Grapefruit	½	130
Grapefruit juice	6 oz	320
Honeydew	1 cup	430
Lima beans	1 cup	720
Milk (whole)	1 cup	350
Mustard greens	1 cup	310
Nectarine	1	410
Orange	1	170
Orange juice	6 oz	380
Papayas	1 medium	710
Parsnips	1 large	610
Peanuts	1 oz	190
Pecans	1 oz	170
Pineapple juice	6 oz	250
Potatoes		
Boiled	2½" round	320
Baked	4¾" long	780
Prunes (dried)	10	750
Prune juice	6 oz	450
Raisins	1 cup	1110
Rhubarb	1 cup	480
Spinach	1 cup	580
Sweet potato	5" long	340
Tomatoes	1	300
Tomato juice	6 oz	410
Walnuts	1 oz	130
Watermelon	1 cup	160

*Values obtained from Nutritive Values of American Foods, in common units. U.S. Department of Agriculture, Handbook 456.

are the amount of renal sodium excretion and the presence or absence of hypertension or congestive heart failure.[4]

The major source of sodium in the normal diet is table salt, however, meat tenderizers, fast food restaurant meals, cured foods, pickled items, and convenience foods (TV dinners, pot pies, canned soups, macaroni and cheese dinners) also contain large quantities of sodium (see Table 15-2). Sodium can also be found in some medications, such as sodium bicarbonate which is used in renal failure to control acidosis.

Sodium restriction plays a large role in helping patients control their fluid intake. With a sodium restriction, thirst decreases and usually results in a spontaneous decrease in fluid intake. Other positive attributes are improving control of blood pressure, edema, and pulmonary congestion.

Calcium and Phosphorus

As the function of the kidney decreases so does the excretion of phosphorus by the kidney and the gastrointestinal absorption of calcium. The excretion of phosphorus is directly related to nephron function. As the number of functioning nephrons decreases there is an increase in serum phosphorus, a decrease in serum calcium, and an increase in the circulating level of parathyroid hormone (PTH) (see Chapter 1). The primary cause of the secondary hyperparathyroidism resulting from this cycle appears to be phosphorus retention. Slatopolsky and associates believe that there should be a proportional reduction of phosphorus intake as nephron function decreases and suggest that this will reduce uremic bone disease.[5]

Early restriction of phosphorus may help avoid or decrease secondary hyperparathyroidism. It is recommended that phosphorus restriction begins when the glomerular filtration rate (GFR) decreases to 50 ml/min or less or the plasma creatinine increases to 3.0–3.5 mg/dl.[6] This should be done even if the serum phosphorus concentration is normal.

Calcium supplementation should be started at the time phosphorus restriction is initiated. Supplementation of calcium is needed due to the low calcium content of the phosphorus-restricted diet and decreased gastrointestinal calcium absorption caused by abnormalities of vitamin D metabolism. The major abnormality is an inability of the kidney to convert vitamin D to its active form of $1,25(OH)_2D_3$.

The achievement of a low phosphorus intake is accomplished through dietary restriction and the administration of phosphate binders. Phosphorus is found predominately in diary products, meat,

Table 15-2
High Sodium Foods*

Food	Serving	mgNa/Serving
A-1 sauce	1 tsp	80
Baking soda	1 tsp	820
Biscuits, canned	1	300
Bologna	1 slice	170
Bouillon cubes	1 cube	960
Bran cereal	1 cup	490
Buttermilk	1 cup	320
Catsup	1 tbsp	560
Cheese	1 oz	200
Cornbread	2½ × 2½"	490
Crackers, saltines	10	310
Hotdog	2 oz	630
Meat tenderizers	1 tsp	1750
Oatmeal, instant	½ cup	200
Olives	10	930
Pickles, dill	1 med	930
Pretzels	10 rings	500
Relishes	1 tbsp	110
Salt	1 tsp	2130
Sausage	2 oz	260
Sauerkraut	1 cup	1760
Soup, canned	1 cup	670–1180
Soy sauce	1 tbsp	1320
Tarter sauce	1 tbsp	140
Teriyaki sauce	1 oz	1150
Tuna, canned in oil	¾ cup	800
TV dinner	1 dinner	280–1400
Worcestershire sauce	1 tsp	50

*Values obtained from Nutritive Values of American Foods, in common units. U.S. Department of Agriculture, Handbook 456 and from Pennington and Church: Bowes Church's Food Values of Portions Commonly Used (ed 13). Philadelphia, Lippincott, 1980.

legumes, chocolate, and nuts (see Table 15-3). Too severe of a restriction of phosphorus can damage the nutritional status of the patient due to the low protein intake. Phosphorus depletion should also be avoided by monitoring the serum phosphorous concentration and maintaining it in the normal range.

Table 15-3
High Phosphorus Foods*

Food	Serving	mgP/Serving
Almonds	1 oz	140
Bran	1 cup	600
Cashews	1 oz	110
Calf liver	3 oz	460
Cheddar cheese	1 oz	140
Ice cream	1 cup	150
Kidney beans	1 cup	260
Lima beans	1 cup	210
Milk, whole	1 cup	230
Milk, chocolate	1 oz	70
Navy beans	1 cup	280
Oatmeal	1 cup	140
Peanuts	1 oz	110
Peanut butter	1 tbsp	60
Pecans	1 oz	80
Puddings		
Chocolate	1 cup	260
Vanilla	1 cup	230
Pumpkin seeds	½ cup	800
Semisweet chocolate	1 oz	40
Split peas	1 cup	180
Sunflower seeds	½ cup	610
Walnuts	1 oz	160

*Values obtained from Nutritive Values of American Foods, in common units. U.S. Department of Agriculture, Handbook 456.

Vitamin and Mineral Therapy

Vitamin supplements are an important part of nutrition therapy due to the restrictions of the renal diet. Predialysis patients are placed on low protein, low phosphorus diets which limit the low-biologic-value protein thus reducing the intake of many essential vitamins and minerals. Patients on dialysis lose water soluble vitamins and minerals during dialysis. The leaching of vegetables to remove potassium also removes water soluble vitamins.

Several of the vitamins and minerals need special consideration when selecting the appropriate vitamin supplement. There have been several studies concerning the need for vitamin B_6 supplementation in chronic renal failure. Kopple and associates have demonstrated evidence of vitamin B_6 deficiency early in progressive renal failure with only a mild or moderate decrease in GFR.[8] This may indicate that other factors besides uremia, dialysis loss, poor dietary intake, or a vitamin B_6 antagonist cause the vitamin B_6 deficiency. It is possible that the normal kidney is needed for the metabolism of vitamin B_6. Kopple recommends 5 mg/day of pyridoxine hydrochloride for pre-dialysis and peritoneal dialysis patients and 10 mg/day for hemodialysis patients and patients taking a pyridoxine antagonist.

The requirement for vitamin D and calcium has been discussed earlier in this chapter and in Chapter 1.

Supplementation of folate is required due to a dietary restriction of fruits and vegetables, loss of folate from the leaching of fruits and vegetables to control potassium intake, and folate losses during dialysis. Supplementation of 1 mg after each dialysis treatment provides a sufficient amount for the dialysis patient.[9]

Ascorbic acid intake is limited in renal failure patients because of the high potassium content of most ascorbic acid-rich foods. Ascorbic acid is also depleted during dialysis. A daily supplement of 100 mg is recommended.[9]

There is evidence of elevated plasma vitamin A levels and retinol binding protein (RBP) in uremia, however, the exact cause is not known.[9] Many of the symptoms of chronic vitamin A intoxication are similar to those of uremia (i.e., elevated PTH, dry skin, bone tenderness, anorexia, generalized weakness, weight loss), and this may be contributing to the clinical findings of uremia.[10] Ellis and associates believe that the vitamin A increase is due to elevated RBP levels rather than decreased excretion, since a decrease in vitamin A intake did not lower vitamin A levels.[10] Vitamin A is less dialyzable since it is a fat soluble vitamin which is protein bound. More research is needed on vitamin A metabolism in uremic patients, but at this point it is recommended that vitamin A supplements not be given to chronic renal failure patients.

Iron stores may be depleted in dialysis patients for several reasons. Antacids, given for control of phosphorus, bind iron and prevent its absorbtion while sodium bicarbonate decreases iron absorption by increasing the pH of the intestinal lumen. The hemodialysis patient may lose more than 50 mg of iron each week in the dialysis tubing and blood sampling. Serum ferritin levels are good indicators of iron stores with diagnostic levels of 30–300 ng/ml.[11]

NUTRITIONAL ASSESSMENT

An initial nutritional assessment of the patient with renal insufficiency with subsequent follow-ups at 6-month intervals will enable the physician and dietitian to formulate an appropriate nutrition plan and evaluate its progress. The initial assessment gives a base line for comparing the subsequent assessments. It is desirable to obtain this base line information before the patient has become sick and lost weight from uremia. This is frequently not possible since many patients are at end stage when diagnosed.

The nutritional assessment can include the following: diet history, anthropometric measurements, visceral protein assessment, and evaluation of the immunologic response. The combination used depends on how complete an evaluation is needed. It is helpful to evaluate several of these parameters since each can be influenced by factors other than diet. An assemblage of these parameters will usually give a good assessment of the nutritional state of the patient.

Diet History

Diet histories give the dietitian basic information about eating habits and an indication of areas which need to be watched in the future. Diet histories must be obtained skillfully and carefully in order to ensure that the information is accurate. The interviewer must ask open-ended questions and not show disapproval to the responses. If the interview is conducted in an open and accepting fashion, acquisition of accurate information is more likely to be obtained.

Anthropometric Measurements

Anthropometric measurements evaluate the somatic protein and fat compartments of the body. Measurements of arm circumference and skin fold thickness determine arm muscle and subcutaneous fat thickness. There is good correlation between the subcutaneous fat thickness with total body fat and arm muscle thickness with total body muscle mass.[12] Measurements are usually taken on the triceps, however, Blumenkrantz and associates advise taking them in three or more places such as triceps, subscapular, thoracic, and suprailiac areas.[13] Multiple measurements minimize sampling errors with the average measurement being more representative.

There are presently no anthropometric standards for chronic renal failure patients. Values obtained from normal controls may be used and a percent of normal can be calculated. The sequential measurements from which the progress of the patient can be followed are of greatest value. Guarnieri found in his patients that subscapular and tricep skin fold thicknesses were inversely correlated with the length of time on hemodialysis suggesting an inadequate caloric intake.[14] Whether appropriate dietary intervention can prevent this problem remains to be seen.

Measurements on hemodialysis patients should be done immediately after the dialysis treatment to minimize interference fom excess body fluid. Anthropometric measurements taken every 6 months enable the dietitian and physician to evaluate if weight changes are muscle, fat, or fluid. It is important to ascertain that progressive protein malnutrition is not being masked by an increase in adipose tissue or fluid.

Some of the plasma proteins, such as albumin and the complement components, are good indicators of the visceral protein status due to their relatively short half-lives. Serum albumin is a readily available measurement and is a more sensitive indicator of protein status than serum total protein concentration. Serum albumin also shows a good correlation with arm muscle circumference indicating parallel effects of nutrition on visceral and somatic proteins.[15] Plasma transferrrin has always been used as an indicator of protein deficiency. A recent study by Milman, however, demonstrates no correlation between serum albumin and serum transferrin in uremic patients due to transferrin's close association with iron metabolism.[16] In uremic patients serum albumin is therefore a better indicator of protein deficiency.

Abnormalities in plasma protein concentrations must be carefully evaluated since their concentrations can be influenced by other factors than the diet. One large factor affecting chronic renal failure patients is hemodilution which may cause false low values. Many diseases which cause renal failure may also change serum complement concentrations independent of nutritional considerations. A sudden decrease in concentration usually does not indicate malnutrition, but a gradual decline over a long period of time usually warrants investigation. There is no correlation between the duration of dialysis and serum protein content.[14]

Immunological Testing

Testing the patient's immunological response is the final nutritional assessment. Decreased cell-mediated immunity is associated with a delay in wound healing, increased sepsis, and an increased morbidity and mortality.[17] The immunological response can be evaluated in two ways. First, by total lymphocyte count and second, by delayed hypersensitivity skin testing using such antigens as mumps, candida, and streptokinase-streptodornase. Protein malnutrition is associated with lymphocyte counts of less than 2000/mm^3 and a lack of response to the skin testing.[15] More research is required in this area in order to determine the relationship between uremia and immunological testing. At this point these tests should be used in combination with the other nutritional assessment procedures.

In the nutritional assessment on chronic renal failure patients a combination of the above techniques is the best indication of the nutritional status. Since there are no standards for this population, sequential changes are again more important than single measurements.

DIETARY COMPLIANCE

Adherence to the renal diet is an important factor in the dialysis regimen and noncompliance can increase hospitalizations and even result in death. The most skillfully and carefully prepared dietary plan is of absolutely no value if not accepted and followed by the patient. The onset of end-stage renal disease is one of the largest disruptions to lifestyle. The necessity of dialysis treatments, frequent loss of employment, dependence on many medications, and severe changes of dietary habits engenders a sense of helplessness. The diet is one of the last aspects of life over which the patient feels he has some control and therefore compliance is often compromised. The renal diet frequently results in a major change in lifestyle for both the patient and his or her family. It requires that certain foods be limited or avoided, restricts fluids, and makes it difficult to eat in restaurants.

Several studies have been done to determine which patients are more susceptible to dietary noncompliance. Blackburn found that compliance decreased as the time on dialysis increased, in spite of an increase in the understanding of the diet.[18] Sand and associates demonstrated that the patient's past lifestyle and current way of living are the most important factors in determining how they will tolerate the demands of dialysis.[19] A study by Procci indicates that patients capable of returning to employment along with students and women capable of performing at least three-fourths of their housework were better dietary compliers than unemployed patients.[20] This study also found that the patient's living conditions made a difference. Patients were better compliers if they lived with a spouse, a financee, and/or children.[20]

Noncompliance may be caused by the fact that the patient frequently does not believe that they are harming themselves. It is hard to understand, for example, that hyperphosphatemia will cause bone disease when they feel no changes in their bones. It is difficult but helpful to attempt to give renal patients a reward for following their diet or to penalize them when they do something wrong.

The more motivated the patient is, the better they do. To help keep the patient motivated, it is important that the staff reinforce good performance and stress the importance of following the diet when they do something wrong. All too often the major focus is on noncompliance and patients are not given encouragement when they have done well.

DIABETICS WITH CHRONIC RENAL FAILURE

Special consideration must be given to the diabetic with chronic renal failure since they must contend with the restrictions of a diabetic diet along with the new restrictions of a renal diet. Some diabetics that reach end-stage renal disease have never been placed on a diabetic diet and many previously have never followed the diet they were given. A typical diabetic renal diet is shown in Table 15-4.

Good control of blood glucose concentration in the diabetic with renal failure is important for several reasons. Hyperglycemia causes an increase in thirst which may lead to fluid overload, hypertension, or congestive heart failure. Using the diet to help control the blood glucose may also decrease the chance of protein malnutrition, since excess insulin therapy causes gluconeogenesis which inhibits protein synthesis.[21] Good control is also important, as in all diabetics, in preventing and/or controlling secondary diabetic complications such as neuropathy, retinopathy, angiopathy, GI disturbances, and skin lesions.

The diabetic is more prone to malnutrition from nausea and vomiting, repeated hospitalizations and gastrointestinal problems. Stress from these problems and from dialysis can increase insulin requirements and may lead to gluconeogenesis with inhibition of protein synthesis.

There are several major changes in the diabetic renal diet from the usual diabetic diet. The sodium restriction eliminates many of the "free" foods. The diabetic would no longer be able to use, for example, dill pickles, soy sauce, steak sauce, or bouillon cubes.

Table 15-4
Diabetic Renal Diet*

Menus
Breakfast
1 egg
1 slice bread with 1 tsp butter and 2 tbs honey
¾ cup dry cereal with 4 oz nondairy creamer
⅓ cup apple juice
½ cup coffee or tea
Lunch
3 oz hamburger
1 hamburger bun
1 cup lettuce with 4 tsp French dressing
1 pear
10 jelly beans
1 cup tea, coffee or water
Dinner
3 oz meat
½ cup mashed potatoes
1 dinner roll with 1 tsp butter
1 cup lettuce with 4 tsp French dressing
½ cup gelatin with strawberries
1 apple cinnamon muffin
1 cup tea, coffee, or water
Snack
¼ cup cottage cheese with ½ cup peaches
4 graham crackers
1 cup Hawaiian Punch

*2600 calories, 90 g protein, 330 g carbohydrate, 90 g fat, 2 g sodium, 1000 mg phosphorous, and 67 mEq potassium.

Several vegetables, which are also considered free in the diabetic diet, now must be counted in the diabetic renal diet due to their potassium content. Starchy vegetables, such as potatoes, are considered a starch serving in the diabetic diet, but are now counted as a vegetable due to the potassium content. Finally, with the elimination of high phosphorus foods, such as milk, cheese, and peanut butter, snacks become very monotonous.

The proportion of carbohydrate, protein, and fat also changes. The usual proportions in the diabetic diet are 45 percent carbohydrate, 20 percent protein, and 35 percent fat which change to 50 percent carbohydrate, 14 percent protein, and 36 percent fat in the diabetic renal diet. The main difference is the decrease in the amount of protein. Complex carbohydrates should be used predominately, however, it may become necessary to use some simple sugars to provide enough calories.

The renal failure diabetic must also be instructed on a different method to treat insulin reactions. In patients without renal failure, orange juice is frequently used, however, due to its high potassium content this must be avoided. Sugar water, honey, or hard candies should be used to treat insulin reactions in the diabetic with renal failure.

PREDIALYSIS NUTRITION

Before 1963 and the work of Giordano, little was known to help improve the symptoms of the predialysis chronic renal failure patient. Giordano in 1963 and Giovanetti, Maggiore and Monasterio in 1964 made it possible to relieve uremic symptoms and postpone the start of dialysis through dietary changes.

These men brought about the first restrictions of protein. Since these studies, many other investigators have experimented with modifications of the Giovanetti and Giordano methods with the same results, an improvement in uremic symptoms. Most of these diets were based on daily intake of 20 g of protein with the remainder of the calories being provided from carbohydrates and fats. A 20-g protein diet is frequently associated with a negative nitrogen balance and the presence of a catabolic state which in the long run will do more harm than the small benefit gained from delaying the start of dialysis. Kopple and associates demonstrated that a 40-g protein diet maintains patients in a better nutritional state than those on a 20-g protein diet.[22] They found that with a 40-g protein diet, renal failure patients were in positive nitrogen balance and uremic symptoms were relieved as well as with a 20-g protein diet.

If patients are in a catabolic state when they start dialysis, the resultant malnourishment compounds the problems caused by the multiple operations, infections, depression, anorexia, nausea, and hospitalizations which frequently occur with the initiation of dialysis therapy. Patients are more likely to withstand these stresses associated with dialysis if they are in neutral or positive nitrogen balance.

There is no general agreement as to when to initiate and how severe protein restriction should be. Protein restriction appears to be of little value before the blood urea concentration is at least 50–75 mg/dl. It presently appears reasonable to restrict protein to 40–60 g when the blood urea nitrogen concentration is elevated above these values and is causing uremic symptoms. Most predialysis patients voluntarily restrict their protein intake, possibly due to a bitter taste that uremia causes in protein foods.

Potassium is usually not a concern in a predialysis patient for two reasons. It is restricted when protein intake is limited and second, potassium excretion does not decrease in proportion to glomerular filtration rate. The predialysis patient usually only needs to be instructed to avoid large intakes of high potassium foods. With the use of diuretics to help relieve hypertension or edema, it may even be necessary to supplement potassium since many of these agents cause increased potassium excretion. This must be done with caution, however, and serum potassium monitored carefully.

Sodium restriction may be important in the predialysis state to help relieve edema and hypertension. The best way to determine the initial sodium prescription is to determine the 24-hour urinary sodium excretion while the patient is at ideal sodium balance. The prescribed intake should approximate this excretion. From this point the patient can be monitored for weight change, edema, hypertension, or signs of sodium depletion to determine if a change in sodium prescription is needed. It is seldom necessary to restrict sodium to less than 2 g/24 hours. If the predialysis patient is in positive sodium balance on a 2-g sodium diet then it is usually better to place the patient on diuretics rather than to impose the severe restrictions of a further reduced sodium intake. Again it must be remembered that some patients are sodium losers and some are sodium retainers.

The changes of uremic bone disease are lessened with early phosphorus restriction. When the glomerular filtration rate decreases to 50 percent of normal or serum creatinine increases above 3, high phosphorus foods such as chocolate, legumes, nuts, and whole grains should be restricted. Phosphate binders should also be started and calcium supplements given if the serum phosphorus is within normal range. Phosphorus intake is automatically further restricted in the predialysis diet when protein intake is limited.

Fluid intake is usually allowed to be taken on an ad-lib basis in the predialysis patient. If the sodium restriction is followed then fluid intake will usually be voluntarily limited. If the patients show signs of water intoxication as indicated by a decrease in serum sodium concentration, the fluid intake should be restricted. A sample predialysis diet can be found in Table 15-5.

HEMODIALYSIS NUTRITION

Once chronic hemodialysis is begun, the diet can be liberalized from the predialysis diet. The goal of the diet remains the same: to provide optimal nutrition while preventing hyperkalemia, hyperphosphatemia, hypertension, and congestive heart failure.

A protein intake of 1 g/kg, with 80 percent being of high biological value, is recommended to maintain the hemodialysis patient in positive nitrogen balance. This is an optimal intake and it appears that most patients do not eat this amount of protein. Blood urea nitrogen concentration can be used as an indicator of intake. If it is low, inadequate protein intake must be suspected. This can be confirmed with urea kinetic studies (Chapter 4) and if present the patient should be encouraged to eat more high protein foods. Protein supplements can also be used but are seldom necessary.

A potassium restriction of 60–80 mEq provides a palatable diet for the hemodialysis patient while avoiding hyperkalemia. If a higher potassium intake is desired, especially during the summer months when fresh fruits and vegetables are available, then the potassium content of the dialysate can be decreased. Patients on digoxin are prone to cardiac arrythmias with low dialysate potassium concentrations and the dialysate potassium should not be lower than 2 mEq/liter in these patients. They must follow a more strict potassium diet. Some potassium can be leached from vegetables by peeling, cutting into small pieces, and soaking for 3–4 hours.

A sodium prescription of 2 g provides a palatable diet and will limit interdialysis weight gains to a reasonable level. This restriction allows no salt in cooking or at the table and requires avoidance of high sodium foods. Emphasis of this restriction is important in order to prevent excessive thirst. Herbs and spices can be used to season food and replace the use of salt.

Fluid intake should be limited to 1 liter/day, which allows a weight gain of 2 kg during the week and 3 kg over the weekend. Weight gains above this frequently cause problems during dialysis such as cramping and hypotension. The daily insensible losses of 500–600 cc can be accounted for as the fluid content found in foods. Patients with daily urine outputs greater than 100 ml may add this volume to their daily fluid intake. The ability of the patient to follow the fluid restriction is

Table 15-5
Sample Predialysis Diet*

Menus
Breakfast
1 egg—fried
¾ cup dry cereal with ½ cup nondairy creamer
½ cup orange juice
1 cup coffee or tea
Snack
Marshmallow rice bar
Lunch
1 oz meat
1 slice bread
1 cup lettuce with French dressing
½ cup pears
ice tea or coffee
Snack
Hard candy
Butter balls
Fondant
Dinner
2 oz meat
½ cup rice with gravy
½ cup broccoli
1 cup lettuce with dressing
½ cup peaches
ice tea, coffee
Snack
½ cup applesauce

*40 g protein, 1 g sodium, 600 mg phosphorus, and 50 mEq potassium.

very dependent on their sodium intake. Most hemodialysis patients will be able to limit their fluid intake appropriately without a specific limitation if they are able to limit their sodium intake and merely instructed to avoid excess fluid intake. Sodium and fluid restrictions appear to be the most difficult aspects of the hemodialysis diet.

Phosphorus intake for hemodialysis patients should be restricted to 800 mg daily and the use of phosphate binders is still required. This restriction requires the avoidance of all dairy products, chocolate, nuts, and legumes. If the intake of high phosphorus food is desired on occasion, extra phosphate binders should be taken after eating those foods. Hemodialysis patients frequently need large amounts of phosphate binders and it often becomes difficult for them to take the prescribed amount. To reduce the number of pills taken, the aluminum hydroxide can be added to applesauce, mashed potatoes, breads, and cookies.

There has been recent research on the use of nutritional therapy to decrease dialysis frequency. Mitch and Sapir demonstrated an improvement in 6 of 7 patients, with some residual renal function, being dialyzed weekly or biweekly by decreasing protein intake and supplementing with essential amino acids.[23]

CAPD NUTRITION

Continuous ambulatory peritoneal dialysis (CAPD) offers a more liberal diet than hemodialysis or intermittent peritoneal dialysis (IPD). Large fluctuations in serum chemistry concentrations do not occur with CAPD since dialysis is continuous. In comparison, intermittent dialysis causes large variations due to the buildup of waste products between treatments. For this reason greater amounts of potassium, phosphorus, sodium, and protein can be taken by CAPD patients without having peak excesses. A sample dialysis diet can be found in Table 15-6.

The most important aspect of the CAPD diet is the protein content. In a recent study by Blumenkrantz it was found that protein losses in CAPD were 8.8 g/24 hours with albumin accounting for 50–79 percent of the protein. There is no correlation between the total outflow volume of dialysate each day and the amount of protein lost.[24]

The CAPD diet should be high enough in protein to replace the dialysate protein loss and to provide enough protein for everyday maintenance. Blumenkrantz feels that 1.2 g of protein for each kilogram of ideal body weight is needed to maintain these patients in a neutral or positive nitrogen balance.[25] In a recent study, however, Gahl speculates from his data that a protein intake of 1 g/kg or less can still maintain patients in an anabolic state or in nitrogen equilibrium.[26] In our clinical experience it appears that although most CAPD patients will not consume 1.2 g/kg of protein even when instructed to do so, many are still capable of at least maintaining their serum albumin concentration within normal range. Protein supplements can be given if indicated by nutritional assessment.

Table 15-6
Sample Dialysis Diet*

Menus
Breakfast
1 egg
¾ cup dry cereal with ½ cup nondairy creamer
1 slice bread with butter and jelly
½ cup orange juice
½ cup coffee, tea, or water
Lunch
3 oz meat
2 slices bread
1 cup lettuce with salad dressing
½ cup pears
1 cup coffee, ice tea, or water
Dinner
4 oz meat
½ cup broccoli
1 cup lettuce with salad dressing
½ cup peaches
1 cup coffee, tea, or water
Snack
½ cup applesauce
½ cup coffee, tea, or water

*80 g protein, 1.5 g sodium, 900 mg phosphorus, and 62 mEq potassium.

When considering caloric intake for CAPD patients, it must be taken into account that calories are absorbed from the dialysate as well as coming from food. Calories absorbed from the dialysate vary according to the glucose concentration in the dialysate and the total number of exchanges per day. The average net glucose absorption from the dialysate is about 200 g/day which accounts for 35 percent of total energy intake.[27] In one study there was a mean weight gain of 7 kg at the end of 1 year of CAPD.[28] Although there are no long-term studies, our clinical impression is that while many patients seem to stabilize their weight after 1 year, some continue to gain weight for long periods of time. To determine the amount of kilocalories available in the dialysate, the volume of solution is multiplied by the glucose concentration and this value is then multiplied by four, since there are 4 kcal/g of carbohydrate. For example, 2000 ml × 4.25 percent glucose dialysate = 85 g CHO × 4 = 340 kcal. While this gives the amount of glucose available, the amount actually absorbed averages 70 percent for 1.5 percent glucose dialysate and 60 percent from 4.25 percent glucose dialysate of that available and varies considerably.[29]

The recommended total caloric intake for a normal adult is 33 kcal/kg of ideal body weight (IBW), 44 kcal/kg in undernourished patients, and 22 kcal/kg in the obese patient. These amounts appear appropriate for the CAPD patient. When the diet is being calculated, the calories absorbed from the dialysate should be subtracted from the total caloric intake wanted and the remaining calories used for food calories.

The CAPD diet should be low in carbohydrates and saturated fatty acids in an attempt to inhibit the increase in plasma triglyceride levels which occurs in this population. The increase is found in the VLDL. It does not appear to be due as much to an increase in the production of VLDL as to a reduction in the metabolic clearance of VLDL.[30] Patients with extremely high triglyceride levels should be placed on a Type IV hyperlipoproteinemia diet with restriction of carbohydrate, cholesterol and alcohol.

Most CAPD patients should be initially instructed on a 2-g sodium diet with no fluid restriction. Patients need to be encouraged to limit sodium and fluid intake if they develop signs of fluid overload such as edema or hypertension. In this way they will not have to increase the number of 4.25 percent exchanges being used, with its resultant increased glucose absorption. Initial instruction should point out this cycle before this problem is encountered.

Potassium cannot be severely restricted because of the need for a high protein diet. Potassium prescriptions of 60–80 mEq allow for the high protein diet and also allow the diet to remain palatable. There is usually very little problem with high serum potassium levels unless the patient is a big eater.

Phosphorus restriction is also more liberal then for hemodialysis patients. Usually patients can be allowed 2 cups of milk and the serum phosphorus concentrations still controlled with aluminum hydroxide.

It is helpful to place patients starting on CAPD on calcium supplements. Serum calcium concentrations frequently increase after 3–6 months and the calcium supplements can be discontinued at this time.[28] Calcium is absorbed from the dialysate with the amount depending on the serum level of calcium, dialysate calcium concentration, and the number of exchanges. Calcium supplements and vitamin D are therefore only given as indicated to maintain a normal serum level of calcium. Patients should also be given a multivitamin to replace water soluble vitamins lost during dialysis.

The sample diets in this chapter illustrate a typical predialysis, dialysis, and diabetic diet. Although it is desirable to avoid simple sugars in diabetics, it is frequently necessary to supplement the diabetic, renal failure diet with simple sugars to provide enough calories as in the sample diet. These menus are samples and many variations are possible.

REFERENCES

1. Giordano C: Use of exogenous and endogenous urea for protein synthesis in normal and uremic subjects. J Lab Clin Med 62:231, 1963
2. Giovannetti S, Maggiore Q: Low protein diet in uraemia. Lancet 1:1000, 1964
3. Reaven GM, Swenson RS, Sanfelippo ML: An inquiry into the mechanism of hypertriglyceridemia in patients with chronic renal failure. Am J Clin Nutr 33:1476–1484, 1980
4. Yium JJ: Determination of diet orders by analysis of lab values. Tex Med 69:114–117, 1973
5. Slatopolsky E, Bricker NS: The role of phosphorus restriction in the prevention of secondary hyperparathyroidism in chronic renal disease. Kidney Int 4:141, 1973
6. Maschio G, Tessitore N, N'Angelo A, Bonucci E, Lupo A, Valvo E, Loschiavo C, Fabris A, Morachiello P, Dreviato G, Giasch E: Early dietary phosphorus restriction and calcium supplementation in the prevention of renal osteodystrophy. Am J Clin Nutr 33:1546–1553, July 1980
7. Schoolworth AC, Engle JE: Calcium and phosphorus in diet therapy of uremia. JADA 66:460–464, 1975
8. Kopple JD, Mercurio K, Blumenkrantz MJ, Jones MR, Tallos J, Roberts C, Card B, Saltzman R, Casciato DA, Swenseid ME: Daily requirement for pyridoxine supplements in chronic renal failure. Kidney Int 19:694–704, 1981
9. Murray MA: Vitamin and mineral needs of chronic hemodialysis patient. Dial Transplan 9:921–924, 1979
10. Ellis S, De Palma J, Cheng A, Capozzalo P, Dombeck D, DiScala VA: Vitamin A supplements in hemodialysis patients. Nephron 26:215–218, 1980
11. Bell JD, Kincaid WR, Morgan RG, Bunce H, Alperin JB, Sarles HE, Remmers AR: Serum ferritin assay and bone-marrow iron stores in patients on maintenance hemodialysis. Kidney Int 17:237–241, 1980
12. Blumenkrantz MJ, Schmidt RW: Managing the nutritional concerns of the patient undergoing peritoneal dialysis, in Nolph KD (ed): Peritoneal Dialysis. The Hague, Nijhoff, 1981, p 281

13. Blumenkrantz MJ, Kopple JD, Gutman RA, Chan YK, Barbour GL, Roberts C, Shen FH, Gandhi VC, Tucker CT, Curtis FK, Coburn JW: Methods for assessing nutritional status of patients with renal failure. Am J Clin Nutr 33:1567–1585, 1980
14. Guarnieri G, Faccini L, Lipartiti T, Ranieri F, Spanquaro F, Giuntini D, Toigo G, Dardi F, Berquier-Vidali F, Raimondi A: Simple methods for nutritional assessment in hemodialysis patients. Am J Clin Nutr 33:1598–1607, 1980
15. Grant A: Nutritional Assessment Guidelines. Seatle, Washington, 1979
16. Milman N: Plasma transferrin and the relation to iron status in patients with chronic uremia. Clin Nephrol 16:314–320, 1981
17. Comty CM: Nutritional assessment in end-stage renal disease. Dial Transplant 10(2):130–134, 1981
18. Blackburn SL: Dietary compliance of chronic hemodialysis patients. J Am Diet Assoc 70:31–37, 1977
19. Wright RG, Sand P, Livingston G: Psychological stress during hemodialysis for chronic renal failure. Ann Intern Med 64:611–621, 1966
20. Procci WR: Dietary abuse in main tenance hemodialysis patients. Psychosomatics 16–24, January 1978
21. Comty CM, Leonard A, Shapiro FL: Nutritional and metabolic problems in the dialyzed patient with diabetes mellitus. Kidney Int 6(1):S51, 1974
22. Kopple JD and Coburn JW: Metabolic studies of low protein diets in uremia. I. Nitrogen and potassium. Medicine 52(6):583–593, 1973
23. Mitch WE, Sapir DG: Evaluation of reduced dialysis frequency using nutritional therapy. Kidney Int 20:122–126, 1981
24. Blumenkrantz MJ, Gahl GM, Kopple JD, Kamdar AV, Jones MR, Kessel M, Coburn JW: Protein losses during peritoneal dialysis. Kidney Int 19:593–602, 1981
25. Blumenkrantz MC, Schmidt RW: Managing the nutritional concerns of the patient undergoing peritoneal dialysis, in Nolph KD (ed): Peritoneal Dialysis, The Hague, Nijhoff, 1981, p 293
26. Gahl GM, Baeyer HV, Averdunk R, Riedinger H, Borowzak B, Schurig R, Becker H, Kessel M: Outpatient evaluation of dietary intake and nitrogen removal in continuous ambulatory peritoneal dialysis. Annals Int Med 94:643–646, 1981
27. Grodstein GP, Blumenkrantz MJ, Kopple JD, Moran JK, Coburn JW: Glucose absorption during continuous ambulatory peritoneal dialysis. Kidney Int 19:564–567, 1981
28. Nolph KD, Sorkin M, :Rubin J, Arfania D, Prowant B, Fruto L, Kennedy D: Continuous ambulatory peritoneal dialysis: Three-year experience at one center. Ann Int Med 92:609–613, 1980
29. Unpublished data of the University of Missouri at Columbia, MO.
30. Blumenkrantz MJ, Schmidt RW: Managing the nutritional concerns of the patient undergoing peritoneal dialysis, in Nolpj KD (ed): Peritoneal Dialysis. The Hague, Nijhoff, 1981, p 284

Judy C. Webb

16

The Administrative Mandate: Effective Utilization of Human, Professional, and Financial Resources

As we enter the third decade of dialysis, the effective and efficient management of a dialysis facility is increasing in complexity. Many different aspects are involved in the administration of a dialysis program. This chapter discusses two facets of the program. The first facet concerns the team approach to the end-stage renal disease (ESRD) patient using a primary nurse system; the second, the reimbursement of the ESRD program through federal funding and the mandate by the government for cost containment.

THE TEAM APPROACH TO THE ESRD PATIENT USING A PRIMARY NURSE SYSTEM

At no time in the history of the provision of health services, has the need for understanding and intelligent interaction with patients been so sharply highlighted as it is in the present. The explosion of scientific knowledge has tended to impersonalize what was once a highly personal service. At the same time, the need for a deeper understanding of psychological problems, social problems, and the specific problems of the individual patients has increased. Due to the tremendous increase in scientific knowledge, no one person can know everything necessary for the provision of high-quality medical care and therefore we have experienced a continuous growth of specialization.

This eventually leads to the lack of capability to view the individual patient as a totality. It has become a challenge for all health care facilities to treat the patient as a totality and to deal with the continuously rising complexity of providing quality health care to a large volume of patients. This is especially true for renal dialysis facilities. One effective way of dealing with these difficulties is to use a team approach.[1]

In recent years, responsibility for providing human services to patients in clinical settings has been shared by a team of professionals. The result of this development and trend has been the promise of a more unified approach to patient care. This approach allows the team to bring together diverse skills and expertise, thus providing high quality, more effective, and better coordinated service for the patient. The team is a collaborative endeavor, combining different skills and expertise of team members to provide the ultimate in patient care. The patient is the center of the team's effort and the purpose for the team's existence.[1]

A primary nursing program is an excellent method of implementing team care delivery. It expands the concept and allows for one person to coordinate each patients care while still maintaining the benefits of the team approach. The objectives of a primary nurse program are:

1. To provide patient-centered care with the patient being the central focus for planning, implementing, and evaluating care.
2. To provide a unified approach to patient care as opposed to a segmented, specialized approach.
3. To provide for continuity of care by the assignment of each patient to one nurse who is responsible for coordinating the full spectrum of services provided to that patient. This includes:
   Total assessment of patient needs.
   Developing a nursing care plan to meet these needs.
   Implementing this care plan.
   Providing, along with other team members, support measures such as counseling, teaching, and consultation.
   Including the patient and the patient's family into the health care team.
   Ongoing evaluation of each step of the nursing process.

In developing and implementing a primary nursing program, it is important for everyone to understand the total concept of the program and how each individual team member will become a part of the program. Primary nursing is a method of delivering nursing care in which one nurse assumes the responsibility for a limited number of patients over a designated period of time. This primary nurse assesses the patient, identifies the patient's nursing needs, develops and implements the plan for meeting those needs. The primary nurse is personally accountable for his or her decisions and actions. The total program revolves around the primary nurse and the success of the program depends on the nurse and his or her capabilities in fulfilling this role. If you were to visualize a wheel, the primary nurse, along with the patient, would be the hub or the main focal point for all communications concerning the patient's care and the coordination of that care, with all other team members and family feeding into that focal point.

Communication

The ultimate success of any team approach to patient care depends on good communication between team members. Primary nurses communicate with the other team members through the following mechanisms: written communication sheets, verbal communication, nursing care plans, and patient care conferences.

The primary nurses' communication process with the team facilities the understanding of the patient's needs by the team members and can help relieve the patient's anxieties during the course of treatment. Team members are better able to assist the patient during treatment on a one-to-one basis by having prior knowledge of the patient's needs. The patient then receives the fullest benefit of all the team members. The primary nurse always remains the number one person responsibile for the patient's care. Although other team members may provide services, the primary nurse is totally accountable for management of the patient's care.

The team care members must meet regularly to discuss the patients' needs. Some meeting should be dedicated to long-term planning of overall objectives of a limited number of patients. Each patient should be thoroughly discussed by the team at least annually and preferably semiannually at these meetings. Separate team meetings should be held regularly to discuss routine care of all the patients and to solve the immediate problems of individual patients. These meetings provide the mechanism for a continual feedback system and give the opportunity for team members to share information relevant to patient care planning. This also helps to provide a common ground for all participants to work toward unified patient care.

The primary nurse does not necessarily have to attend all meetings concerning the patient if the head nurse or charge nurse is there to receive feedback. It is then their responsibility to relate the significant changes in planning and treatment to the primary nurse. As each team member—social worker, dietitian, nurse clinician, physician, primary nurse, and so on—provides direct and immediate communication, the communication cycle completes itself and all team members remain informed of the patient's management. During the dialysis treatment the charge nurse accompanies the physician on patient rounds and relays information to the primary nurse to further coordinate and provide optimum patient care management.

Since the communication process is such an integral part of the program, it is important to ensure communication internally. To enhance the transmission of exchanging of information a primary nurse communication form can be used (see Fig. 16-1). This form will be filled out by the charge nurse as he or she rounds with the physician, or by any team member when communicating patient needs. Upon completion, it is given to the primary nurse who then makes the necessary changes in the patients care plan.

Kardex, physician orders, discharge summaries, social service, and dietary notes are also a means of communication by providing up-to-date information as to changes in the patient's treatment, etc. Although the primary nurse should be in charge of the patients actual dialysis treatment as often as possible, scheduling limitations make it impossible for this to occur all the time. The assigned staff dialyzing the patient need to communicate with the care team. Although this can be achieved by direct verbal communication during rounds or sooner if necessary, it will still need to be written for documentation. A special section of the dialysis flow sheet can be designated for this purpose.

Specific Duties of the Primary Nurse

Primary nurses are responsibile for providing total, comprehensive, continuous patient–clinical care. Essential components of their responsibility are coordinating all aspects of patient care and communicating relevant information to the physician, other team members, and families.

The specific duties of the primary nurse are outlined in Table 16-1 in the progression beginning with day one through a 6-month course of care. The duties are divided into the following sections: (1) admission day, (2) weekly, (3) monthly, (4) 6-monthly (see Table 16-1).

When a patient requires hospitalization, the primary nurse pre-

Name: _____

Patient Name: _____
Date: _____
Dialysis Changes:
Target Weight: _____ Dialysate: _____
Dialyzer: _____ Duration: _____
Anticoagulation: _____ Ultrafiltration: _____
Other: _____
Medication Changes: _____
Lab Needed: _____
Dialysis Time Changed: _____ Date: _____
  Time: _____ Reason: _____
Hospitalized: _____ Transfer form needed: _____
Discharged from Hospital: _____
Hospital Records Needed: _____
Social Service Problem: _____
Dietary Problem: _____
Patient Educator: _____
Nurse Clinician: _____
Physician: _____
Place form in Head Nurse's office when changes are complete.

Figure 16-1. Primary nurse communication form.

pares transfer information to accompany the patient and when the patient returns to the unit the primary nurse receives and reviews the transfer information from the hospital and makes appropriate changes in the patient's care plan.

The quality of care should be regularly monitored by formal assessment, periodic random cross-checking, and peer review. This should be arranged with the knowledge of the whole team for mutual benefit and not as something potentially ominous and threatening.

The family plays an important part in the patient's understanding

Table 16-1
Primary Nurse Duties

First Dialysis Day	Weekly	Monthly	Six-Month
Obtain, if possible, referral information prior to the patient's arrival	Assesses patient problems, subjective, and objective, and dialysis goals, update Kardex	Checks medication list with patient every month	Reviews summary of hospitalizations for completeness
Prepares chart and sees the patient on the first day to do initial evaluation; identifies needs or problems and takes appropriate action	Reviews physician orders assures orders have been carried out assures verbal orders have been cosigned	Reviews with patient every month how to check patency of vacular access on a daily basis	Evaluates patient's understanding of dialysis, refers to nurse clinician if patient can benefit by further education
Initiates and performs first dialysis	Reviews lab results and takes appropriate action	Assesses patient, reads progress notes, and writes a monthly summary	Reviews with patient education material: fistula care hypotension emergency, on-call policy
Identifies immediate needs and communicates to the appropriate person, i.e., social worker, dietitian, and physician	Writes progress note when needed	Thins dialysis flow sheets; place in permanent file	Completes nursing information for 6-month team care conference
Obtains and informs patient of dialysis schedule			
Writes progress notes at end of the dialysis			

and acceptance of his illness as well as in his overall treatment. It is therefore extremely important that the primary nurse/family relationship begin as soon as possible. Families should be included in the teaching aspects of the patient's care whenever feasible. Family conferences provide a means for discussion of different aspects of the patient's illness, and also provide the opportunity to express to the family ways that they can be supportive to the patient. These conferences can be the responsibility of various members of the team—the primary nurse, nurse clinician or patient educator, depending on the organization of the particular renal program and the patient's level of knowledge about end-stage renal disease.

It is helpful for the primary nurse to alternate patients every 6 months to broaden the care given.

The Role of the Team

An essential aspect of the team is the ability of professionals to work together, whether or not they are of the same profession. Differences in opinions, status, and interlocking roles can easily lead to conflict between team members, thus reducing the effectiveness of the team. Problems more often arise between different professions rather than within a certain profession. The reason for this generally is that the professional is often not aware of the specific competencies and roles of members of different professions.

Strong positive relationships between team members are an important determinant of the team's ability to achieve their goals and objectives. Conflict among professionals seriously interferes with collaborative efforts. Language barriers and noncommunication also impede the team's ability to function effectively. The team's ability to handle such barriers may determine its ultimate effectiveness. To avoid role ambiguity and stereotypes, each individual team member needs to communicate with other professionals regarding their roles and professional identity. Example:

> If the nurse's professional role is confusing to others, then the roles of other professionals may be equally unclear to the nurse. The nurses may have stereotypes of other professionals, or may not understand them simply because of a lack of contact and experience with them.[2]

In most circumstances, team members come together with certain ideas about their own roles and the roles of other professionals on the team. Perceptions may differ considerably from one professional to the next. Although some differences are unavoidable, extreme dissonance among team members impedes the movement of the team and prevents the team from providing the optimum in patient care.

One method of helping team members understand and appreciate each others role in the overall care of the patient is to have a series of inservice programs by the team members. Each discipline (nurse, social worker, physician, dietitian, administrator, technician, etc.) prepares and gives a 1-hour talk describing the basic philosophies and methods of their professions.

Another area in which problems may arise is that of professional territoriality. Of all factors mentioned, this is the hardest to deal with and find a media with which all team members are willing to establish reasonable parameters. Conflict among team members mainly results from ambiguous and overlapping roles. Individual team members may be confused about their own roles due to filling several different roles concurrently. Personalities, professional competencies, and the role each member assumes in the team can cause frustration in delineating which action is appropriate. Role ambiguity or role confusion arise from team members filling several different kinds of roles simultaneously. A composite of feelings, both professional and personal must be discussed and conflicts resolved on an individual basis for the team to work effectively.[1]

The most prevalent problem for the ESRD team centers involve these overlapping responsibilities and the inability of individual team members to handle the conflict. The decision of one team member to overlap from one area into another must be done discreetly while keeping in mind the job responsibilities of others. Territorial conflicts can be prevented by defining roles by job description; establishing goals and objectives for each specialty; clarifying overlapping roles; role assignments; and by educating team members in the different specialities and their functions.

Teamwork depends on the full utilization of each individual team member's capabilities. Maximum use of these capabilities enhances the effectiveness of the team.

The success of any team is dependent on the desire of each member to work with the other toward a common goal. The patient and his or her health problems are the point of departure and focus of all activities of the team. Among the team members there must be recognition, acceptance, and understanding of the goal; knowledge of the capabilities and responsibilities of each member; and coordinated planning and evaluation of activities with provision for complete two-way communication.

If the staff is to successfully meet the needs of the patient, there must be teamwork. Basic to any team is the fact that each member can and does make a substantial contribution, although the levels of education, preparation, and experience may be extremely varied.

One of the main reasons for using the team approach to patient care is to enlist the broad spectrum of knowledge of many specialists. One specialist's area or profession does not encompass a broad enough knowledge base to deal adequately with all problems that an ESRD patient will encounter. By using the team approach, we integrate the diverse skills of several professions, thus giving us the capabilities of better serving the ESRD patient.

Once the team concept is working in a clinical setting, its continued success depends on the motivational level of each individual team member. In order for a team member to achieve a high level of performance he or she must be a self-motivator. It is extremely hard to motivate others, but an environment can be conducive to producing the desired effect from our employees.

A leader can help others obtain satisfaction by giving recognition to individuals for the work they are doing. It is important for a leader to listen. Leaders should allow individuals opportunities for achievement, make the work challenging, and help each person learn new skills and improve old ones; show trust in each person's capabilities by delegating as much responsibility as possible; and should provide opportunities for advancement within the job or to another level.[3]

THE ESRD MEDICARE PROGRAM

On September 30, 1972, the Senate passed an amendment to the Social Security bill, extending Medicare coverage to patients with ESRD. The wisdom of this amendment has since been frequently questioned but no one doubts that it is here to stay. The makings of the ESRD program began in 1960, when it first became possible to prolong life by performing dialysis. At this time dialysis was extremely costly and was provided on a very limited basis. The average annual cost for each patient was approximately $40,000. While the technology for treatment of ESRD was available, lack of money was an obstacle preventing the treatment of large numbers of people. Committees were developed to decide who would make the best candidate for dialysis. This problem prompted the Senate into introducing a program, based primarily on humanitarian motives, to provide federal funding for the majority of patients. The tremendous growth and increase in the cost of the program has caused the federal government to question the wisdom of their decision.

Twice in the nine-year existence of the program, changes or amendments have been made in the Social Security Act, under which the original program was adopted (see Fig. 16-2).

In the late 1970s, approximately 48,000 dialysis patients were being treated at a cost of one billion dollars annually in contrast to a cost of 250 million in the early 1970s. The average annual cost for a patient in 1982 was about $28,000 compared to $40,000 ten years previously. The cost for each treatment has decreased in spite of inflation and the increase in total cost has been entirely due to the fact that the dialysis population has increased immensely.[5]

After the federal government began paying for dialysis, more and more patients were chosen for dialysis, allowing patients who, in the past had not been given the opportunity to extend their life. Because of the high cost of the total program, once again the question is surfacing, should there be tighter controls on who are chosen for dialysis? Should it be only patients who can most benefit from dialysis medically, and are able to lead productive lives? At this stage, there is no turning back and the federal government will not and should not put a price tag on a human life. Who or what can determine that a 70-year-old grandmother is not leading as productive a life as a 25-year-old patient?

CONTROLLING THE COST OF DIALYSIS

Beyond these philosophical considerations, the mandate by the federal government is cost containment. Without extremely efficient administration, dialysis programs in general may be in financial trouble. Administrators will need to make shifts in policies to stimulate or encourage cost control. It appears that the most difficult problems administrators will face in the next decade are inflated costs and major budgetary cutbacks. At the same time, clinics are expected to be more productive and to provide high-quality care.[6]

An analysis of the total scope of a program needs to take place and areas defined for potential targets for cost reductions. There are three particular areas in dialysis units that account for the majority of expenditures. They are overhead, personnel, and supplies.

High overhead usually stems from poor utilization of existing facilities. Economizing, along with effective management, are the two strongest adversaries of high overhead expenses. Constant monitoring

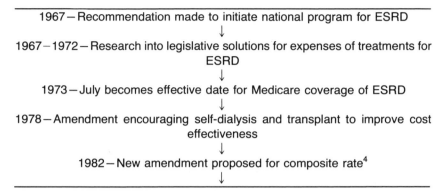

Figure 16-2. Chronology of the legislative background involved in the ESRD program.

of expenses, both indirect and direct, on a timely basis are essential to curtail runaway cost and to keep one cognizant of total expenses.[7,8]

Personnel and labor costs can be addressed from several different perspectives. Effective utilization of staff is of prime concern because of the potential yield of cost effectiveness. Using the primary nursing concept in a facility is extremely helpful for cost effectiveness because the care is of high quality; the person most prepared and best equipped to perform does so on a continuing basis for the same patients. In addition, turnover of nursing staff is decreased because of job satisfaction, and, finally, professional nurses do the job for which they are paid so "unproductive" time decreases dramatically.[3] The primary nurse concept provides the nurse the opportunity for giving the patient special attention. By utilizing other staff to clean machines and perform other functions, primary nursing provides the opportunity for the best utilization of personnel.

Another perspective that can be examined is the scheduling of patients and staff. Scheduling can provide a chance to use many innovative ideas to optimize staffing, give patients a better choice of treatment times, plus it can potentially reduce the need for new staff.

The optimal scheduling pattern for patients and staff for an individual dialysis unit is dependent on the total number of patients, the number of dialysis stations available, the percentage of patients who need special scheduling consideration because of employment and other factors. Plans such as four, 10-hour shifts each week for the staff should be considered.

Supply cost is a substantial portion of the overall cost of dialysis, and therefore much can be gained by being very prudent about supply expenses. One major way to reduce supply cost is to purchase competitively, making sure that supplies are being made available in the most economical package. Be creative, develop contacts, and shop around until a supplier is willing to deal on an economical basis. There are several other ways to reduce supply cost, among them reuse of dialyzers and in-house production of dialysate.

Reuse of Dialyzers

If the reimbursement rate is lowered as projected, multiple use of dialyzers could definitely become a necessity in order for many of the present dialysis facilities to continue in successful operation. At this point in time, dialyzer reuse is not an accepted practice in many dialysis facilities. It has, in fact, become a very controversial issue with some fractions strongly opposing reuse. There are very little relevant data, however, to support the negative aspects. Because of the tremendous need for cost savings in today's world of high inflation, it is imperative that minds be kept open and alternative solutions evaluated carefully and not discarded because of hypothetical possibilities.[9]

Many positive results in dialyzer reuse has been achieved in the last few years. Studies have shown that multiple use of dialyzers can be used effectively over long periods of time with no related suspicious clinical symptoms.[10] Lanning reports 16 years of experience with reuse without any apparent detriment to patients.

At the University of Missouri, our reuse program has been in existence for approximately 1.5 years with no significant incidents. Our only problems dealt directly with a small population opposed to reuse. To minimize these types of problems and increase patient acceptance of reuse, all of our patients were given a letter several weeks prior to the initiation of our reuse program. This letter described the reasons for the need to reuse dialyzers, our sincere belief that with our proposed program that reused dialyzers were at least as safe and as efficient as new dialyzers and asked for their comments. All of their questions were answered by the physicians and staff in an open and honest manner. All of the in-center dialysis patients are required to participate in the program. Those who do not want to be treated with reused dialyzers are given the opportunity to use new dialyzers on home dialysis or transfer to another dialysis unit. None of the patients chose these alternatives and to our knowledge all of our patients are comfortable with our reuse program. The average use of each dialyzer is at present approximately five to six times. This has established a cost savings for our 50-patient clinic of $113,000 each year. We feel very confident about the safety and efficiency of reused dialyzers, but continue to monitor our program carefully. The ideal situation would be cheaper dialyzers which will make reuse unnecessary but until that time, dialyzer reuse can be safely and effectively done as long as very high standards of control are utilized.

On-Site Dialysate Concentrate Preparation

Another source of potential cost savings to a facility is the preparation of dialysate concentrate at the dialysis unit. The continuous spiraling price of concentrate has actually doubled over the last 2 years. This type of inflationary factor forces facilities to attempt to deal more effectively with an item that is necessary to dialysis.

Over the last few years, some dialysis facilities around the country have been able to produce dialysate concentrate in a very cost-effective manner.

Since a major factor in the cost of dialysate is transportation and since even in dialysate concentrate the majority of the weight is water, on site preparation can substantially reduce costs by preventing the need to transport large amounts of water long distances. An additional advantage of local dialysate concentrate production is that the formula can be easily determined by the local unit. This is frequently difficult with commercial suppliers.

Safe, efficient production of dialysate concentrate is a major endeavor. It is probably not cost effective for units treating less than 50 patients. Continuous monitoring and adequate testing are essential. The details of setting up a program are beyond the scope of this text but for a 50-patient dialysis unit, $5,000–$10,000 each year can be saved by the on-site production of dialysate concentrate.

REFERENCES

1. Ducanes AJ, Golin AK: The interdisciplinary health care team. Germantown, Maryland Aspen Systems Corporation, 1979
2. Stueks AM: Working together collaboratively with other professions. Community Mental Health J 1, 4:316–319, 1965
3. Kron Thora: The Management of Patient Care (ed 5). Philadelphia, Saunders, 1981
4. Iglehart JK: Health policy report. New Eng J Med, 306:492–496, 1982
5. Lourie EG, Hampers CL: The success of medicare's end stage renal disease program. New Eng J Med 305:434–438, 1981
6. Kolata GB: Dialysis after nearly a decade. Science 208:473–476, 1980

7. Day L: Incentive reimbursement for outpatient dialysis. Contemp Dial 2:9,90–91, 1980
8. Day L: The reimbursement rate issues. Contemp Dial 2:18–20, 1981
9. Cotler D: The food and drug administration's position on kidney reuse. Dial Transplant 9:31–32, 1980
10. Lanning J, Winterich C, Zuanaich N: Multiple use of hollow fiber dialyzers in a free-standing center. Dial Transplant 9:36–38, 1980

SUGGESTED READINGS

1. Hampers CL, Hager EB: The delivery of dialysis services on a nationwide basis—Can we afford the non-profit system? Dial Transplant 8:417–423, 1979
2. Diaz-Buxo JA, Chaneller JT: Home dialysis—The best alternative? Dial Transplant 9:813–814, 1980
3. Wagstaff L: A model for team work in medical education and health care. SA Med J 25:916–917, 1978
4. Wilson MR: Are quality of care and cost containment mutually exclusive? Contemp Dial 2:10–14,55, 1981
5. Day L, Blagg C: Composite rate reimbursement NPRM. Contemp Dial 3:12–16, 1982
6. Schweiker RS: The age of competition in health care. Contemp Dial 3:25,28,42, 1982
7. Ney R: The ESRD medicare program—A clarification. Dial Transplant 10:227–230, 1981
8. Crystal R: The health care financing administrations position on re-use. Dial Transplant 9:23–26, 1980
9. Ogden D, Kopec G, Guy M: Cost effectiveness of multiple dialyzer use. Dial Transplant 10:407–411, 1981
10. Vercellini G, et al: Re-use of dialyzers. Dial Transplant 7:350–359, 1978

Index

Acetaminophen (Tylenol), 62
  intoxication with, 279–280
Acetate dialysate, 95–98, 130, 131
  blood pressure and, 137
  for peritoneal dialysis, 197
  in children, 242
Acetate infusion fluid, in
  hemofiltration, 224, 226
Acetazolamide, 64
Acetohexamide (Dymelor), 67
Activated partial thromboplastin time
  (APTT), 131–132
Activated whole blood coagulation
  time (ACT), 132–134
Adolescent dialysis patients, 252
Air detector, 111
Alcohol intoxication, 280–281
Aldosterone, 18
Alkaline phosphatase, monitoring
  serum concentrations of, 8
Allen-Brown shunt, 146–148
Alprenolol, 65
Aluminum, in dialysate, 89
Aluminum intoxication, dialysis
  dementia associated with, 29–30
Amantadine (Symmetrel), 67
Amikacin (Amikin), 59
Amino acids, 336
  for acute renal failure, 226–267

Aminoglycosides, 58–59
Amitriptyline (Elavil) intoxication,
  278
Amoxicillin, 60
Amphetamine intoxication, 279
Ampicillin, 60
Analgesic nephropathy, 44
Analgesics, 62–63
  intoxication with, 279–280
Ancobon (flucytosine), 62
Androgens, for anemic patients,
  13–14
Anemia, 10–14
  androgens for treatment of, 13–14
  dialyzer residual loss of blood and,
    103
  folic acid deficiency, 13
  iron deficiency, 12
  iron overload associated with,
    14–15
  treatment of, 12–14
Anergy, cutaneous, 15–16
Aneurysm, as complication of
  arteriovenous access, 161
Angiography, for evaluation of
  arteriovenous fistulas and internal
  arteriovenous shunts, 163
Angiotensin, 18
Anorexia, 25

371

Antacids, phosphorus binding, 5, 51–52
Anthropometric measurements, 343–344
Antiarrhythmic agents, 65
Antibiotics, 58–62
 aminoglycoside, 58–59
 cephalosporin, 59–60
 penicillin, 60
 sulfonamide, 60–61
 tetracycline, 61
Anticoagulants, 131. *See also* Heparin
Anticoagulation, 131–134
Anticonvulsants, 65
Antidepressant tricyclic amine intoxication, 278
Antihistamines, 65–66
Antihypertensive agents, 49–50, 63–64. *See also specific medications*
Antiinflammatory agents, 66
Antineoplastic agents, 67
Antithrombin III deficiency, thrombosis of vascular access and, 159
Apresoline (hydralazine), 49
APTT (activated partial thromboplastin time), 131–132
Arrhythmias. *See also* Antiarrhythmic agents
 potassium in dialysate and, 92–93
Arsenic poisoning, 281
Arsine poisoning, 281
Arterial line, pressure monitor on, 110
Arteriolar nephrosclerosis, 48
Arteriovenous fistula, internal, 77–78, 144, 149–151
 in children, 250
 declotting, 159–160
Arteriovenous shunts
 external, 144–149
 internal, 144, 151–154
 declotting, 159–160
Ascorbic acid, 342

Aspirin, 62
 intoxication with, 279
 for thrombosis of vascular access, 159
Assessment, for patient education, 293–296
Asterixis, in uremic encephalopathy, 27
Atherosclerosis, 19
Atromid-S (clofibrate), 68
Azathioprine (Imuran), 67

Barbiturate intoxication, 275–276
Base, in dialysate, 95–98, 130–131
 peritoneal dialysis, 197
B cells, 15
Beliefs about health, 298–299
Benadryl (diphenhydramine), 65–66
Beta-adrenergic blocking agents, 49
Bicarbonate dialysate, 95–98, 130–131
 for peritoneal dialysis in children, 242
Bleomycin, 67
Blood access. *See also* Vascular access
Blood flow, peritoneal, 165–168
Blood leak detector, 110
Blood loss, 103
 in the dialyzer and blood tubing at the end of dialysis, 13
Blood-membrane interaction, 101–102
Blood pressure. *See also* Hypertension; Hypotension
 control of, 48–50
Blood pump, 111
Blood urea nitrogen (BUN), morbidity and, 121–122
Blood volume
 extracorporeal, 103
 residual, 103
Body water, total, 122
Body weight, target, 134–136
Bone biopsies, 9–10
Brethine (terbutaline), 68–69

Bromergocryptine, 35
Buselmeier shunt, 146, 250

Calcium
  in dialysate, 93–94, 129–130
  intake of, 339
  metabolism of
    abnormalities in, 1–9
    monitoring, 7–9
    phosphorus retention, 2–3
    parathyroid hormone resistance, 5
    treatment of, 5–7
    vitamin D metabolism, 4–5
  in peritoneal dialysis fluid, 197
Calcium carbonate, 6
  supplementation of, 6
    in continuous ambulatory peritoneal dialysis, 354–355
  in peritoneal dialysis, 205
Caloric intake, 336–337
  for continuous ambulatory peritoneal
    dialysis patients, 353
  peritoneal dialysis and, 203–204
Cannulation
  of femoral vein, 155–156
  of subclavian vein, 156–158
CAPD. *See* Continuous ambulatory peritoneal dialysis
Captotril, 50
Carbamazepine (Tegretol), 65
Carbenicillin (Geopen), 60
Cardiac arrhythmias. *See* Arrhythmias
Cardiac failure: high-output, as complication of vascular access, 162–163
Cardiovascular abnormalities, 17–24. *See also* Atherosclerosis; Hypertension; Myocardial dysfunction; Pericarditis
  increased morbidity and mortality rates from, 19
Cardiovascular system, in drug intoxication, 272

Catapress (clonidine), 49–50
Catheters
  for hemodialysis in infants and children, 249
  in peritoneal dialysis, 180–188
    acute peritoneal dialysis catheters, 181
    break-in techniques, 183, 185
    in children, 240–241, 243
    chronic peritoneal dialysis catheters, 183–187
    troubleshooting malfunctions, 187
  for single-needle dialysis, 115
Cation exchange resins, for acute renal failure, 264
Ceclor (cefador), 60
Cefadroxil (Duricef), 60
Cefadyl (cephapirin), 60
Cefamandole (Mandol), 60
Cefazolin (Kefzol), 60
Cefoxitin (Mefoxin), 60
Cell-mediated immunity, 15–16
Cellophane membranes, 100–102
Cellulose acetate membranes, 101, 102
Central nervous system, 27–28
Cephalexin (Keflex Dista), 60
Cephalosporins, 59–60
  for peritonitis, 210–212
Cephalothin (Keflin), 60
Cephapirin (Cefadyl), 60
Cephradine (Velosef), 60
Charcoal hemoperfusion in drug intoxication, 274. *See also* Drug intoxication
Children, dialysis for, 231–253
  causes of renal failure in, 232–233
  and hemodialysis, 245–251
    acute hemodialysis, 245, 248–249
    chronic hemodialysis, 249–251
    vascular access, 248–250
  indications for, 234–239
    acute renal failure, 235–236
    chronic renal failure, 236–239

Children, dialysis for *(continued)*
 neonatal renal failure, 239
 peritoneal dialysis, 240–245
  acute renal failure, 240–242
  chronic renal failure, 242–245
  psychological problems, 251–252
Chloral hydrate intoxication, 276
Chloramines
 in the dialysate, anemia and, 13
 in dialysate water, 89
Chlordiazepoxide (Librium)
  intoxication, 277
Chlorpheniramine (ChlorTrimetron),
  65–66
Chlorpromazine (Thorazine) intoxication, 277
Chlorpropamide (Diabinase), 67–68
Chlorthalidone, 64
Cimetidine (Tagamet), 68
Cistaplin (Platinol), 67
Clearance, in peritoneal dialysis, 171
Clofibrate (Atromid-S), 68
Clonidine (Catapress), 49–50
Cloxacillin, 60
Coil dialyzers, 105, 107
Collodian membranes, 71, 100
Communication, team approach to patient care and, 359–360
Computerized roentgenography, monitoring the mineral content of bone by, 9
Concentration gradient, diffusive transport and, 85
Conductive transport, 85–86
Conductivity of the dialysate, 110
Congestive heart failure, 20
Constipation, 26
Continuous ambulatory peritoneal dialysis (CAPD), 79, 174, 179, 189–190. *See also* Peritoneal dialysis
 in children, 238, 244, 245
 dialysate flow rate in, 169–170
 dialysate for, 198
 nutrition in, 352–355
 peritonitis and, 208–213

Continuous cycle peritoneal dialysis (CCPD), 192
 in children, 244
Convection, in peritoneal dialysis, 170
Convective transport, in hemofiltration, 219–220
Copper, in dialysate, 89
Corticosteroids, 66
Cost of dialysis, 366–369
Cramps, during dialysis, 139–140
Cuprophan membranes, 101
Cycler, in peritoneal dialysis, 190–191
Cyclophosphamide (Cytoxin), 67

Darvon (propoxyphene), 62
 intoxication with, 280
Decadurobulin (nandrolone decanoate), 14
Declotting vascular access
 in children, 249
 of external shunts, 147
 of an internal arteriovenous fistula, 159–160
Defense mechanisms, 299–302
Dementia, dialysis, 29–30
Demerol (meperidine), 63
 intoxication with, 280
Denial, 300–301
Depakene (valproic acid), 65
Desferrioxamine, 15
Diabetics
 dietary management for, 346–348
 on peritoneal dialysis, 199–200
Diabinase (chlorpropamide), 67–68
Dialysate
 in hemodialysis, 86–100
  base used in, 95–98, 103–131
  calcium in, 93–94, 129–130
  chloramines in, anemia and, 13
  conductivity of, 110
  glucose in, 98, 100
  magnesium in, 94–95
  potassium in, 92–93, 129
  sodium in, 90–92, 138

temperature of, 90, 110
water preparation for, 87–90
in peritoneal dialysis, 188–198
  alteration of peritoneal
    physiology by, 175–176
  automated systems, 192–195
  buffer, 197
  calcium concentration, 197
  continuous ambulatory
    peritoneal dialysis (CAPD),
    189–190
  cycler for, 190–192
  flow rates, 169–170
  glucose concentration, 195
  magnesium, 197
  manual peritoneal dialysis,
    188–189
  osmolality, 176
  osmotic pressure, 172
  pH of dialysis solutions, 176
  potassium, 197
  semi-automated devices for,
    190–192
  sodium concentration, 195, 197
  techniques for exchanging
    dialysis fluid, 188–195
  temperature, 176
Dialysate concentrate, on-site
  preparation of, 369
Dialysis. *See* Hemodialysis;
  Peritoneal dialysis
Dialysis dementia, 29–30
Dialysis disequilibrium syndrome,
  28–29
Dialysis index, 120
Dialysis machines, 107–111
  monitoring functions, of 109–111
Dialysis prescription, 119–141
  dialysate, 128–131
  duration and frequency of dialysis,
    128
  for patients starting on chronic
    hemodialysis treatments,
    140–141
  symptoms during dialysis and,
    136–140

total amount of dialysis treatment,
  119–124
Dialyzers, 100–107
  blood loss in, 13
  choosing, 124
  coil, 105, 107
  configurations of, 105
  cost of, 104
  currently available, 124–127
  evaluation of, 102–104
  hollow fiber capillary, 107
  membranes of, *See* Membranes
  plate, 105–107
  reuse of, 368–369
  ultrafiltration coefficient of, 103
Diazepam (Valium) intoxication, 277
Dicloxacillin, 60
Dietary management (diet therapy),
  335–353. *See also* Nutrition
  in acute renal failure, 266–267
  calcium and phosphorous intake,
    339–340
  caloric intake, 336–337
  for children, 251
  compliance with renal diet,
    345–346
  for diabetics, 346–348
  in early and moderate renal
    insufficiency, 45–48
  immunological testing, 344–345
  nutritional assessment, 343–345
  potassium intake, 337
  predialysis nutrition, 348–350
  protein restriction, 335–336
  sodium intake, 337, 339
  vitamin and mineral therapy,
    341–342
Diet history, 343
Diffusion, in peritoneal dialysis, 170
Diffusive transport, 84–85
Digitalis, 64
  potassium concentrations in
    dialysis and, 92–93
Digitoxin, 64
Digoxin (Lanoxin), 64
Dihydrotachsyterol, 7

Dilantin (phenytoin), 65
Diphenhydramine (Benadryl), 65–66
Dipyridamole, for thrombosis of vascular access, 159
Diquat ingestion, 282
Disequilibrium syndrome, 28–29
  in children, 248
Disopyramide (Norpace), 65
  intoxication, 283
Diuresis, forced, in drug intoxication, 273–274. *See also* Drug intoxication
Diuretics, 64
  as antihypertensive agents, 49
Doriden (glutethimide), 63
  intoxication, 276
Doxepin (Sinequan) intoxication, 278
Drug intoxication, 271–284
  alcohol, 280–281
  amphetamine, 279
  analgesics, 279–280
  arsenic and arsine, 281
  forced diuresis in, 273–274
  hemofiltration in, 272–275
  herbicides, 282
  insecticides, 282
  mushrooms, 283
  pulmonary care in, 271–272
  sedatives, 275–276
  tranquilizers, 277–278
Duricef (cefadroxil), 60
Dymelor (acetohexamide), 67

Education of the renal patient. *See* Patient education
Elavil (amitriptyline) intoxication, 378
Electroencephalographic (EEG) changes, in uremia, 28
Emotional reactions to illness, 299–302
Endocrine abnormalities, in chronic renal failure, 31–36
  pancreatic hormones, 33–34
  sexual dysfunction, 34–36
  thyroid function, 32–33

End-stage renal disease (ESRD), 179
  in children, 238
Erythropoiesis inhibitors, 11
Erythropoietin, decreased production of, 10
Ethacrynic acid, 64
Ethambutal (Myambutol), 61–62
Ethanol intoxication, 280–281
Ethchlorvynl (Placidyl) intoxication, 278
Ethylene glycol ingestion, 281
Eutonyl (paragyline) intoxication, 278

Femoral vein, cannulation of, 155–156
Ferritin, serum concentration of, 12
Flucytosine (Ancobon), 62
Fluid balance, 134–136
Fluid intake, 350–351
  in continuous ambulatory peritoneal dialysis, 354
  in predialysis patients, 349–350
Fluid removal
  hypertension controlled by, 135–136
  hypotension and, 137, 138
Fluoxymesterone (Halotestin), 14
Fogarty catheter, declotting shunts with, 147
Folic acid deficiency, anemia caused by, 13
Folic acid supplementation, 342
Follicular-stimulating hormone (FSH), 35
Furadantin (nitrofurantoin), 58
Furosemide (Lasix), 64
  for acute renal failure, 263–264

Garamycin (gentamicin), 59
Gastric acid secretion, 25–26
Gastric lavage, 272
Gastrin, 25–26
Gastroenterocolitis, 25
Gastrointestinal system, in chronic renal failure, 25–26
Gentamicin (Garamycin), 59

Geopen (carbenicillin), 60
Glomerulonephritis, 44
Glucagon, 33–34
Glucose
  in dialysate, 98, 100
  in peritoneal dialysis fluid, 195
  for pediatric patients, 241
Glucose metabolism 33
Glucose tolerance (or intolerance), 33–34
Glutethimide (Doriden), 63
  intoxication, 276
Gore-Tex catheter, 186
Granulocytes, 16
Growth hormone, 34

Halotestin (fluoxymesterone), 14
Hematoma, subdural, 27
Hemodialysis.
  for acute renal failure, 264–266
  cost of, 366–369
  in drug intoxication. *See* Drug intoxication
  hemofiltration compared to, 219–220, 223–229
  history of, 71–79
  in infants and children. *See* Children, dialysis for
  principles and mechanics of, 83–116
    dialysate. *See* Dialysate
    dialysis machines, 107–111
    dialyzers, 100–107
    semipermeable membranes, 83
    solute transport, 84–86
    ultrafiltration, 83–84
  single-needle, 111–116
  symptoms during, 136–140
    hypotension, 137–139
    muscle cramps, 139–140
  ultrafiltration in, 84
Hemofiltration, 219–229
  in acute renal failure, 266
  convective transport in, 219–220
  in drug overdoses, 272–275. *See also* Drug intoxication
  equipment for, 222–223
  fluid removal, tolerance in, 224
  infusion solution for, 220
  length of the treatment with, 223
  norepinephrine in, 227
  peripheral resistance in, 225–226
  postdilution versus predilution, 221–222
  sodium in, 226–227
  ultrafiltration in, 220–221
  for uncontrollable hypertension, 227–229
Hemolytic-uremic syndrome, in infancy and childhood, 232, 235–236
Heparin
  anticoagulation response to, 131
  dosage of, 132
  loading dose of, 132
  monitoring administration of, 132–133
  regimens of, 133–134
  replacement dose of, 132–133
Hepatic comea, hemofiltration in, 275
Herbicide ingestion, 282
Hernias, peritoneal dialysis and, 201, 213–214
Hollow fiber capillary dialyzers, 107
Hydralazine (Apresoline), 49
Hyperalimentation
  in acute renal failure, 267
  in peritoneal dialysis, 207
Hyperkalemia, in acute renal failure, 264
Hyperprolactemia, 35
Hypertension, 17–19. *See also* Antihypertensive agents
  atherosclerosis and, 19
  in children, 251
  fluid removal for control of, 135–136
  hemofiltration for uncontrollable, 227–229
  treatment of, 48–50
Hypersplenism, in anemic patients, 13

Hypoglycemia, 34
Hypotension
 during dialysis, 137–139
 in drug intoxication, 272
Hypothermia, in infants and small children undergoing hemodialysis, 248
Hypothyroidism, 32

Ibuprofen (Motrin), 66
Imipramine (Tofranil) intoxication, 278
Immunologic abnormalities, in chronic renal failure, 15–16
Immunological testing, 344–345
Imuran (azathioprine), 67
Indomethacin, for pericarditis, 24
Infants, *See* Children, dialysis for
Infection
 in acute renal failure, 267
 of hemodialysis accesses, 160–161
INH (isoniazid), 61
Insecticide poisoning, 282
Insulin, 33, 68
 in peritoneal dialysis solutions, 207–208
Iron
 absorption of, 12
 deficiency of, 12, 342
 overload of, 14–15
Iron dextran, 12
Isocarboxazid (Marplen) intoxication, 278
Isoniazid (INH), 61
Isopropyl alcohol intoxication, 281

Keflex (cephalexin), 60
Keflin (cephalothin), 60
Kefzol (cefazolin), 60

Lactate dialysate, for peritoneal dialysis, 197
 in children, 242
Lanoxin (digoxin), 64
Lasix (furosemide), 64
Learning theories, 319–320

Lee White clotting times, 131
Librium (chlordiazepoxide) intoxication, 277
Lidocaine, 65
Lifestyle of the patient, peritoneal dialysis and, 201–202
Lincomycin (Lincocin), 61
Locus of control, 297–298
Loniten (minoxidil), 50
Lopressor (metaprolol), 49
Luteinizing hormone (LH), 34–35

Magnesium, in dialysate, 94–95
Mandol (cefamandole), 60
Mannitol
 for acute renal failure, 263–264
 for hypotension in hemodialysis, 138
Marplen (isocarboxazid) intoxication, 278
Mass transfer area coefficient (MTAC), 172
 nitroprusside used to increase, 176–177
 in peritoneal dialysis for children, 242
Medicare, 365–366
Medications. *See also specific types and names of medications*
 in chronic renal failure, 55–69. *See also specific medications*
 analgesics, 62–63
 antiarrhythmic agents, 65
 antibiotics, 58–62
 anticonvulsants, 65
 antihistamines, 65–66
 antihypertensive agents, 63–64
 antiinflammatory agents, 66
 antineoplastic agents, 67
 digitalis, 64
 diuretics, 64
 sedatives and tranquilizers, 63
 dosage adjustment, 58
Mefoxin (cefoxitin), 60
Membranes (semipermeable membranes), 83

blood interaction with, 101–102
cellophane, 100–102
cellulose acetate, 101, 102
collodion, 71, 100
cuprophan, 101
peritoneal, 168–169
   adequacy of, 199
   visceral and parietal components of, 166
permeability of, 84–85
polyacrylonitrile, 101
solute transport across, 84–86
thrombogenicity of, 103–104
Meperidine (Demerol), 63
   intoxication with, 280
Meprobamate (Miltown), 63
   intoxication, 277
Metabolic acidosis
   dialysis disequilibriuim syndrome and, 28–29
   treatment of, 52–53
Metaprolol (Lopressor), 49
Methanol intoxication, 280–281
Methaqualone (Quaalude) intoxication, 277–278
Methicilln (Staphcillin), 60
Methimazole (Tapazole), 68
Methotrexate (Mexate), 67
Methyprylon (Noludar) intoxication, 278
Metolazone (Zaroxolyn), 64
Mexate (methotrexate), 67
Middle molecular clearance, 120–121
Miltown (meprobamate), 63
   intoxication, 277
Mineral supplements, 341–342
   in peritoneal dialysis, 205, 207
Minipress (prazosin), 49
Minoxidil (Loniten), 50
Molecular weight, diffusive transport and, 85
Monitoring
   anticoagulation, 131–132
   calcium and phosphorus metabolism, in chronic renal failure, 7–9

conductivity of the dialysate, 110
heparin administration, 132
parathyroid hormone concentrations, 8
pressure on arterial line and venous line, 110
temperature of dialysate, 110
Monoamine oxidase inhibitors, intoxication with, 278
Motor nerve conduction velocity (MNCV), in uremic peripheral neuropathy, 30
Motrin (ibuprofen), 66
Moxalactam, for peritonitis, 212–213
Muscle cramps, during dialysis, 139–140
Mushroom poisoning, 283
Myambutol (ethambutal), 61–62
Myocardial dysfunction, 19–21
Mysoline (primidone), 65

Nafcillin, 60
Nalidixic acid (NegGram), 58
Nandrolone decanoate (Decadurobulin), 14
Naproxin (Naprosyn), 66
Narcotic intoxication, 280
Narcotics, 62–63
Nardil (phenelzine) intoxication, 278
Nausea, 25
Nebcin (tobramycin), 59
NegGram (nalidixic acid), 58
Neonates, renal failure in
   causes of, 234
   indications for dialysis, 239
Neostigmine (Prostigmin), 68
Nephropathy
   analgesic, 44
   obstructive, 44
Nephrosclerosis, arteriolar, 48
Nephrotic syndrome, 19
Neurologic abnormalities, in chronic renal failure, 26–27
Neuropathy, peripheral, 30
Neutron activation analysis, 8–9

Neutropenia, blood-membrane
    interaction and, 101–102
Nialamide (Niamid) intoxication, 278
Nitrofurantoin (Furadantin), 58
Nitroprusside, 63–64
    as vasodilator in peritoneal
        dialysis, 176–177
Noludar (methyprylon) intoxication,
    278
Norepinephrine, in hemofiltration,
    227
Norpace (dispyramide), 65
    intoxication, 283
Nutrition. *See also* Dietary
    management
    in acute renal failure, 266–267
    continuous ambulatory peritoneal
        dialysis, 352–355
    hemodialysis, 350–352
    peritoneal dialysis and, 200,
        202–208
        calcium and vitamin D, 205
        calories, 203–204
        hyperalimentation, 207
        insulin, 207–208
        phosphorus, 205–206
        potassium, 206–207
        protein, 204
        vitamins and minerals, 205, 207
    predialysis, 348–350
Nutritional assessment, 343–345

Obstructive nephropathy, 44
Osmolality, oif peritoneal dialysis
    dialysate, 176
Osteitis fibrosis cystica, 9
Osteosclerosis, 9
Osteodystrophy, renal, 9–10
    in children, 250–251
Osteomalacia, 9
Osteoporosis, 9
Oxacillin, 60

Pancreatic hormones, 33–34
Paragyline (Eutonyl) intoxication,
    278
Paraquat ingestion, 282

Parathyroid hormone
    monitoring serum concentration of,
        8
    phosphorus metabolism and, 2, 3
    resistance to the action of, 5
    vitamin D metabolism and, 4
Parnate (tranylcypromine)
    intoxication, 278
Patient care, team approach to,
    357–365
Patient education, 45, 287–331
    assessment of patients and,
        293–296
    background of, 288–289
    barriers to, 315–319
    in chronic illness, 290–296
    difficulties in, 294–295
    evaluation of programs of,
        329–331
    goals of a predialysis renal
        education program, 302–309
        anticipated outcomes, 307–309
        educational mechanisms,
            305–306
    implementation of program of,
        319–329
        background of adult learning
            theory, 319–320
        emotional suggestions and
            considerations, 325
        families and significant others,
            education of, 327–328
        life experiences, 324
        presenting overviews of dialysis
            treatments, 328–329
        principles of adult learning,
            320–321
        readiness to learn and problem-
            oriented learning, 324–325
        self-directed learning, 321–324
        structural suggestions and
            considerations, 326–327
    planning the program of,
        309–315
        developing educational
            objectives, 311, 314–315
        modular format, 310–311

psychosocial issues in, 297–302
  beliefs regarding illness,
    298–299
  emotional reactions to illness,
    299–302
  locus of control, 297–298
  steps in, 292–293
Penicillin G, 60
Penicillins, 60
Pentose phosphate shunt, 13
Peptic ulcers, 26
Pericardectomy, 24
Pericardial friction rub, 22–23
Pericardial tamponade, 23
Pericardial window, 24
Pericardiocentesis, 23–24
Pericarditis, 21–24
  dialysis-associated, 21–22
  therapy of, 23–24
  uremic, 21–22
Peripheral neuropathy, 30
Peritoneal anatomy and histology,
  165–167
Peritoneal blood flow, 165–168
Peritoneal capillaries, 165
Peritoneal dialysis
  for acute renal failure, 265, 266
  catheters in, 180–188
    acute peritoneal dialysis
      catheters, 181
    break-in techniques, 183, 185
    chronic peritoneal dialysis
      catheters, 183–187
    troubleshooting malfunctions,
      187
  contraindications to, 198–199
  diabetics on, 199–200
  dialysate in, 188–198
    alteration of peritoneal
      physiology by, 175–176
    automated systems, 192–195
    buffer, 197
    calcium concentration, 197
    continuous ambulatory
      peritoneal dialysis (CAPD),
      189–190
    cycler for, 190–192

flow rates, 169–170
glucose concentration, 195
magnesium, 197
manual peritoneal dialysis,
  188–189
osmolality, 176
osmotic pressure, 172
pH of, 176
potassium, 197
semi-automated devices for,
  190–192
sodium concentration, 195, 197
techniques for exchanging,
  188–195
temperature, 176
  dynamics of, 172–174
  efficiency of, 170–172
  factors controlling, 167–170
    blood flow, 167–168
    dialysate flow, 169–170
    membrane, 168–169
  fluid removal during, 84
  history of, 78–79, 179–181
  integrated approach to the patient
    in, 214–215
  lifestyle of the patient and,
    201–202
  limiting factors in use of, 177–178
  manual, 188–189
  nutrition and, 200, 202–208
    calcium and vitamin D, 205
    calories, 203–204
    hyperalimentation, 207
    insulin, 207–208
    phosphorus, 205–206
    potassium, 206–207
    protein, 204
    vitamins and minerals, 205, 207
  patient characteristics and,
    198–202
  in pediatric patients, 231, 240–245
    acute renal failure, 240–242
    chronic renal failure, 242–245
  peritonitis and, 177–178, 199,
    208–213
    diagnosis, 209–210
    organisms, 209

peritonitis and *(continued)*
  treatment, 210–213
  tunnel and exit infections, 209
  pulmonary function and, 200–201
  schedule for, 177
  vasodilators in, 176–177
Peritoneal membrane, 168–169
  adequacy of, 199
  visceral and parietal components of, 166
Peritonitis, peritoneal dialysis and, 177–178, 199, 208–213
  diagnosis, 209–210
  organisms, 209
  treatment, 210–213
  tunnel and exit infections, 209
Permeability, in peritoneal dialysis, 170
Phenelzine (Nardil) intoxication, 278
Phenobarebital, 63
Phenothiazine intoxication, 277
Phenytoin (Dilantin), 65
Phosphate binders
  for children, 250–251
  in hemodialysis, 352
Phosphorus binding antacids, 5, 151–152
Phosphorus intake, 339–340
  in peritoneal dialysis, 205–206
Phosphorus metabolism
  abnormalities in, 1–3
  monitoring of, 7–9
  normal, 2
  treatment of, 5–6
Phosphorus restriction, 50–52, 349, 351–352
Phosphorus retention, 51
Placidyl (ethchlorvynl) intoxication, 278
Plate dialyzers, 105–107
Platelet aggregation, thrombosis of vascular access and, 159
Platelet function, abnormalities of, 16–17
Platinol (cistaplin), 67
Polyacrylonitrile membranes, 101
Postcapillary sphincters, 165

Potassium
  in dialysate, 92–93, 129
  in the diet, 337
  in peritoneal dialysis fluid, 197
    for pediatric patients, 241
Potassium intake, 349, 350
  in continuous ambulatory peritoneal dialysis (CAPD), 354
  in peritoneal dialysis, 206–207
Prazosin (Minipress), 49
Primary nurse system, 357–365
Primidone (Mysoline), 65
Problem-oriented learning, 324–325
Procainamide (Pronestyl), 65
Prolactin, 35
Promazine (Sparine) intoxication, 277
Pronestyl (procainamide), 65
Propoxyphene (Darvon), 62
  intoxication, 280
Propranolol, 49, 65
Propylthiouracil, 68
Prostaglandins, hypertension and decreased secretion of, 18
Prostigmin (neostignime), 68
Protein catabolic rate, urea generation and, 121–123
Protein intake, 121–122, 335–336
  of children, 251
  in continuous ambulatory peritoneal dialysis (CAPD), 352, 354
  in peritoneal dialysis, 204
Protein restriction, 45–46, 53, 335–336
  in hemodialysis, 350
  in predialysis patients, 348–349
Psychological problems, of children on chronic dialysis, 251–252
Psychosocial issues, in patient education, 297–302
  beliefs regarding illness, 298–299
  emotional reactions to illness, 299–302
  locus of control, 297–298
Purdue column-disk catheter, 186
Pyelonephritis, 44

Quaalude (methaqualone)
  intoxication, 277–278
Quinidine, 65
Quinine intoxication, 283
Quinine sulfate, for muscle cramps,
  139

Ramirez shunt, 145–146, 148
Recirculating, single-pass (RSP)
  dialysis machines, 107–109
Recirculation of blood, in single-
  needle dialysis, 114–115
Red cells
  increased destruction of, 11
Regional heparization, 134
Renal failure, acute, 259–268
  definition, 259
  in infants and children
    causes of, 232–233
    indications for dialysis, 235–236
  pathogenesis of, 260–262
  patient education in, 289–290
  prognosis for, 267–268
  treatment of, 262–267
    dialysis, 264–266
    diuretics, 263–264
    hyperkalemia, 264
    infection, 267
    nutrition, 266–267
Renal failure, chronic, 1–69
  in children
    causes of, 233–234
    indications for dialysis, 236–239
  conservative management of,
    43–53
    blood pressure control, 48–50,
      135–136, 227–229
    diet therapy, 45–48, 335–353
    education of the patient, 45,
      287–333
    initiating replacement therapy,
      53, 140–141
    metabolic acidosis, treatment of,
      52–53
    phosphorus control, 50–52
  medications in, 55–69. *See also
    specific medications*
    analgesics, 62–63
    antiarrhythmic agents, 65
    antibiotics, 58–62
    anticonvulsants, 65
    antihistamines, 65–66
    antihypertensive agents, 63–64
    antiinflammatory agents, 66
    antineoplastic agents, 67
    digitalis, 64
    diuretics, 64
    sedatives and tranquilizers, 63
  systemic manifestations of, 1–36
    anemia, 10–14
    calcium metabolism, 1–9
    cardiovascular abnormalities,
      17–24
    constipation, 26
    endocrine abnormalities, 31–36
    gastrointestinal manifestations,
      25–26
    hematologic abnormalities,
      10–17
    hypertension, 17–19
    immunologic abnormalities,
      15–16
    myocardial dysfunction, 19–21
    neurologic abnormalities, 26–27
    pericarditis, 21–24
    phosphorus metabolism, 1–3
    phosphorus retention, 2–3
    vitamin D metabolism, 1, 4–7
Renal failure index, 262–263
Renal osteodystrophy, 9–10
  in children, 250–251
Renal transplantation, 214, 215
  in children, 238–239
Renin, 18
Restless leg syndrome, 31
Retinol binding protein (RBP), 342
Rocaltrol (1,25 Vitamin D_3), 6–7
Role conflict, patient education and,
  318–319

Salicylate. *See* Aspirin
Scholl's solution, 52
Scribner shunt, 145
  in infants and children, 248–249

384 • Index

Sedatives, 63
  intoxication, 275
Self-directed learning, 321–324
Semipermeable membranes, 83
  blood interaction with, 101–102
  cellophane, 100–102
  cellulose acetate, 101, 102
  collodion, 71, 100
  cuprophan, 101
  peritoneal, 168–169
    adequacy of, 199
    visceral and parietal components of, 166
  polyacrylonitrile, 101
  solute transport across, 84–86
  thrombogenicity of, 103–104
Sexual dysfunction, in chronic renal failure, 34–36
Sieving coefficient, 85–86
Silastic-Teflon shunt, 144–145
Sinequan (doxepin) intoxication, 278
Single-needle dialysis, 111–116
Small molecular weight clearance, 121, 123
Sodium
  in dialysate, 90–92, 138
  in hemofiltration, 226–227
  in peritoneal dialysis fluid, 195, 197
Sodium bicarbonate, for acute renal failure, 264
Sodium intake, 46–48, 337, 339
  in continuous ambulatory peritoneal dialysis (CAPD), 354
  in hemodialysis, 350
  in predialysis patients, 349
Sodium nitroprusside, as vasodilator in peritoneal dialysis, 176–177
Solute transport, 84–86
Sparine (promazine) intoxication, 277
Sphincters, postcapillary, 165
Spironalactone, 64
Spleen, in anemia, 13
Splenectomy, in anemic patients, 13
Square meter-hour hypothesis, 120, 121
Staphcillin (methicillin), 60

Staphylococcus aureus infections, 161
Stelazine (trifluoperazine) intoxication, 277
Stenosis, as vascular access complication, 160
Stress ulcers, in acute renal failure, 268
Subclavian vein, cannulation of, 156–158
Subdural hematoma, 27
Sulfamethoxazole, 60–61
Sulfonamides, 60–61
Sulfoxazole, 60–61
Surface area, in peritoneal dialysis, 170–171
Symmetrel (amantadine), 67

Tagament (cimetidine), 68
Target weight, 134–136
T cells, 15
Team approach to the end-stage renal disease (ESRD) patient, 357–365
Teflon tubing, 77, 144–145
Tegretol (carbamazepine), 65
Temperature, of dialysate, 90, 110
Tenckhoff peritoneal dialysis catheter, 180, 183–184, 241
Terbutaline (Brethine), 68–69
Testosterone, 36
Tetracyclines, 61
Theophylline intoxication, 283–284
Thiazides, 64
Thiocyanate, 64
Thomas shunt, 146–148
Thorazone (chlorpromazine) intoxication, 277
Thrombosis
  as complication of vascular access, 158–159
  external shunts and, 147
Thyroid hormones, 32–33. *See also individual hormones*
Thyroid stimulating hormone (TSH), 32, 33
Thyroxin binding globulin (TBG), 32
Thyroxine, 32–33

Index • 385

Ticorcillin (Ticar), 60
Tobramycin (Nebcin), 59
 for peritonitis, 210, 212
Tofranil (imipramine) intoxication, 278
Toronto-Western Hospital peritoneal dialysis catheter, 184
Total body water, 122
Tranquilizers, 63
Transplantation. *See* Renal transplantation
Tranylcypromine (Parnate) intoxication, 278
Triamterone, 64
Tricyclic drug intoxication, 278
Trifluoperazine (Stelazine) intoxication, 277
Trimethoprim, 60–61
Tubular necrosis, acute. *See* Renal failure, acute
Tylenol (acetaminophen), 62
 intoxication, 279–280

Ulcers
 peptic, 26
 stress, in acute renal failure, 268
Ultrafiltrate, in peritoneal dialysis, 171
Ultrafiltration, 83–84
 in hemofiltration, 220–221
Ultrafiltration coefficient, 103
Urea generation, 121–123
Uremia
 disequilibrium syndrome and, 28, 29
 electroencephalographic changes in, 28
 endocrine abnormalities and, 31–32
 peripheral neuropathy associated with, 30
Uremic cardiomyopathy, 20
Uremic encephalopathy, 27
Uremic pericarditis, 21–22

Valium (diazepam) intoxication, 277
Valproic acid (Depakene), 65

Vancomycin (Vancocin), 61
Vascular access, 77–78, 143–163
 angiographic evaluation of, 163
 complications of, 158–163
  aneurysm, 161
  clotted AV fistula, 159–160
  high-output cardiac failure, 162
  infection, 160–161
  stenosis, 160
  thrombosis, 158–159
 external arteriovenous shunts, 144–149
 immediate, 154–158
  femoral vein cannulation, 155–156
  subclavian vein cannulation, 156–158
 in infants and children, 248–250
 internal arteriovenous fistula, 144, 149–151
 internal arteriovenous shunts, 144, 151–154
Vascular disease, peritoneal dialysis and, 214
Vasoconstriction, 18
Vasodilators
 in hypertension, 49
 in peritoneal dialysis, 176–177
Velosef (cephradine), 60
Venous line
 air detector on, 111
 pressure monitor on, 110
Vital Assists single-needle device, 112–115
Vitamin B_6 supplementation, 342
Vitamin D metabolism, 1, 4–7
 treatment of abnormalities in, 5–7
Vitamin D supplementation, 6–7
 in peritoneal dialysis, 205
Vitamin supplements, 341–342
 in peritoneal dialysis, 205, 207
Vomiting, 25

Warfarin, for thrombosis of vascular access, 158–159
Water. *See also* Total body water
 for dialysate, 87–90

Weight gain
  in continuous ambulatory
    peritoneal dialysis (CAPD),
    353–354
  in hemodialysis
    hypotension and, 138

middle molecular clearance and, 121

Zaroxolyn (metozalone), 64
Zinc deficiency, 35–36